AF213565

pour cou quil i a grant
peril. Et li doit on do
ner a boire aigue ou
sient grec ⁊ dates se
ront cuites. ⁊ se li do
nes trois fois ou quatre
se mestiers est. ou plus.
Ou vous li dounes iii
de rue .ii. drames. en
vin tiede. ou vis de
sauine. ou boire cha
nele ⁊ waranche en
vin. Et se ele est cras
se si se couche a dens.
⁊ tienes les ienous vi
ers la tieste ⁊ ait .i.
cousin souz le ventre
Car si faitement demo
rer. fait toutes femes
plus legierement deli
urer. Et quant ele se
ra deliuree. si le doit
on baignier. ⁊ recon
forter de bounes via
des. Et se dolours ⁊ au
tres maladies lor a
uienent. si facent me
decines qui a lor ma
ladies safierent. li .xx.
chapitres. coment vos
deues lenfant warder
puisquil est ne de mere.

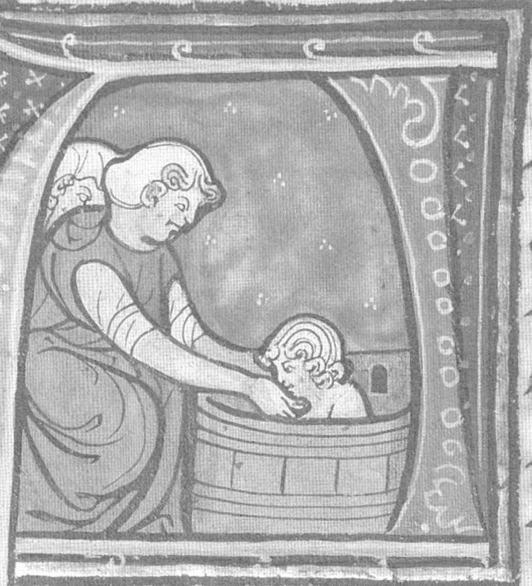

pries
cou que
li en
fes se
ra ne.
⁊ la fe
me de
liure
e. Si vous estuet sauo
ir coment vous le de
ueres garder. Si tost
com il iert nes le co
uient enuoleper en
roses broiees. meslees
a sel delie. Et deues tr
enchier le boutenil
au res de quatre pains
Et metre sus poudre
de sanc de dragon. ⁊
sarcacol. ⁊ de comin.

Visualizing Household Health

Medieval Women, Art, and Knowledge in the *Régime du Corps*

JENNIFER BORLAND

The Pennsylvania State University Press
University Park, Pennsylvania

Publication of this book has been supported by a Samuel H. Kress Foundation Grant from the International Center of Medieval Art.

Library of Congress Cataloging-in-Publication Data
Names: Borland, Jennifer Regan, author.
Title: Visualizing household health : medieval women, art, and knowledge in the Régime du corps / Jennifer Borland.
Description: University Park, Pennsylvania : The Pennsylvania State University Press, [2022] | Includes bibliographical references and index.
Summary: "Examines several illustrated copies of the late medieval health guide known as the Régime du corps, demonstrating how the manuscripts' depictions of household care highlight female-dominated expertise within the domestic sphere"—Provided by publisher.
Identifiers: LCCN 2021038343 | ISBN 9780271090597 (cloth)
Subjects: LCSH: Aldobrandino, da Siena, –1287. Régime du corps—Illustrations. | Medicine, Medieval—Europe. | Medical care—Europe—History—To 1500. | Women—Health and hygiene—Europe—History—To 1500. | Historiated initials—Europe—History—To 1500.
Classification: LCC R141 .B66 2022 | DDC 610.94—dc23
LC record available at https://lccn.loc.gov/2021038343

Copyright © 2022 Jennifer Borland
All rights reserved
Printed in Korea
Published by The Pennsylvania State University Press,
University Park, PA 16802-1003

The Pennsylvania State University Press is a member of the Association of University Presses.

It is the policy of The Pennsylvania State University Press to use acid-free paper. Publications on uncoated stock satisfy the minimum requirements of American National Standard for Information Sciences—Permanence of Paper for Printed Library Material, ANSI Z39.48–1992.

Frontispiece: Newborn care. The Bute Painter, *Le Régime du corps*, ca. 1285 (fig. 25).

To Barbara Hagan and Suzanne Lewis,
incredible women who have provided endless
encouragement and inspiration

and also to Dad, who I think would be proud

Contents

List of Illustrations ix

Acknowledgments xiii

Introduction 1

1. The Visual Language of the *Régime du corps* 17
2. The Illustrated Manuscripts and Their Audiences 61
3. The Medical Context for the *Régime du corps* 93
4. Household Management, Status, and the Care of the Body 123

Conclusion 157

Appendix 1: Summary of Illustrated Copies 161

Appendix 2: Scenes Depicted in Each Illustrated Copy 163

Appendix 3: Known Manuscript Copies of the Régime du corps 169

Notes 174

Bibliography 192

Index 205

Illustrations

1. Bloodletting. British Library, Sloane 2435, fol. 11v 3
2. Ears. Universitätsbibliothek Leipzig, Cod. Haen. 3478, fol. 67v 9
3. Pregnancy. Biblioteca Apostolica Vaticana, Reg.lat.1256, fol. 37v 10
4. Fish. Bibliothèque nationale de France, Arsenal 2894, fol. 91v 10
5. Wine. British Library, Sloane 2435, fol. 44v 11
6. Cider and vinegar. British Library, Sloane 2401, fol. 55v 12
7. Hair. Bibliothèque nationale de France, Arsenal 2510, fol. 29v 13
8. Wet nurse scene. British Library, Sloane 2435, fol. 28v 18
9. Wheat. British Library, Sloane 2435, fol. 42r 22
10. Pepper. Bibliothèque nationale de France, Fr. 12323, fol. 130r 23
11. Mulberries. British Library, Sloane 2435, fol. 46r 23
12. Making beer and cider. Cambridge University Library, Ii.V.11, fol. 51r 24
13. Eye treatment. Bibliothèque nationale de France, Fr. 12323, fol. 103r 25
14. Copulation. British Library, Sloane 2435, fol. 9v 28
15. David and Bathsheba. Morgan Library & Museum, M.638, fol. 41v 29
16. Complexion. British Library, Sloane 2435, fol. 37r 30
17. The Visitation. J. Paul Getty Museum, Ludwig IX 3 (83.ML.99), fol. 63v 31
18. Mouse, mole. British Library, Royal 12 C XIX, fol. 37r 32
19. Stag, hare, rabbit, bear. British Library, Sloane 2435, fol. 48v 33
20. Initial *C*(olor), with artist mixing colors. British Library, Royal 6E VI–6E VII, fol. 329r 34
21. Scholar lectures to students. Yale Medical Library, MS 28, fol. 57r 35
22. Annunciation, Visitation, and Nativity with surgical scenes. British Library, Sloane 1977, fol. 2r 36
23. Women presenting breast diseases to surgeon. British Library, Sloane 1977, fol. 7v 37
24. Vomiting. British Library, Sloane 2435, fol. 21r 39
25. Newborn care. Bibliothèque nationale de France, Arsenal 2510, fol. 25v 41
26. Wet nurse scene. Bibliothèque nationale de France, Fr. 12323, fol. 97r 42
27. Wet nurse scene. British Library, Sloane 2435, fol. 28v 46
28. Woman breastfeeding newborn. Biblioteca da Ajuda, Cod. 52-XIII-26, fol. 49r 48
29. Woman breastfeeding newborn. Universitätsbibliothek Leipzig, Cod. Haen. 3478, fol. 54v 48
30. Newborn care. Cambridge University Library, Ii.V.11, fol. 34v 50
31. Newborn care. British Library, Sloane 2401, fol. 37v 50
32. Newborn care. Morgan Library & Museum, M.165, fol. 44r 52
33. Copulation. Bibliothèque nationale de France, Fr. 12323, fol. 78r 53
34. Copulation. Bibliothèque nationale de France, Arsenal 2510, fol. 9r 53

35. Copulation. Morgan Library & Museum, M.165, fol. 17r 55

36. Copulation. British Library, Sloane 2401, fol. 16v 55

37. Copulation. Biblioteca da Ajuda, Cod. 52-XIII-26, fol. 16v 55

38. Pregnancy. Bibliothèque nationale de France, Fr. 12323, fol. 95v 56

39. Woman presenting breast disease to surgeon. Montpellier, Bibliothèque interuniversitaire, H 089, fol. 22r 57

40. Cupping. British Library, Sloane 2435, fol. 14r 59

41. Cheese. Bibliothèque nationale de France, Fr. 12323, fol. 128r 62

42. Cheese. British Library, Sloane 2435, fol. 69r 63

43. Cheese. Cambridge University Library, Ii.V.11, fol. 77r 64

44. Bathing. British Library, Sloane 2435, fol. 8v 69

45. Grain. Bibliothèque nationale de France, Arsenal 2510, fol. 39v 71

46. A man holding an axe above his head. J. Paul Getty Museum, 46 (92.MK.92), fol. 188v 72

47. Purging. Bibliothèque nationale de France, Fr. 12323, fol. 84v 74

48. Diagrams of the influence of the moon on the Earth. Bibliothèque nationale de France, Fr. 12323, fol. 55v 76

49. Phases of the moon and the influence of the sun and moon on the Earth. Bibliothèque municipale de Rennes, 593, fol. 76r 77

50. Millet, rice. Cambridge University Library, Ii.V.11, fol. 49r 80

51. Farro, bran Morgan Library & Museum, M.165, fol. 65r 82

52. Pregnancy. British Library, Sloane 2401, fol. 36v 84

53. Pregnancy. Biblioteca da Ajuda, Cod. 52-XIII-26, fol. 47r 86

54. Pregnancy. British Library, Sloane 2435, fol. 27v 94

55. Teeth. Bibliothèque nationale de France, Fr. 12323, fol. 104v 95

56. Frontispiece of master with students. Universitätsbibliothek Leipzig, Cod. Haen. 3478, fol. 2r 96

57. Liver. Morgan Library & Museum, M.165, fol. 59v 96

58. Bloodletting. Bibliothèque nationale de France, Fr. 12323, fol. 80r 97

59. Cupping. Bibliothèque nationale de France, Fr. 12323, fol. 83r 97

60. Cupping. Morgan Library & Museum, M.165, fol. 24r 98

61. Diagram of veins. Bodleian Library, Oxford, Ashmole 399, fol. 19r 107

62. Anatomy, female reproductive system. Bodleian Library, Oxford, Ashmole 399, fol. 15v 108

63. Doctor and students. British Library, Harley 3140, fol. 32v 109

64. Urine wheel in almanac. Rosenbach Library, 1004/29, fol. 9v 110

65. Physician with urine-flask attribute. *The Hours of Jeanne d'Evreux*, fol. 65v 111

66. Apothecary shop. British Library, Sloane 1977, fol. 49v 112

67. Diagram of *fistula-in-ano* and tools. British Library, Add. 29301, fol. 25r 113

68. Zodiac Man. Wellcome Library, 8932, fol. 5r 117

69. Vomiting. Bibliothèque nationale de France, Arsenal 2510, fol. 17v 124

70. Vomiting. Bibliothèque nationale de France, Fr. 12323, fol. 89v 125

71. Vomiting, with woman aiding. Morgan Library & Museum, M.165, fol. 33r 126

72. Cupping, administered by a woman. Bibliothèque nationale de France, Arsenal 2510, fol. 13v 133

73. Cupping, administered by a woman. British Library, Sloane 6, fol. 177v 135

74. Cupping, administered by a woman. Bodleian Library, Oxford, Laud Misc. 724, fol. 96v 136

75. Complexion. British Library, Sloane 2435, fol. 37r 142

76. Heart. Bibliothèque nationale de France, Fr. 12323, fol. 105v 143

77. Pregnancy. Morgan Library & Museum, M.165, fol. 42r 144

78. Vomiting. Cambridge University Library, Ii.V.11, fol. 26v 144

79. Old cheese. Bibliothèque nationale de France, Nouv. acq. lat. 1673, fol. 59v 147

80. Watermelon, cucumber. Bibliothèque nationale de France, Nouv. acq. lat. 1673, fol. 38v 148

81. Theriac. Bibliothèque nationale de France, Lat. 9333, fol. 51v 149

82. Frontispiece with pharmacy scene. IRHT-CNRS, Bibliothèque municipale de Besançon, 463, fol. 1 150

83. Purging. British Library, Sloane 2435, fol. 16r 152

84. Purging. Bibliothèque nationale de France, Arsenal 2510, fol. 15v 153

85. *Bas-de-page* defecation scenes. Trinity College, Cambridge, B.11.22, fol. 73r 154

Acknowledgments

My appreciation must first go to those have been instrumental in helping me work on this book throughout its long development, reading and re-reading the text, facilitating momentum, cheering me with humor, and reminding me why we do this work. This book would simply not exist without Louise Siddons, a treasured colleague, collaborator, and friend for more than twenty years. Thank you for your generosity, collegiality, and devotion to this project. Sarah Kyle's close reading, thoughtful feedback, and infinite kindness throughout the process have made this book so much better. Thanks as well to Rachael Cullick for her regular writing sessions, delivering consistent optimism and serenity over coffee and then over Zoom. Cassidy Petrazzi was instrumental in helping me manage the permissions and organization of my images, while also giving me much-needed encouragement in the final stages. I am so grateful to each of you for your constant support and enthusiasm.

Many wonderful scholars have contributed to this book by reading chapters or other sections, giving me feedback on other projects related to it, or providing general support and encouragement. My thanks to Tracy Chapman Hamilton, Jack Hartnell, Kathleen Kennedy, Amanda Luyster, Asa Mittman, Mariah Proctor-Tiffany, Benjamin Tilghman, and Theresa Tyers, who all provided excellent feedback along the way. The project was sustained by an invaluable network of colleagues and mentors, including Irene Backus, Lucy Bailey, Rebecca Brienen, Jennifer Brown, Shirin Fozi, Eliza Garrison, Emily Graham, Karen Greenwalt, Suzanne Lewis, Liz Roth, Alexa Sand, Sally Schuh, Karl Whittington, and Shaoqian Zhang. Angie Bennett, Holly Crocker, Mary Kate Hurley, Nicole C. Kirk, and Allie Terry-Fritsch—members of a fantastic online writing group—provided inspiration and motivation at an especially critical moment. Much appreciation goes to the many scholars who provided feedback at conferences over the years, especially at the meetings of the Gender and Medieval Studies Group. I am grateful to Monica Green for introducing these manuscripts to me while I was still a graduate student; my book is unquestionably built on the foundation of her extensive body of scholarship. The feedback from external reviewers greatly improved this book, and I am grateful for their time and consideration. And I will never be able to say enough thanks for the wisdom, perspective, and laughter provided by my beloved Material Collective crew: Marian Bleeke, Rachel Dressler, Martha Easton, Anne Harris, Asa Mittman, Karen Overbey, Nancy Thompson, Benjamin Tilghman, and Maggie Williams—you all rock.

Residential fellowships at the University of Pennsylvania and Rice University provided me with the time and resources to concentrate on researching and writing this book. As a Mellon Postdoctoral Fellow at the Penn Humanities Forum, I benefited greatly from the robust conversations and feedback I received, from both the other fellows in my cohort—Chiara Cillerai, Johanna T. Crane, Sindhumathi Revuluri, and Andrew Witmer—and the many other scholars whom I met that year, especially Emily Hage, Jennie Hirsh, Timothy McCall, and Elly Truitt. Jennifer Conway and Sarah Varney also contributed to creating a remarkable environment for the fellows. Thank you as well to Holly Pittman and the rest of the Department of the History of Art for such generosity in welcoming back an alumna. Wonderful connections and conversations also took place at the Humanities Research Center at Rice University, and I am especially grateful to Melissa Bailar, Farès el-Dahdah, Linda Neagley, and Diane Wolfthal for fostering such collegiality during my year there.

The research and publication of this book have also been supported with grants from the International Center of Medieval Art, the Samuel H. Kress Foundation, Oklahoma Humanities, and the National Endowment for the Humanities. At Oklahoma State University, support came from the College of Arts and Sciences, the Vaughn Vennerberg Chair of Art fund, and the Department of Art, Graphic Design, and Art History. This project would not have come to fruition without the support of the Oklahoma State University Library, as well as the generosity of those at the British Library, the Bibliothèque nationale de France, the Morgan Library and Museum, the Cambridge University Library, the Bodleian Library, the Rosenbach Library, and many others.

Thank you to the marvelous Eleanor Goodman for her encouragement, pragmatism, and infinite patience, and to the many other fantastic people at Pennsylvania State University Press for getting this book out into the world, including Maddie Caso, Laura Reed-Morrisson, and Regina Starace, as well as Nancy Evans of Wilsted and Taylor Publishing Services and Candace Hyatt.

I would like to acknowledge the previous publications upon which sections of this book are based. Chapter 1 is derived in part from the article "Freeze-Framed: Theorizing the Historiated Initials of the *Régime du corps*," published in *Word & Image* in 2016; chapter 2 is based on the chapter "Female Networks and the Circulation of a Late Medieval Illustrated Health Guide," in *Moving Women, Moving Objects (400–1500)*, edited by Tracy Chapman Hamilton and Mariah Proctor-Tiffany (Brill, 2019).

I am also incredibly grateful to family members who stayed upbeat about this project, cheered me on, and helped me finish it under unexpectedly challenging circumstances. I am especially grateful to my mother, Jane, who has over the years provided so much support, including countless hours spent reading to her grandchild over Skype to facilitate the final phase of this book's completion. Thanks as well to Barbara, Kris, Bill, Jay, Rebecca, Robb, Heather, and Jess. I reserve special gratitude for my long friendship with Heather Olson, a fellow writer whose generosity and perspective enrich my life every day. I had just started the research for this project when my father, John, passed away, but I know he would be so happy about the end result.

Finally, no one has lived with the persistent presence of this book more than Benjamin and Eleanor. Their endless encouragement, patience, and love made it possible, and I hope they are proud of what we accomplished together.

INTRODUCTION

At first glance, the historiated initial in figure 1 seems to be typical of a deluxe manuscript from the late thirteenth or early fourteenth century. An elaborately decorated capital *V* is articulated in vivid blue pigment, complemented by flourishing details in red and white, abundant gold leaf, and whimsical, curling decoration. There is even a doglike beast's head emerging from the letter's upper right ascender. Yet, if we look closely, it reveals a distinct and unexpected activity. The small space, just a couple of inches across, provides limited room for the depiction of figures and thus logically includes only two in the confined area. We see two rosy-cheeked men: on the left, a seated figure dressed in a red tunic, his head uncovered and his left sleeve rolled up; on the right, a standing figure wearing a shorter, blue tunic that reveals his gray stockings and a simple white coif. The man on the right holds a scalpel to the arm of his patient, which he cradles with his left hand; as the recently cut vein drips blood into a bowl on the ground, the smiling patient looks away. This initial depicts the act of bloodletting, a relatively common treatment in the Middle Ages for all kinds of conditions and ailments.[1]

This historiated initial is among the many that appear in several illustrated copies of a health guide frequently called the *Régime du corps*, or "regimen of the body," also sometimes referred to as the *Livre de physique* (book of medicine) or *Régime de santé* (regimen of health).[2] It is one of the seventy-two illuminated initials that accompany the text of the *Régime* in a manuscript now at the British Library in London (Sloane MS 2435); the manuscript is one of seven known copies with historiated initials in a corpus of more than seventy manuscripts that contain at least a partial text of the *Régime*. Sloane 2435 unexpectedly combines luxurious materiality—not unlike that of bibles and psalters—with depictions of the everyday maintenance of health. Its sparse yet extravagant images are remarkably rich in details that indicate how issues including class, gender, and authority may have played out in the medical treatment of the time.

According to the text's prologue, the ambitious countess of Provence, Beatrice of Savoy (1207–1265), enlisted her personal physician to create a health handbook,[3] presumably in anticipation of Beatrice's travel to see her four daughters, all of whom were the present or future queens of England, France, Germany, and Sicily. Purportedly written by Aldobrandino of Siena in 1256, this health guide was one of the first medical texts to be written in French rather than Latin, and it would become popular and influential: it was translated into at least four other languages and existed in dozens of surviving copies that were made during the next two hundred years. Aldobrandino's text was essentially a compendium of small excerpts culled from various established medical sources that were associated with the training of physicians in universities, including Isaac Judaeus's *Universal Diets*, the work of Constantine the African, and especially Avicenna's *Canon of Medicine*. Presented in a concise, general, and accessible tone, the resulting text seems less directed toward professional practitioners than toward those who oversaw households, albeit quite elite households. The advice it offers was intended for the maintenance of health and the treatment of minor illnesses in the home, serving as a kind of self-help guide.

The illustrated *Régime* manuscripts are not the kinds of books most often studied in medieval art history. They are not bibles, prayer books, or other devotional works; they do not contain especially conventional or expected iconography; they rarely have large, full-page illuminations; their medical content is not highly technical or particularly specific; their patrons or original users are often unknown. Yet they have many other aspects that make them important for historical study: they are luxury objects, secular art, encyclopedic compendia, repositories of privileged knowledge, health-care guides, tools of household management, examples of gift giving, family heirlooms, records of fashion trends, and documents of social stratification. When considered in just one of these contexts, they may seem inadequate, unremarkable, peculiar, or out of place. But as manuscripts that rest more comfortably at the intersection of multiple categories, they bring specific aspects of late medieval life into focus. The illustrated copies of the *Régime* speak to an elite interest in health care through the movement of canonical medical texts into the domestic sphere. They also offer insights into the role of the household in health-care management, asserting the complexities of care of the body that remain largely undocumented. Moreover, they demonstrate the potential sophistication of historiated initials, which, despite their simple organization and relatively small size, can communicate the intricacies of social status, relationships, emotions, and temporality. The manuscripts of the *Régime* are many things at once. Exploring what happens when these genres or spheres of knowledge intersect, and what we can learn from such overlaps, is a primary concern of this book.

Despite the fact that these manuscripts engage with so many different facets of medieval culture, scholars have primarily dealt with them from a single perspective and in a selective way: as part of a textual tradition, as medical manuscripts, or as medical imagery. While the illustrated manuscripts have not received sustained study as a group, the text of the *Régime* that survives in extant manuscripts has been

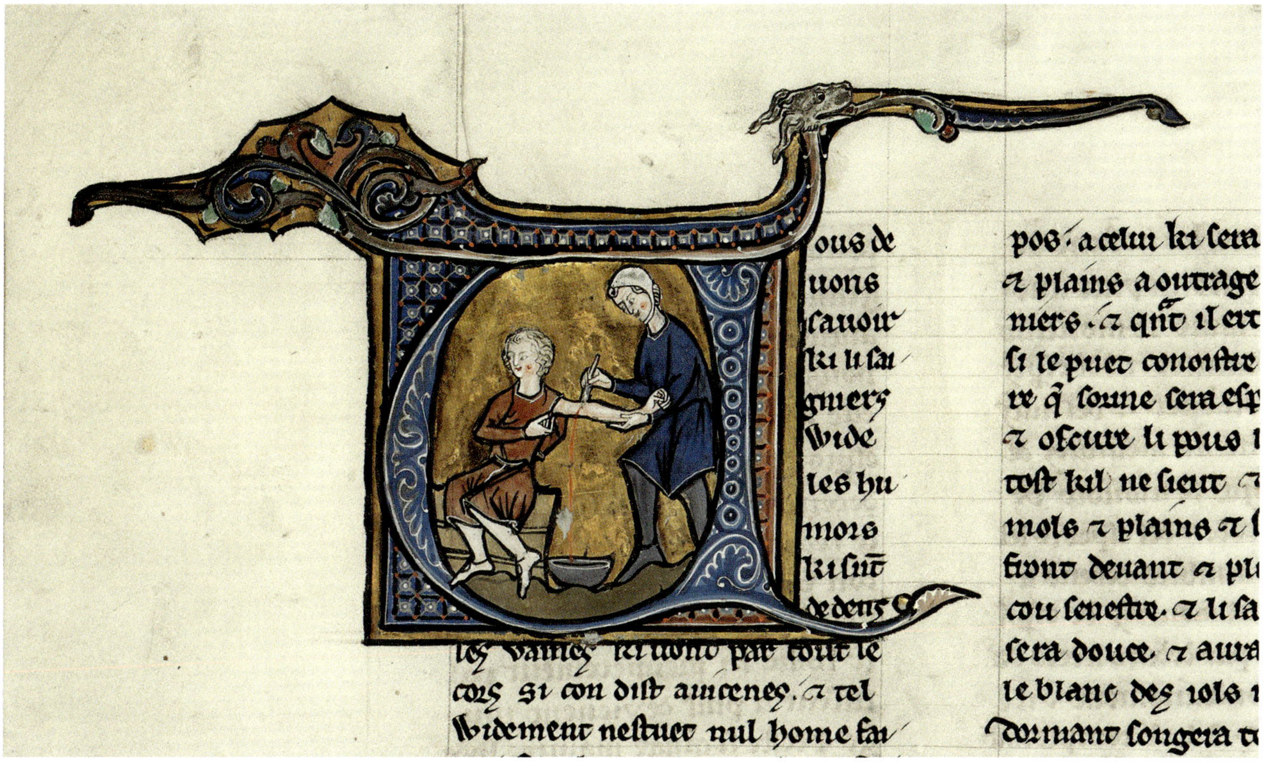

Fig. 1
Bloodletting. *Le Régime du corps*, ca. 1265–70. British Library, Sloane MS 2435, fol. 11v, detail. © The British Library Board.

more thoroughly considered, most notably in Louis Landouzy and Roger Pépin's 1911 transcription of the *Régime du corps*.[4] This indispensable work provides an introductory essay discussing the context and significance of the *Régime*, a catalogue of known manuscripts at the time, and a transcription based on Bibliothèque nationale de France Fr. 2021, thought to be the earliest version of the text.[5] Many of the most important conclusions about the *Régime*—that it was written by Aldobrandino for Beatrice in 1256, that it is one of the first medical texts to be written in French, and that it plays a role in the vernacular explosion of the thirteenth century—are established here by Landouzy and Pépin. Since then, scholars including Françoise Fery-Hue, Marilyn Nicoud, and Sebastiano Bisson have contributed to the work of Landouzy and Pépin by identifying additional copies and expanding a discussion of the literary tradition in multiple languages (see also appendix 3).[6] Along with Fery-Hue, scholars such as Paul Meyer, Kathleen Sewright, Theresa L. Tyers, and Luís Campos Ribeiro have also published work that digs more deeply into specific manuscripts, while Monica H. Green and Peter Murray Jones have considered the broader implications of the *Régime* tradition from perspectives that include women's medicine and the visual culture of medicine.[7] As a prime example of the popular genre of regimen texts that were based on an established medical canon but likely created for lay readers, Aldobrandino's work for Beatrice facilitated the consideration of academic medicine in the domestic realm.

While the *Régime* images are of a genre sometimes dismissed for presenting inaccurate or oversimplified representations of medical procedures and other activities related to health care, they are also remarkably rich in other types of information. For example, in the bloodletting scene from Sloane 2435, the clothing and headwear of the practitioner suggest that he is not a physician; this correlates with what we know about medieval bloodletting practices, which were traditionally administered by barbers (and later surgeons, or barber-surgeons) even when recommended by physicians. It is true that the composure of the sitter, as well as the extremely tidy nature of the wound and dripping blood, suggest an idealized portrait of this relatively common activity. But this image successfully demonstrates the content of the chapter, while also displaying the particular aesthetics associated with historiated initials in all kinds of manuscripts from this period: simplicity for the sake of clarity, and room for embellishments to further accentuate the status of the book as a whole.

The illustrated manuscripts of the *Régime*—not only their text but also their images—provide important evidence for thinking through the complex points of crossover between the different spheres of late medieval medical care. The *Régime du corps* is a reflection of household health practices while also being informed by academic medicine. The illustrated copies often defy our preliminary expectations, in part because they are difficult to fit squarely into existing categories of knowledge. They are genre-bending books, existing at once as medical texts, encyclopedias, household guides, and women's books. Indeed, while their audiences were not exclusively made up of women, many of these copies can be associated with female users and the households they likely managed. These books illuminate women's agency within the sphere of the home, contributing to a richer understanding of healing practices as performed in the domestic sphere. In such spaces, female networks revised traditional medicine for their own purposes. My book argues that gender is essential to understanding the *Régime* and its images, illuminating for the first time the readers of these manuscripts, the impact these books had on the care of the body within the home, and, more broadly, the roles for women's work within the medieval household.

Gendering Audience and Use

The model of dissemination implied by the *Régime*'s prologue, which suggests that distribution was made possible by the movement of women, provides a central framework for my consideration of the illustrated copies, including what role women and their households had in their production and what kinds of audiences might have had access to them. By taking this methodological cue from the manuscripts themselves, I aim to consider the contexts of these books through the perspectives of such likely commissioners.[8] Undetermined patronage is often quite common for women's books, in part because archival and documentary material for both object and owner is often less substantial. As a result, my project is deeply informed by work in medieval gender studies that has explored women as patrons, owners, and readers of medieval books.[9] Such likely audiences are suggested in the domestic context that we see illustrated in these manuscripts, illuminating a sphere of knowledge that oversaw much of household health.

Not much is known about Aldobrandino of Siena, an Italian who worked in France; later in his life he is thought to have lived in Troyes and apparently died there in 1287.[10] He seems to have worked primarily for Beatrice, though he may have served as physician to Louis IX and his wife, Margaret of Provence, as well.[11] He is most often discussed as an example of a thirteenth-century author writing in the vernacular (in this case, French), and he is often paired with Brunetto Latini as an educated Italian who wrote early vernacular texts in French.[12] The earliest copies of the *Régime* are written in Walloon, a dialect associated with northern France (rather than the Provençal language of Beatrice's home region), and as a result some scholars have speculated that Aldobrandino had a northern scribe.[13]

More, however, is known about Aldobrandino's audience. The *Régime du corps* is one example of the genre known as "regimen literature" that was popular by the thirteenth century. Some regimen literature was written for very specific patrons, and some was much more broadly conceived and disseminated; Aldobrandino's *Régime du corps* has been positioned somewhere between these two types.[14] This could be the result of the particular circumstances of the text's commissioning. Although Aldobrandino may have been the personal physician of Beatrice of Savoy and apparently worked for her for most of his career, his text was not intended exclusively for her, but for her to share with her daughters. Although these daughters cannot be directly tied to the illustrated copies, their movement is constructive for thinking through how these books came to be. This new vernacular and domestically oriented collection of medical material moved quickly throughout Europe, possibly as each daughter brought the text into her home and introduced it to a new audience.

The extensively illustrated manuscripts of the *Régime* were constructed to be on a par with other types of books commissioned by royal patrons of the period, in that they likewise served as examples of luxury, literacy, and cosmopolitanism as they moved between owners and across lands. Thinking about these manuscripts as having "object itineraries" draws particular attention to their movements, and potentially the movements of their users and owners, over time, even when we cannot know all the details of that trajectory. This approach is central to the 2019 volume *Moving Women, Moving Objects (400–1500)*, edited by Tracy Chapman Hamilton and Mariah Proctor-Tiffany, which considers women as instigators for the movement of medieval objects.[15] Proposed in a 2015 volume edited by anthropologists Rosemary A. Joyce and Susan D. Gillespie, the concept of an "object itinerary" builds on the ideas of new materialism, object-oriented ontology, and Igor Kopytoff's "object biography."[16] In their volume, the object itinerary model is used to explore the routes "by which things circulate in and out of places where they come to rest or are active."[17] They advocate for the "object itinerary" over the "object biography" initially proposed by Kopytoff in his 1986 essay on the cultural biography of things.[18] Kopytoff's assertion is that objects—more precisely, commodities—can be seen as having "life histories" analogous to the life of a person.[19] Joyce and Gillespie acknowledge the powerful force of this notion, now an established concept in anthropology, but they also point out a number of issues with this construction.[20] There are limits to thinking about objects in the circumscribed time frame of a finite human life; our understanding of the nature of objects and how they work is obscured by such personification.[21]

The benefits of thinking about itineraries, on the other hand, are manifold. According to Joyce and Gillespie: "Examining the itineraries of things requires consideration of technologies for circulation; of impediments and facilitators of movement; of natural and cultural transformations along the way; of whether objects travel intact or incomplete, with others or alone; of the landscapes that result from the places linked through their travels; and of the value of circulating objects for the production and reshaping of cultural relations that separate people, as well as for those that connect persons, places, and things across space and time."[22] By putting "even partial and collective objects into context as segments of potentially unending itineraries," this approach allows us to make use of the fragmentary information about each *Régime* manuscript despite the absence of original patrons or owners.[23] It encourages the consideration of each manuscript's life beyond the initial period of construction and encapsulates the longer temporal and spatial trajectory of these books. Medieval access to such objects was not only the privilege of the initial commissioner or owner; several generations of families and their wider households, including both men and women, would have made up the audiences for these books. And of course, if we think about how medieval books, and many other household belongings, moved around over the course of their lives, key instances in the movement of those items would have been the result of women relocating for marriage or making gifts to family members, including sisters and daughters.[24]

Facets of my arguments in the following chapters are also informed by historical approaches like social history that are broadly employed within interdisciplinary fields like medieval studies. For example, in lieu of the identification of specific commissioners or owners for these illustrated *Régime* copies, it is often possible to narrow down their patronage or ownership to a small group of people, or at least to make a case for the social group in which the manuscript was made. Establishing the late medieval audiences interested in texts like the *Régime* contributes to a better understanding of these books. The shared characteristics evident across this group of manuscripts imply strong connections among them; these connections are further strengthened by the clear familial networks across Europe, but especially across the English Channel, that they represent. Indeed, these manuscripts encourage investigation into and actively invite speculation about producers, commissioners, and users.

While this book focuses on the illustrated copies of the *Régime*, the owners and readers of those manuscripts are not necessarily identical to the readership for the larger textual tradition. The breadth of the potential audiences for the text of the *Régime* is also implied in appendix 3, a list of currently known copies of the text. Even though the text is part of a vernacular textual tradition that is often associated with the burgeoning interest in medicine and science by lay readers, the *Régime du corps* was clearly also of interest to some academic readers. This broader group of manuscripts includes academic volumes that were likely intended for physicians or scholars; the *Régime* appears alongside Roger Frugardi's surgical text, work by the Montpellier doctor Bernard de Gordon, or urology texts.[25] This combination of texts may have been collected in part to educate physicians on the health-care information that was commonly of interest to lay readers, providing such readers with strategies for communicating complex theories to their patients. There are also manuscripts with a devotional focus that suggest a religious audience, including texts such as the Psalms, the Life of St. Margaret, hymns, or other types of prayers alongside the *Régime*.[26] Such copies reinforce the intertwined nature of prayer, medical treatment, and everyday practices for addressing health and well-being. For these reasons, it is a futile project to attempt to summarize what the usual reader for the *Régime* text might have looked like—indeed, the most accurate statement would be that there are numerous different audiences for this text.

Women were undoubtedly participants in manuscript culture broadly conceived, but their role as an audience for specifically medical manuscripts is less established. Indeed, in much of her work, historian Monica H. Green has convincingly demonstrated that many medieval obstetric and gynecological textual traditions were developed for male academic readers while being explicitly unavailable to women.[27] She argues that, as women's medicine became of interest to medical professionals, its traditions were coopted by the masculine medical establishment. Even when considering female ownership of medical texts, Green concludes that very few such texts were owned or read by women.[28] But regimen texts like the *Régime du corps* were a different, albeit related, health tradition, one that was likely more accessible to a wider range of potential audiences.[29] Green's foundational work on women's health care in the context of learned medicine grounds my study and is complemented by additional scholarship that considers less established forms of health-related textual traditions, such as recipes and general regimens such as the *Régime du corps*. For example, Monserrat Cabré and Theresa L. Tyers focus on forms of everyday health care that are inherently difficult to trace and employ approaches that aim to get at these somewhat ephemeral traditions. Cabré argues that recipes, often left unconsidered when made as marginal or ancillary notes in manuscripts, are key to understanding the traditions of health management in the domestic sphere, often orally transmitted practices communicated between women.[30] Tyers's approach has been to carefully consider the texts compiled in specific manuscripts, looking at the "internal logic" and offering compelling evidence for a focus on health concerns pertinent to household use.[31] Elaine Leong's work on household medicine in early modern England, although admittedly focused on later sources from the seventeenth century, provides another excellent model for thinking about this significance of knowledge creation in the domestic sphere.[32] Such work supports my emphasis on women's roles in domestic health care in relation to the illustrated copies of the *Régime*.

Although we cannot determine precisely why this text would have developed a strand of illustrated manuscripts, the pictorial tradition nevertheless provides an additional perspective into the activities and interactions associated with household health care. Even if the patrons and owners of the illustrated copies were not always also readers of the books they owned, the illustrated copies convey rich commentary regarding contemporary practices especially pertinent to women, starting with the noblewomen for whom the texts may have been created. By considering the object itineraries of these books across a larger network of time and space and by reconstructing as much as possible their trajectories from initial creation to where they are today, we in essence trace the paths of Beatrice's four daughters.

Illustrating the *Régime du corps*

Within the surviving illustrated copies, this study focuses on a specific subgroup of copies that employ historiated initials, exploring the visual language shared among these manuscripts as well as the compelling communicative power the historiated initial format offers. I discuss these manuscripts in two chronological groupings, a division that makes sense in terms of place of production as well as dating and aligns with certain affinities evident between the manuscripts within each group. Three were created in the late thirteenth and fourteenth centuries (British Library Sloane MS 2435, Bibliothèque nationale de France Fr. 12323, and Bibliothèque nationale de France Arsenal MS 2510), and four date from the fifteenth century (British Library Sloane MS 2401, Cambridge University Library Ii.V.11, Morgan Library MS M.165, and Ajuda Cod. 52-XIII-26).

Among the three earlier illustrated manuscripts of the *Régime*, Sloane 2435 was likely made by an identified artist, the "Aldobrandin Master," in northern France between 1265 and 1270. Seventy-two images appear with the *Régime* in this manuscript, one of the earliest copies of the text to survive, and they share distinct similarities with BnF Fr. 12323, which was made later, probably around 1350 in Paris. Neither of these copies has been directly linked to specific patrons or early owners. The third copy in this group is Arsenal 2510, likely made ca. 1285 in northern France. This manuscript's date is more concrete because it has been attributed to the Bute Painter, a fairly well-known artist working in cities such as Cambrai, Tournai, Lille, and Saint-Omer in the 1270s and 1280s. Arsenal 2510 is aesthetically unique, with a smaller number of images that display notable innovation.

The latter group of illustrated manuscripts includes four known copies that are all dated to the fifteenth century and reflect significant affinities with one another. They all have a similar number of images, around 140, and contain comparable subject matter in many of their scenes. Cambridge Ii.V.11 and Morgan MS M.165 were likely both made in Rouen around 1440–50. Sloane 2401 shares much with these two copies and likely has a similar origin. The fourth example exhibiting this extensive program of

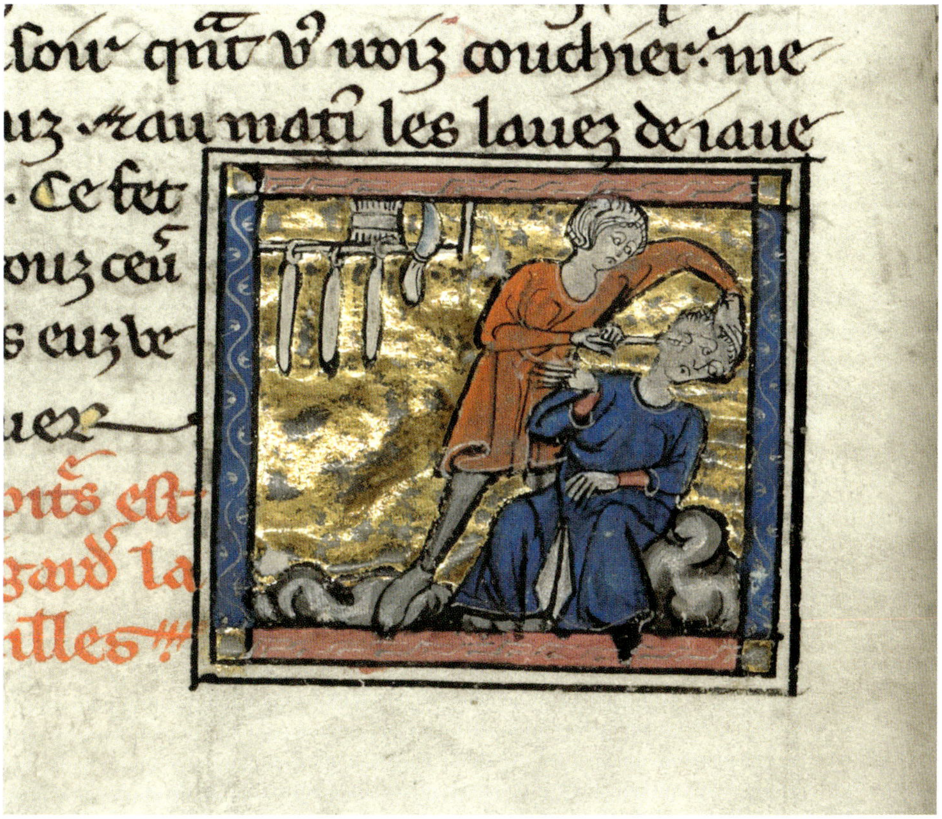

Fig. 2
Ears. *Le Régime du corps*, ca. 1270–1300. Universitätsbibliothek Leipzig, Cod. Haen. 3478, fol. 67v, detail. Universitätsbibliothek Leipzig.

historiated initials is Ajuda 52-XIII-26, which has been dated to around 1470–80 and tied to specific artists working in Bruges: primarily the Master of the Harley Froissart (Philippe de Mazerolles), possibly with additional work by the Master of the London Wavrin. All four seem to have been made on the Continent in cities such as Rouen and Bruges but are then linked to English owners within a few decades of production.

Some additional *Régime* manuscripts exist with illustrations in formats different from the focus of my book. Although I do not deal with them in depth, further information can be found in the appendices. These manuscripts include a group of twelve that display either a single introductory initial or frontispiece, rather than an extended program of illustrations. Furthermore, three other manuscripts contain image programs that differ significantly from the copies with historiated initials: Universitätsbibliothek Leipzig Cod. Haen. 3478, Biblioteca Apostolica Vaticana MS Reg.lat.1256, and Bibliothèque nationale de France Arsenal MS 2894. Leipzig Cod. Haen. 3478 is a late thirteenth- or early fourteenth-century manuscript, likely made in France; the *Régime du corps* is its only text.[33] The illustration program includes thirty-five images, slightly larger than most historiated initials in terms of proportion on the page. Although its scenes are not contained within letters, rectangular frames of similar scale to initials confine tight spaces, which are integrated into the text block, and

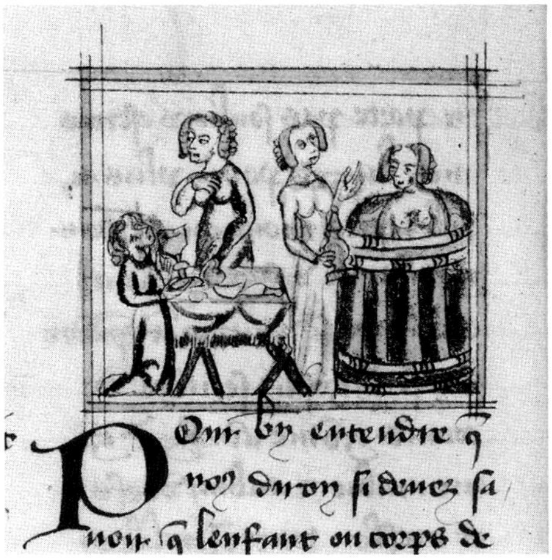

Fig. 3
Pregnancy. *Le Régime du corps*, fifteenth century. Biblioteca Apostolica Vaticana, Reg.lat.1256, fol. 37v, detail. © 2021 by permission of Biblioteca Apostolica Vaticana, Rome.

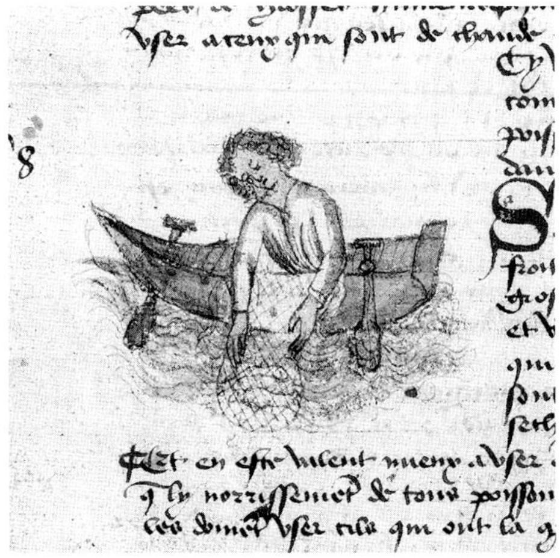

Fig. 4
Fish. *Le Régime du corps*, fifteenth century. Bibliothèque nationale de France, Arsenal MS 2894, fol. 91v, detail. © Bibliothèque nationale de France.

the simplicity of the scenes is evocative of historiated initials as well (fig. 2). I occasionally reference this copy because of some of these formal similarities to copies with historiated initials.

The two other versions, Reg.lat.1256 and Arsenal 2894, are later copies from the fifteenth century. The twenty-one images in Reg.lat.1256 are limited to part 1 of the *Régime* text.[34] Although they are contained within frames, the limited palette and light wash share little with the aesthetics of the other copies (fig. 3). Arsenal 2894 contains eighty-one loosely sketched but colored images without frames at all. The manuscript's text is an amalgamation of different medical treatises and various pieces of the *Régime*, and its images, including several diagrams, correspond to a variety of texts (fig. 4).[35] Although in-depth analysis of each of these manuscripts goes beyond the scope of this book, they represent the diversity and expansiveness of approaches to illustrating the *Régime* and offer opportunities for continued research by scholars.

The relatively large corpus of *Régime* manuscripts includes dozens that are unillustrated, even as we acknowledge the robust illustrative tradition upon which my book is focused. Many are in a humbler form than the illustrated copies, indicating that the text itself was of interest to a variety of audiences ranging from physicians to clergy to other individuals or households.[36] It seems clear, therefore, that the text was seen as useful in a variety of incarnations. While we can never be absolutely certain as to why some copies were illustrated and others were not, the relative consistency in the historiated initial programs indicates a shared purpose for those images in that smaller group of books. As such, we might ask what new content the illustrations brought to those copies, what types of audiences would have been interested in that content or messaging, and what seems to be missing in copies without such extensive illumination. I argue that the illustrated copies offer an additional visual narrative as evidence of domestic health care, one that is not present in the unillustrated versions of the text. Aside from the obviously pronounced ostentation of a book filled with energetic and provocative scenes that are encased in embellished and glittering decorative letters, the images packed much more information into these books—information that relates specifically to the domestic context in which those copies circulated. What is conveyed in those images is essentially what this entire book is about.

Depicting Health Care

Each copy I discuss contains dozens of historiated initials, ranging from totals of thirty-seven to 149, which introduce chapters and most often contain a simple scene of activity. While the illustrated *Régime* manuscripts all have unique characteristics and stylistic idiosyncrasies, their images share a general compositional format.[37] Most of the illustrated copies of the *Régime* do not include larger, full-page images or images other than initials, except for the occasional embellished expansion of letter elements with hybrid creatures (as in Sloane 2435) or a single frontispiece on a larger scale. The initial, therefore, establishes a form that is shared across this diverse group of illustrated *Régime* manuscripts and the many images within them, setting up a type of engagement with the reader that facilitates intimate looking as much as it does reading.

The bloodletting scene from Sloane 2435 described at the beginning of this introduction provides a glimpse of the variety and inventiveness to be found in this group of illustrated manuscripts. The historiated initials range in topic, format, and pictorial strategy; they include images that feature various treatments or consultations, household activities such as food and drink production or preparation, and simple representations of specific animals and plants essential to a healthy lifestyle. The animal and plant images, in which a creature or substance is often depicted in isolation, parallel medieval manuscript traditions of bestiaries and medical herbals, though in the sections of the *Régime* that deal with such fauna and flora we also see various chapters represented with people in the act of production. For example, a guilty-looking monk sneaks a taste of wine in an image from Sloane 2435 (fig. 5), and two men stir apple mush in a cider-making scene from Sloane 2401 (fig. 6, top initial).

Other household activities, such as bathing, sleeping, or copulation, are captured with nuance and inflected with commentary despite being depicted in compact and concise scenes. Body parts are often represented with a patient being treated for an ailment in that part of the body. The particularly innovative artist of Arsenal 2510, known at the Bute Painter, tackles these potentially boring topics with eye-catching perspective, as seen in his image for the chapter on hair (fig. 7); his scene for the chapter on vomiting is also

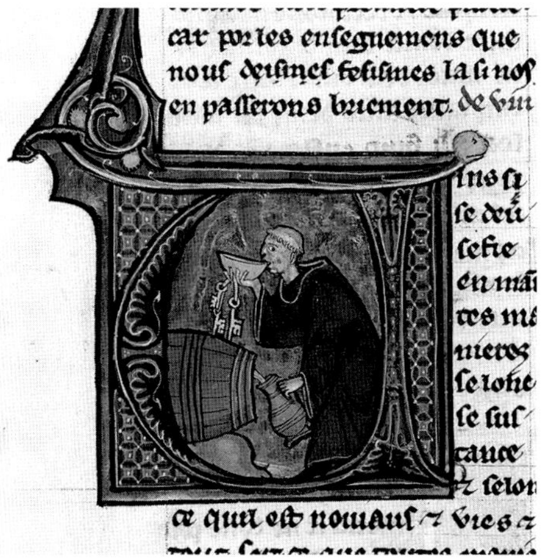

Fig. 5
Wine. *Le Régime du corps*, ca. 1265–70. British Library, Sloane MS 2435, fol. 44v, detail. © The British Library Board.

Régime du corps that are the focus of this book, including basic codicological information, the number of historiated initials, and other texts included within the same manuscripts. The second appendix lists the specific illustrations included in each of those manuscripts, allowing for an instant comparison of their pictorial programs. And the third includes a list of all the known manuscripts that include the *Régime* text in part or in whole (seventy-five at the time of publication), along with some basic information about those manuscripts, offering some sense of an answer to questions about the shape of the *Régime*'s tradition beyond the illustrated copies alone.

The illustrated *Régime du corps* manuscripts were filled with images, often spectacular scenes embellished with many colors and gold leaf. These books were clearly expressions of status, luxurious objects intended to reflect the social position, wealth, and learning of their owners. At the same time, however, much more can be gained from these books than merely their economic significance. Complicating the narrative of these books as solely status objects, I instead approach them as useful tools that both encouraged and displayed household habits of care, practices that are especially pronounced in the historiated initials themselves. Consequently, the illustrated scenes in these manuscripts are transformed into compelling evidence for women as active agents within the household, enacting multiple types of care that would have taken place within the home. Alongside the academic medicine of learned physicians, a wide variety of paths were available to facilitate good health, and many of those were based in the domestic sphere. The *Régime*'s images, this book contends, provide a unique view of this expanded world of health care, broadening notions of medical community and asserting a more human-focused view of medicine based on daily care of the body.

THE VISUAL LANGUAGE OF THE *RÉGIME DU CORPS*

I

In one of the more arresting scenes depicted in the illustrated *Régime du corps* manuscripts, two women stand opposite each other. One woman bares her breast, while the other reaches out to touch the exposed extremity (fig. 8). This image depicts the evaluation of a wet nurse, and, as we look more closely, further details illuminate our understanding of this exchange. The woman on our left, who holds out her breast for examination, is dressed in less refined clothing, while the woman on the right is clearly the more elite of the two. The woman on the left offers up her breast with one hand, while her other hand gestures in acquiescence; in contrast, the figure on the right evokes power both through her somewhat aggressive grabbing of the other woman and through her other hand's gesture of authoritative direction, or even admonition.

This scene of wet nurse selection is one of inherent inequality, inequality that is visually explicated through careful use of clothing, gesture, and touch by the image's designer. The image expresses power relations based on class but also implies a certain anxiety around the selection of a wet nurse and her subsequent care of the child. The nuanced associations reproduced in this exchange reveal the remarkable sophistication of the often seemingly basic images in the *Régime*. Such sophistication is also evident in the open-ended ambiguity of some scenes, which speak to the very real state of uncertainty in medieval health care on the ground.

That complexity is in some degree a result of the format used in these manuscripts. In some respects, they resemble any number of other later medieval manuscripts, with folios that have both text and image, often with embellished letters and other marginal decoration, and many chapters punctuated by historiated initials containing scenes of activity. The pigments and gold leaf, as well as the various drawing styles, seem to reflect what we also frequently see in manuscripts of the thirteenth through the fifteenth centuries: bibles, books of hours, chronicles, psalters, and encyclopedias. Without question, the *Régime du corps* manuscripts reflect the aesthetics,

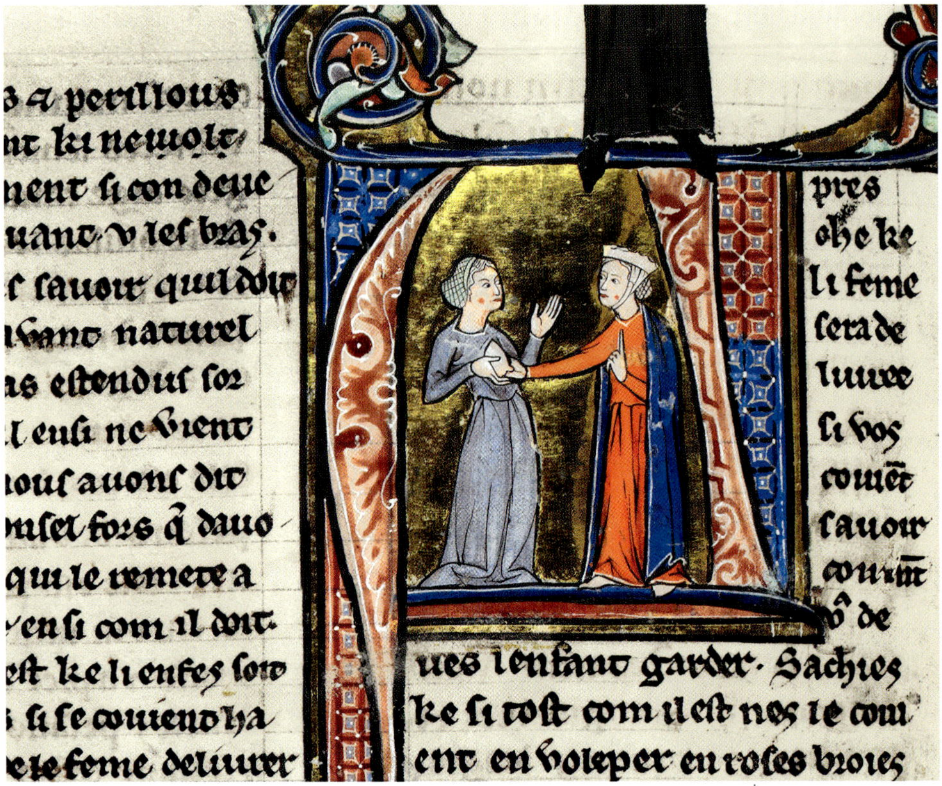

Fig. 8
Wet nurse scene. *Le Régime du corps*, ca. 1265–70. British Library, Sloane MS 2435, fol. 28v, detail. © The British Library Board.

forms, and styles of their period, and in many ways that context is clearly evident in them. At the same time, however, these books demonstrate how many of these conventional building blocks can be combined and employed in new ways. The books reveal a wide range of strategies on the part of the designers to select a scene for the initial letter that introduces each chapter, strategies that help us better understand how these books might have been used, and how those decisions might have directly affected that use. Here we see the bringing together of models with nuance and subtlety and, when such sources were unavailable, originality and innovation.

The *Régime* manuscripts that exclusively display historiated initials are just as sophisticated as better-known books of the period, if not more so, for how they reflect serious consideration of form as well as content. Despite the small spaces within which the creator had to work, the historiated initials of the *Régime* manuscripts hold a remarkable amount of information—not only about what is happening in the scene, but also regarding aspects such as authority, status, and narrative nuance. Throughout these manuscripts, brief snapshots of action in progress are used to imply further activity and events; the apparent simplicity of images in an encyclopedic compendium are far more complex than they initially appear.

The narrative ambiguity displayed in many of the *Régime* images allowed the users to move beyond the books' diagnosis and treatment and into the physical realities of their own time and place. Although the *Régime* images are narratively independent, each as a single episode has the potential to be part of its own narrative, admittedly one that is largely left unillustrated, in what scholars have described as "monoscenic" or "monophase" pictures.[1] In some ways, these treatment scenes operate like other medieval narrative images. However, as single images that are not part of a narratively connected sequence of several scenes, they also demonstrate some of the limitations of traditional narrative interpretation. Elsewhere I have asserted that such single-scene images function in a way similar to the cinematic freeze-frame, which is able to conjure for the viewer the moments before and after as well as that which has been captured.[2] The freeze-frame allows for the possibility of multiple futures, futures imagined by the viewer, who is engaged to help construct the narrative instigated by the captured image. In the case of the *Régime du corps* and its focus on health, the viewer is encouraged not only to create imaginatively the image's outcome but also, possibly corporeally, to experience or even facilitate that outcome in the real world.

The potentiality of a freeze-framed scene uniquely hinges not just on its form but also on the specifics of the scene's content and the particular moment that has been captured. When the content is medical or practical in nature, it engages the viewer beyond a simple mental construction of narrative. An unresolved scene both allows and encourages audience participation, providing a point of departure for the viewer to create ideas about the possible conclusion of the depicted activities. Thinking about the historiated initial as a freeze-frame emphasizes how a single scene of action in progress can create even more narrative potential than a pictured series of scenes, and how it does so expressly by engaging the viewer to make those imaginative leaps. The viewer's "filling-in" action selects a specific choice among a multitude of options, all of which may lead to different outcomes; in the case of medical treatment, these outcomes will potentially take place in the actual, physical world.

The images of these manuscripts present unique commentary about social relationships that is not evident in the text alone. My focused discussion around the depictions of wet nurses serves as a key example of such visuality, in which touch or its absence impacts how intimacy or gestures of power are indicated. The subtleties of these visualized interactions communicated incredible depth and complexity to the users of these books, nuancing their understanding of the *Régime* text while bringing far more content to contemplate with each chapter. The scenes provided numerous inflections that informed the reader's thinking about the status of each figure, their roles in each scene, and the parallels that might be noticed across the manuscript's pictorial program.

In efficient, economic ways, the images delivered to book users information about a wide variety of relationships that occurred in these domestic encounters, potentially offering guidance for how to negotiate situations, anticipate new experiences, and exert one's own authority. The negotiations of power implied in these scenes do not always align with traditional modes of gender, class, or intellectual status. Within the social sphere of the household, the circumstances of caring for bodies often disregard conventional status and hierarchies.[3] As such, the unresolved narratives in these initials engaged the reader and moved them into the real world, forcing them to consider the unknowns of health care in the realm of reality.

Text and Image Relationships in the *Régime du corps*

The types of subjects we find illustrated in these versions of the *Régime du corps* align to a certain degree with the four main sections of the text: following the Prologue, the first part deals with general dietetic aspects for preserving health; the second with care for different parts of the body; the third with "simples" or remedies that include food and beverage recommendations; and the fourth, a short section, with physiognomy. Part 1, on aspects of preserving one's health, has twenty-one chapters, including those on topics such as drinking, air, sleeping, bathing, sex and reproduction, care of an infant, purging, cupping, and bleeding. The images in these chapters tend to depict scenes in which these activities take place or treatments are administered. In the scenes of treatment, we usually see two people, a patient and a practitioner. The second part, on care for different parts of the body, is presented in eight chapters, which include subjects such as the eyes, the ears, and the hair. This section also often includes images of two people, one administering a treatment to another. The third part focuses on remedies, with up to 136 sections on grains, beverages, meat, birds, legumes, fruits, herbs, fish and dairy, and spices. Throughout this section, we see a variety of subjects in the accompanying images, ranging from one or two people involved in the activity of preparing a particular substance to more static images that depict a particular animal, plant, or spice. The last part, on physiognomy, contains twenty-seven very short chapters. This section essentially lists various characteristics that would ostensibly allow one to know the nature of an individual by their external complexion or appearance and is usually accompanied by only one or two images, including that of a physician facing and gesturing toward a nude man and nude woman, presumably in the process of assessing their visible characteristics.

One of the results of the widespread dissemination of the *Régime*, as indicated by the large body of existing copies, is that different redactions developed over time. Landouzy and Pépin acknowledged four different redactions, and Fery-Hue builds on their distinctions to identify Redaction A, Redaction B, a mixed redaction, and an abridged redaction.[4] Sloane 2435 includes Redaction B, and BnF Fr. 12323 contains the mixed redaction. Arsenal 2510, which has the fewest historiated initials of the copies on which I focus, also includes the abridged redaction. The fifteenth-century copies contain a popular variation of Redaction B known as "roger male branche," which includes that phrase in the chapter on sorghum, further emphasizing the connection between the manuscripts in that group.[5] The sample chapter titles I provide here are from Redaction B.

The condensed nature of Aldobrandino's text resulted in general suggestions but without a great amount of specificity, and certainly nothing as detailed as a recipe. For example, the chapter on copulation, "To live with a woman" (*d'abiter avoec femme*), emphasizes setting up conditions for successful procreation in terms of food, sleep, and other factors and focuses on determining the best moment in the digestive process and amount of rest. The chapter begins by addressing a male reader, stating, "He who has sense and discernment should devote his understanding and all of his efforts to learning how one should cohabit with a woman."[6] Much of the advice in this section concerns food and drink before and after intercourse, especially for the male partner; the chapter concentrates on the man's health as the key to successful procreation. This theory is hardly unique to Aldobrandino; he refers to commonly held ideas based on Galenic philosophies that ascribe the greater life-giving force to the man's semen while the woman is characterized primarily as a vessel.[7] In fact, he names ʿAlī ibn al-ʿAbbās al-Majūsī (known in the Latin West as Haly Abbas) and Galen in his text as authorities on this topic.[8]

Another chapter in part 1 of the *Régime*, on bathing (*du baignier*), does not give a single guideline for frequency but instead includes instructions that consider different seasons, eating (before or after bathing), and bathing at different ages. In another, later chapter on caring for the body at all ages (*comment on se doit garder en iiii aages et tarder de viellece et soi maintenir jovenes*), Aldobrandino discusses bathing at different stages of the life cycle: for pregnant women, newborn babies, children, the middle-aged, and the old.[9] Indeed, much of the timing discussed in the *Régime du corps* seems to be in terms of the life cycle rather than of the daily or monthly basis that we might expect based on the astrological medicine of the period.

In the chapter on caring for a woman during pregnancy (*comment la feme se doit garder quant ele est ençainte et comment ele se doit delivrer*), broader practices of health maintenance are adjusted for such unique circumstances, including recommendations to avoid bleeding or purging during the earlier and later parts of a pregnancy; these procedures are deemed acceptable, however, during the fourth and fifth months.[10] The pregnant woman is encouraged toward some foods and away from others, discouraged from bathing until the last few weeks, and instructed to avoid extreme emotional stresses and seek out joy.[11] The chapter also provides some suggestions for drinks, perfumes, and steeped baths as the delivery time approaches, as well as care for the woman after she gives birth, or in the case of a stillbirth. The next chapter deals with caring for a newborn (*comment on doit garder l'enfant quant il est nés et d'eslire et connoistre la norrice pour l'enfant norrir et garder*) and covers cleaning, swaddling, nursing, and when to wean.[12] Much of the chapter is dedicated to the selection of a wet nurse based on a range of characteristics, including her age, physical condition and appearance, habits, breasts, and milk quality, as well as how to maintain her health once she is nursing.

Part 3 of the *Régime*, on "simples," focuses on foods and drinks for good health. These chapters are generally descriptions of the substances and their humoral characteristics (wet or dry, cold or hot), as well as what they are good for or the conditions they might be used to treat. The text also suggests what one might want to look for in terms of choosing a good version of the item, how it looks, the age of the substance,

en sante caude et sece u cau
de et moiste u froide et sece u
froide et moiste si se diuseferont
li signe si con dit vous avons
et cascuns u sera les coses con
traires a se naturel complexi
on et por savoir les quels sunt
especiaus medicines dou cuer
si le vous nomerons. Ce sunt
jagonsses. or. argent et bouglo
se et basilicum qui porte une
flourete noire ce sunt coses te
prees ki confortent le cuer.

Coses caudes por user
a ceus qui ont le cuer
froit si est zidoare
muse. ambre. sore soie. saffran
girofles siloes. melise. carda
mom. cubebes foille de cetr
inde enula. Coses froides por
user a ceux qui lont caut si st
pelles. margerites canfre san
dales blances. rouges. coral
blans et rouges. roses. carabes
et pode. terre sigillata. et pomes.
et coriande. sec. et vert. ce sunt
les coses apres pour le cuer
maintenir en sante. Or vous
meterons fin a ceste secunde
fin partie et ne vous en par
lerons plus por ce que qui set les
principaus membres des quels
nous vous avons parle gar
der en sante il saura garder
les autres membres legiere

ment. [illegible] la tier
ce partie ki vous enseigne
ra le nature de toutes coses
ki convienent [illegible]
[illegible]

Li premiers sera de toutes ma
nieres de bles et dou pain con
en fait.

Li secons de toutes manieres
de buverages.

Li tiers de toutes cars.

Li quars de tous leums

Li .v. de tous fruis.

Li .vi. de tous poissons.

Li .vii. de toutes manieres
derbes.

Li .viii. de toutes manieres
dues. de fromages. de lait.

Li .ix. de toutes espices. Li pre
miers cap. de tos bles et pre
mierement dou forment.

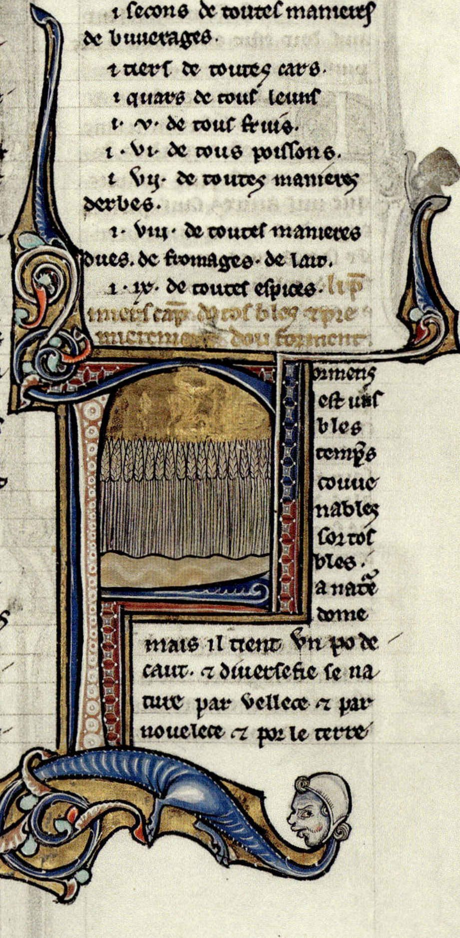

Formens
est uns
bles
temprés
couve
nables
sor tos
bles.
A nature
donne
mais il tient un po de
caut. et diversefie se na
ture par vellece et par
novelece et por le terre

and the different types that may exist. It does not, however, include more complex compounds or recipes, nor are the serving suggestions, preparations, or amounts very specific. Sometimes there are suggestions for how one might want to consume a substance. For example, eggs are most nourishing when "eaten with good spices, such as cinnamon, pepper and ginger, and with meat," than when eaten with cheese.[13]

Many chapters, especially those in part 3 on remedies, simply depict the item or substance that will be covered in that chapter and only occasionally contain human figures. These include various plants, animals, foods, and spices. For many of the plants depicted, the designers have rendered a small piece of a field with a handful of stalks or leaves, such as the image of wheat from Sloane 2435 (fig. 9). Despite the ornate decoration and coifed hybrid creature of the letter's frame, the grain is depicted with characteristic simplicity and even abstraction. Spices like pepper are frequently shown as a substance presented within a container such as a large sack (fig. 10). Chapters on meat, poultry, and fish are indicated with an image of the live animal, before slaughter, and thus in general show a strong affinity with the medieval bestiary tradition.[14]

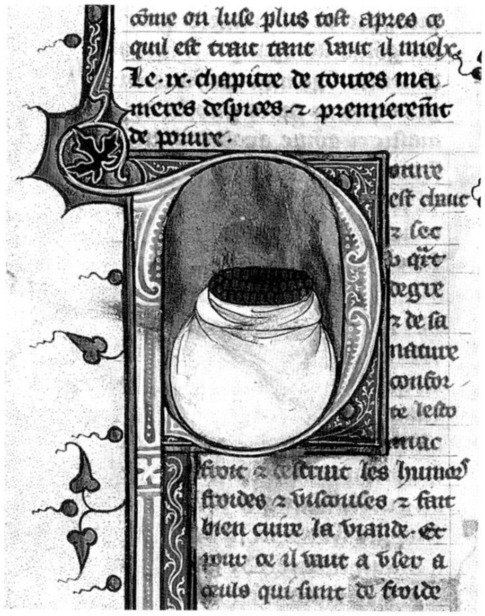

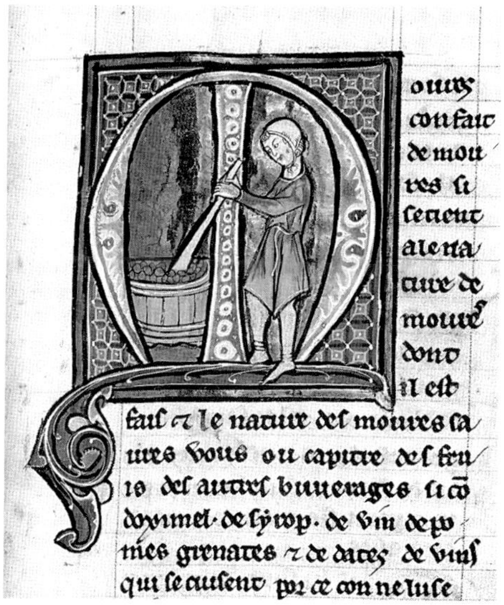

Fig. 9 (opposite)
Wheat. *Le Régime du corps*, ca. 1265–70. British Library, Sloane MS 2435, fol. 42r. © The British Library Board.

Fig. 10
Pepper. *Le Régime du corps*, fourteenth century. Bibliothèque nationale de France, Fr. 12323, fol. 130r, detail. © Bibliothèque nationale de France.

Fig. 11
Mulberries. *Le Régime du corps*, ca. 1265–70. British Library, Sloane MS 2435, fol. 46r, detail. © The British Library Board.

Other foods and beverages are illustrated with scenes of their production, as in the case of beer and cider. In Sloane 2435, a man is shown stirring a vat that contains mulberries (fig. 11). In the later group, several manuscripts also show some of the activities involved in making such products. The scenes of cider- and beer-making appear together on the same folio in both the Morgan and Cambridge manuscripts, and similar scenes are depicted in Sloane 2401 as well. In the Cambridge manuscript, the first initial shows a man with a hat bending over to put logs into a fire underneath the left-hand vat, with a second vat to the right; in the second initial, two men stand behind a wooden trough that angles up across the space; they hold large stirring sticks submerged in the bumpy apple mash that is in the trough, with two barrels in the foreground (fig. 12).

mieulx lui fait mais quil ne boiue a oultrage car le boire a oultra
ge fait mal ou foye & au cerueau et aux nerfs et fait gouttes et
fait les membres trambler & fait lomme deuenir paralitique & aucune
fois fait lomme mourir soubdainement et pource fait bon congnoistre
la nature de chascun selon ce quil aime et luy fait mieulx sil le doit user.

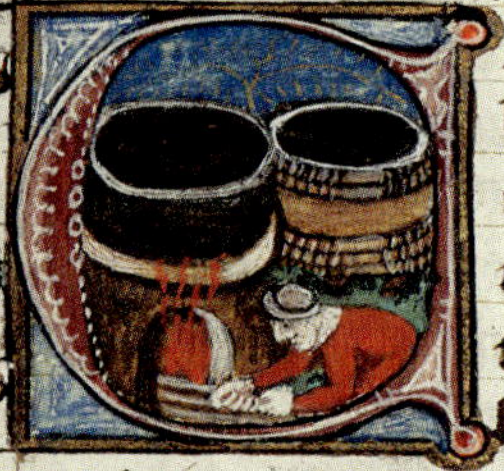

Ceruoise est une maniere de **de ceruoise.**
buurage que len fait de aueine & de froument
et dorge mais celle qui est daueine & de froument
vault mieulx pource quelle enfle ne ne fait
tant de ventosite. Mais de quelque chose quelle
soit faicte ou daueine ou dorge ou de froument
elle fait male teste et enfle la fourcelle & fait mauuaise alaine
et mauuaises dens & remplist de grosses fumees le cerueau. Et
pource que auec le vin la boit elle enyure legierement mais elle a
nature de faire lomme orine et bien oriner et de faire blanche char
et souefue. Et ceruoise qui est faicte de seigle ou de pain de seigle ou
il a mente & ache sur toutes autres ceruoises est la meilleur. De

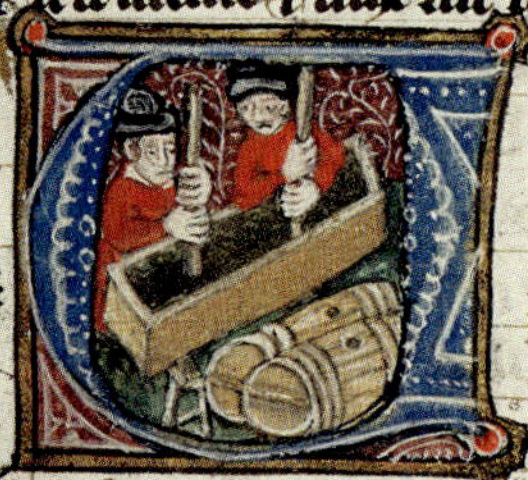

Vin qui est fait de pommes **vin de pommes.**
meures si est chault & moiste attrempement
mais il nest pas sain a user pource quil en
fle et engroissist la fourcelle & estoupe les
voies du foye & du pulmon mais il a nature
de engressier & de donner assez nourrissement
et vault especialment a ceulx qui ont la poitrine aspre et seiche
et qui ne peuent legierement cracher. Et se tel vin est fait de pom
mes aigres il tient nature de vin aigre et vault moult a ceulx
qui ont la cole amere & la fourcelle et qui ont le foye eschauffe.
Et toutes gens pourroient en este tel vin user quant il fait grant
chault. Verius que len fait de roisins qui ne sont pas meurs et de

Part 2 of the *Régime* covers a number of body parts, several of which are visualized only in the Arsenal manuscript. The image of "Hair" from this manuscript is particularly engaging, showing the foreshortened body of a person lying on a table, the top of their head facing the viewer and the hair falling down in flowing waves, while a second figure touches the long tresses (see fig. 7). The clarity and straightforwardness of this image belies the complexity and originality of its composition, which uses an unusual perspective to most clearly feature the body part under discussion. More frequently across the manuscripts, these body parts are illustrated with scenes in which a person with an ailment is treated by a practitioner. In BnF Fr. 12323, for example, the chapter on the eye shows a seated man looking upward to receive medication; the physician stands next to him and holds an inverted flask over the patient's face, presumably to pour some of a liquid into his eye (fig. 13). This more active approach for scenes in the body-part chapters of the second section of the *Régime*, in which a treatment is shown in progress, is similar to what we see for many of the scenes in part 1.

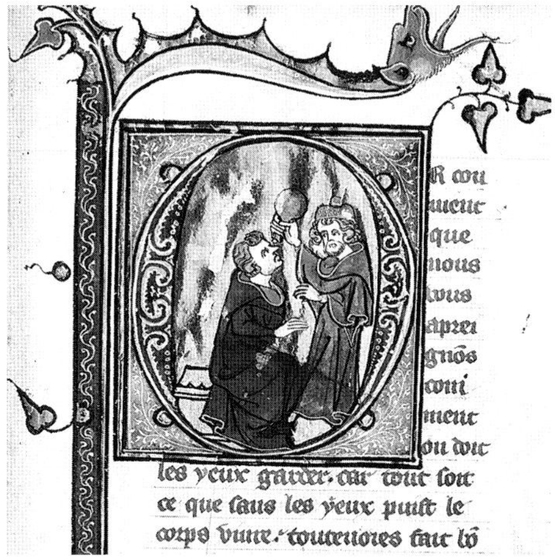

Fig. 12 (opposite)
Making beer and cider. *Le Régime du corps*, ca. 1450. Cambridge University Library, MS Ii.V.11, fol. 51r. Reproduced by kind permission of the Syndics of Cambridge University Library.

Fig. 13
Eye treatment. *Le Régime du corps*, fourteenth century. Bibliothèque nationale de France, Fr. 12323, fol. 103r, detail. © Bibliothèque nationale de France.

Although many of the topics and substances covered in the *Régime du corps* are included because the authorities cited by Aldobrandino discuss them, it is worth noting that many also indicate the elite audience he intended for his text. For example, the *Régime* includes many spices that were expensive and used only in upper-class households, including cinnamon, cloves, pepper, ginger, and saffron.[15] Such an elite audience is also worth keeping in mind in any assessment of Aldobrandino's contribution to medieval medicine. While it may seem that there is very little original material within the *Régime*, especially given its reliance on canonical sources, Landouzy and Pépin point out that this approach was commonly adopted by many medieval medical writers; furthermore, they argue that his efforts to create a French text that condensed known practice and authorities in fact introduced these ideas to a new and wider readership, making a significant contribution to the tradition.[16] In the words of Faith Wallis, "[t]he fact that Aldobrandino wrote in the vernacular reflects both the courtly milieu in which he worked and the appetite of the literate laity of the thirteenth century for didactic literature."[17] Although the abundant surviving copies of the text suggest a much wider readership than perhaps originally intended, it is clear that the upper-class audience reflected in the creation and content of the *Régime* aligns with the types of audiences who would have been patrons and owners of the illustrated copies.

Broader Visual Language

The illustrated *Régime* manuscripts have been underexplored by modern scholarship in part because they do not fall into any one pictorial tradition. Instead of seeing them as out of place, however, we are better positioned to understand them if we consider how they exist specifically at the intersections of numerous contexts. This is demonstrably clear when we consider the visual languages and systems carried out on their pages. Although these *Régime* manuscripts lack full-page illuminations and instead display small, simple scenes within historiated initials, their format and its resonances are exceedingly appropriate for incorporating ideas from a wide range of models as well as original new designs. These manuscripts were not created in isolation, and the artists and designers responsible for their creation would have made full use of existing models. Furthermore, these works are clearly in dialogue with various stylistic trends of the periods in which they were made.

The copies illustrated with historiated initials are generally of a similar size: Sloane 2435 is the largest, at 295 × 190 mm, or 11.6 × 7.5 inches, and Arsenal 2510 is the smallest, at 232 × 165 mm, about 9.1 × 6.5 inches (see appendix 1). Therefore, they are neither huge volumes laborious to manipulate nor handheld books intended for portability in a purse or pocket. They were sized to be easy to handle; in today's terms, their dimensions are a little smaller than a conventional piece of 8.5 × 11-inch paper, and a little larger than a paperback novel. This consistency is evident in the historiated initials, which are all of relatively small scale: a couple of inches in width and height, under 50 mm in each direction. Although these manuscripts are not precisely scaled to fit in the hand like books of hours, the scenes within them remain remarkably small and finely detailed.

The initials in these manuscripts reflect careful appropriation of artistic conventions, including period style, as well as innovative tactics when invention is required. For instance, the excessive gold leaf and other luxurious materials used in the production of these manuscripts are powerful indications of the wealth and position of the commissioners as well as the intended recipients. In Sloane 2435, most of the backgrounds of the scenes in the initials are gilded, as are the frames of the letters; the color palette is relatively diverse, and the figures' faces and bodies are tinted with pinks and reds and clearly defined with delicate brushstrokes. The Aldobrandin Master created figures that seem appropriately sized for the space they are given in the initial, and they generally have bodies that are in proportion. The figures in BnF Fr. 12323 seem a little clunkier than those in Sloane 2435, with noticeably large heads and hands that succeed in bringing attention to the abundant gestures throughout the manuscript; these figures also wear more specific garments and headgear, suggesting that in the context in which the manuscript was made, clothing was particularly important for the communication of status. Arsenal 2510 has a limited color palette of primarily blues, pink, red, and white; the figures are articulated through black lines drawn over white painting; and there is use of gold in the body of most of the letters. The aesthetics of

Arsenal 2510 demonstrate a number of characteristics evident in manuscripts associated with the Bute Painter, whose unique style depicts bodies in unusually dramatic positions, accentuated through gesture and expressiveness through bold lines and simplified compositions, along with an affinity for blue and pink tones.[18] Style is often a useful tool for identifying an individual artist's work, especially an artist as singular as the Bute Painter, but stylistic variances across a group of manuscripts also facilitate a better understanding of how these copies of the *Régime* relate to one another.

Both form and style offer insights into the relationships that exist between the later copies and broader traditions of the fifteenth century. The aesthetics of Cambridge Ii.V.11 not only are characterized by the use of luxurious materials through abundant gold and rich, varied colors but also reflect less refined artistry through the volume's bulky figures, which do not quite seem to fit in the spaces into which they have been placed. The images in Morgan MS M.165 are very similar to those in the Cambridge manuscript. In contrast, however, the Morgan shows different embellishments around the letters, suggesting separate details of production as well as artwork that, despite a characterization of the artist as "mediocre," seems more precise and less claustrophobic than what we see in the Cambridge images.[19] In Ajuda 52-XIII-26, two artistic styles have been identified by scholars: a more stylized, linear approach attributed to the Master of the Harley Froissart (Philippe de Mazerolles) and a more naturalistic style evoking greater depth and volume by a second artist, possibly the Master of the London Wavrin.[20] Both styles make use of extensive color and gold in the initials. Furthermore, a unique characteristic of this copy is the intermittent use of camaïeu for some images; using monochromatic tints, which are primarily green in this manuscript, camaïeu creates an effect similar to grisaille. The muted colors, simple descenders and margins, and lack of gold illumination of Sloane 2401 stand out among the other fifteenth-century examples, all of which are decidedly more luxurious in materials—though it seems more refined in some fine details as well as less crowded. Sloane 2401 seems simplest in terms of color palette and has no gold; the Morgan is richer in colors, patterns, and gold; and Cambridge has some gold on the frames and has the most ornate borders, with plants, many of which are gold, too, rather than just line work.

The group of manuscripts produced in the fifteenth century may reflect some influence of the thirteenth- and fourteenth-century illustrations, but in all the later cases the program has been expanded significantly, including scenes or topics left unillustrated in the earlier versions. The iconography of these manuscripts, if it came from preexisting models, was likely drawn from a wide range of manuscript genres. The *Régime* manuscripts engage with several illustrated genres, including bibles and literary texts, bestiaries and herbals, and illustrated medical and scientific manuscripts (their relationship with medieval medical illustration is explored more fully in chapter 3). While the images of the *Régime* manuscripts sometimes demonstrate very direct engagement with models from a variety of common manuscript types, they also exhibit important distinctions and differences from some of these possible sources and comparisons.

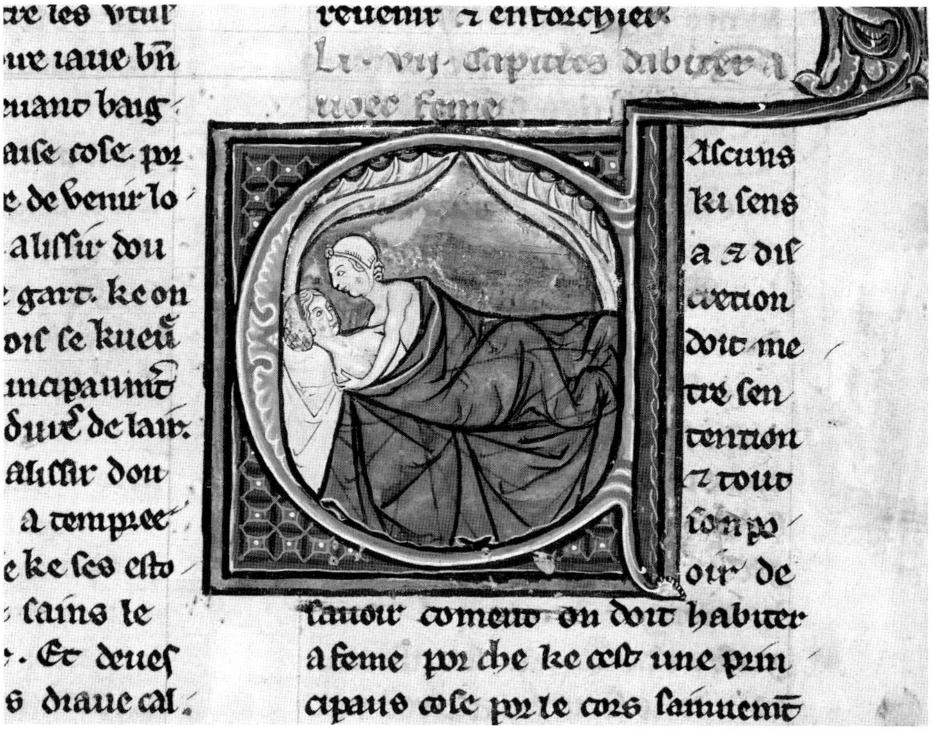

Fig. 14
Copulation. *Le Régime du corps*, ca. 1265–70. British Library, Sloane MS 2435, fol. 9v, detail. © The British Library Board.

Fig. 15 (opposite)
David and Bathsheba. The Crusader Bible, 1240s. The Morgan Library & Museum, MS M.638, fol. 41v, detail. The Morgan Library & Museum, New York. Purchased by J. Pierpont Morgan (1867–1943) in 1916.

Furthermore, the clear adherence to some of these illustrative traditions or pictorial sources brings into focus the *Régime* images that do not appear to be based on models.

The scene of the couple in bed demonstrates the breadth of potential sources available to the makers of the *Régime* (fig. 14). Copulation may seem incongruous with the piety often assigned to medieval art, but this scene appears in a remarkable variety of contexts in thirteenth- and fourteenth-century manuscript production, especially made in and around the region of Paris. One obvious parallel is the depiction of David's sin of adultery with Bathsheba, found in many illustrated bibles (fig. 15). This scene also appears in romance literature, such as the *Roman de la Rose*, and in scientific treatises such as Aristotle's *De generatione*.[21]

The generic nature of this scene's content clearly lends itself to repetition across a wide range of contexts, but alongside such direct references as the copulation scene, other depictions in the *Régime* hint at more subtle inferences to external pictorial traditions. For example, a depiction of a practitioner's touch may have evoked the healing miracles of Christ. The trope of Christ-as-physician has been suggested for other types of medical manuscript illustration, including British Library Sloane MS 1977, where the layout combines surgical scenes with episodes from the life of Christ.[22] In another case, the conversation between two women about skin care in the relevant chapter of the *Régime*, like the scene in Sloane 2435, may derive from models depicting the Visitation, when the Virgin Mary greets her cousin Elizabeth (figs. 16–17). Such proximate models indicate that the illustrated *Régime* manuscripts were fully part of the

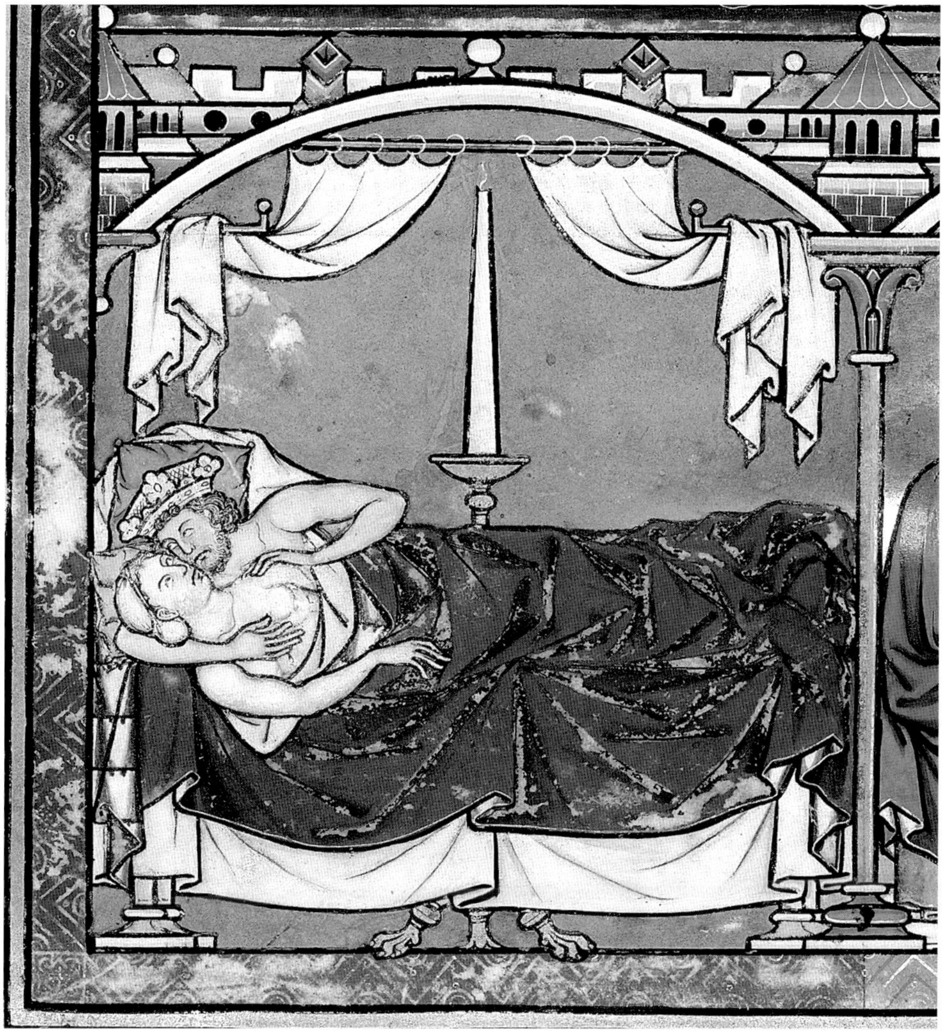

broader medieval manuscript culture and were often created alongside manuscripts more commonly associated with the period, such as bibles and prayer books. Patrons likely saw these copies of the *Régime* as complementary to their collections, bringing forth household health as an important part of ensuring both physical and spiritual well-being.

Bestiaries and herbals are also visual traditions with which the *Régime* clearly converges. Static, encyclopedic depictions of plants, animals, or food appear primarily in the third part of the *Régime*. The repetition of animal images in part 3 creates a kind of zoological compendium much like those found in bestiaries: lists of animals and their attributes with a moralizing component similar to fables, which were often illustrated. More than one hundred manuscripts, produced in several languages across Europe for several centuries, have been traced to this tradition.[23] The Latin versions are most abundant; they are commonly dated to the late twelfth or thirteenth century, often

ens dens ⁊ es gencives ⁊
ki face les gencives enfler
⁊ queles soient prestes de
recevoir les fumees qui vi
enent de le forcele ⁊ dautre
part ⁊ si fait froter font pl⁹
mal que bien.

Pour garder les dens
prendes une once de
corne de cerf arse et
semence de tamarís ⁊ ciperi
⁊ roses ⁊ piquenart de cas
cun autant ⁊ saugeme une
quarte douce ⁊ en faites por
re delie ⁊ le metes en .i. sa
cet v en un drapiel ⁊ en fro
tes les dens ⁊ apres les la
ves de bon vin caut ceste por
re garde ⁊ conforte mlt les
dens ⁊ les gencives. En cor
prendes le racine de titimaul
⁊ le faites boulir en vin et
dou vin v ele sera cuite vos
laves le bouce .ij. fois v .iij.
le mois car cest une cose qui
fait bone alaine de bouce ⁊
garde les dens de dolours ⁊
dautre maladies. si condist
a iunecennes. En cor por les gē
cives ⁊ les dens blancir p̄n
nes marbre blanc ⁊ coral blāc
⁊ os de sece ⁊ saugeme ⁊ encēs.
⁊ mastic. de cascun igaument
⁊ en faites porre delie ⁊ le me
tes en .j. sacet de toille ⁊ en fro
tes les dens ⁊ de bon vin les
laves apres ⁊ apres les frotes
dun drapiel descarlate.

En cor por les gencives
qui volentiers sai
nent ⁊ por les dens
blancir ⁊ por faire bone a
laine p̄nnes galie musquete
⁊ pume marine sel rosti ⁊ cor
ne de cerf arse de cascun .iiij.
drames ⁊ alun ⁊ nitre ⁊ pu
me grenate gale balaustie
de cascun .ij. drames ⁊ pindie
spic costb. lin. aloes tandamo
de cascun une drame ⁊ en fai
tes porre delie ⁊ en frotes les
dens.

Se vous voles remo
voir laacement des
dens qui souent avi
ent masces porcelaine ama
des avelonnes froumage rosti
⁊ vin caut tenir en le bouce ⁊
sel ⁊ toutes coses caudes ostēt
ces maladies. li .v. cap quant
on doit garder le visage.

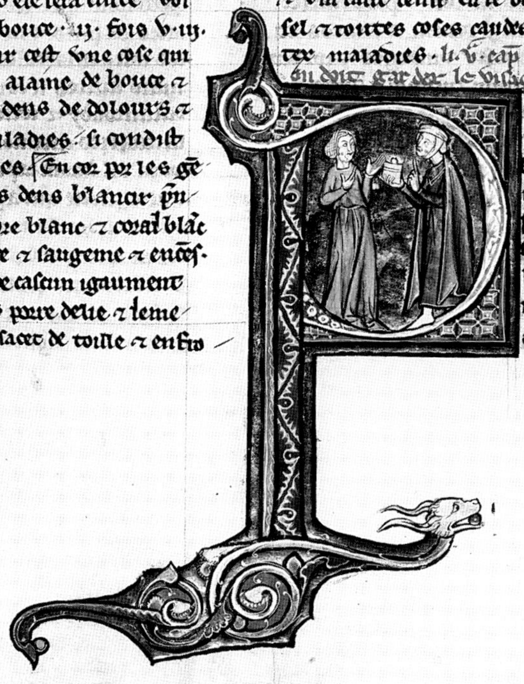

Pour
plus
brie
ment
parler
si vos
laisse
rons
a dire

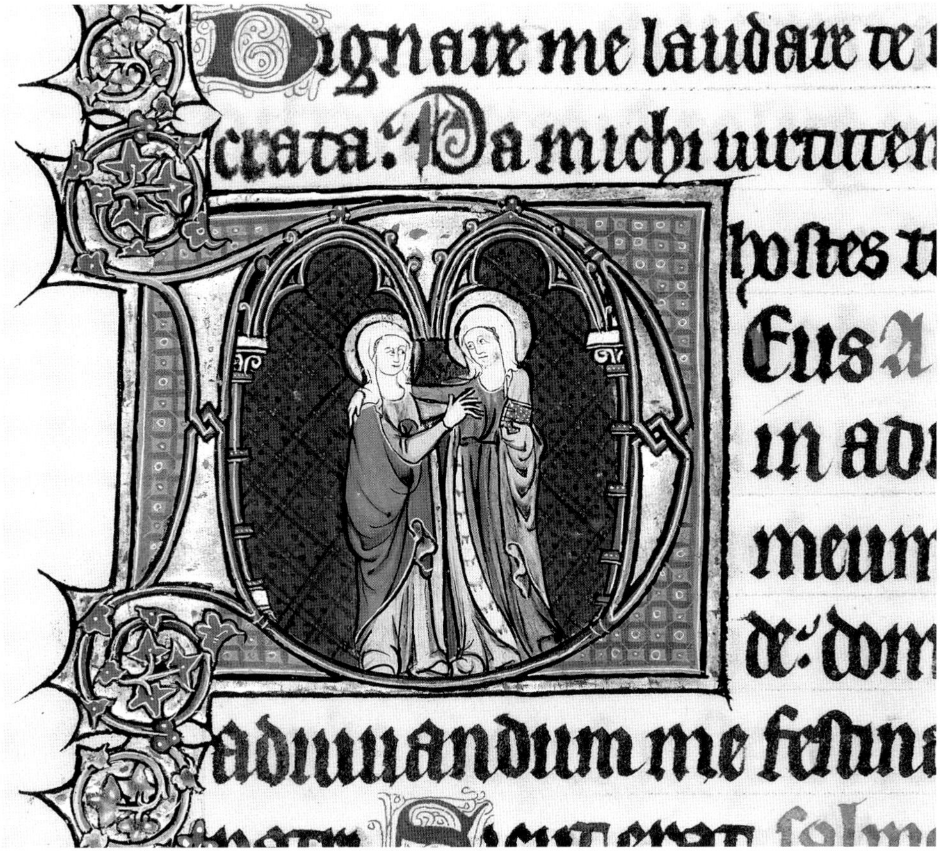

Fig. 16 (opposite)
Complexion. *Le Régime du corps*, ca. 1265–70. British Library, Sloane MS 2435, fol. 37r. © The British Library Board.

Fig. 17
The Visitation. The Ruskin Hours, ca. 1300. The J. Paul Getty Museum, MS Ludwig IX 3 (83.ML.99), fol. 63v, detail. Digital image courtesy of the Getty's Open Content Program.

illustrated, and especially popular in England. Although the aesthetics of these examples and the *Régime* animals may differ, the long history of bestiaries as a genre was likely familiar to many involved with manuscript production at this time. The images in British Library Royal MS 12 C XIX, a bestiary from the early thirteenth century, are representative examples in which animals are often depicted without any background and contained in circular frames (fig. 18).

Bestiary sections were sometimes included within medicinal herbals that listed plants with their attributes and benefits, an independent but robust textual tradition with a long pictorial legacy stretching back to at least the sixth century.[24] In one miscellany of medical and herbal texts from the late twelfth century, images of animals and images of plants are both included in the same manuscript.[25] The linking of animals to a wider collection of medicinal substances makes their appearance in the *Régime* logical as well. The long traditions of illustrated bestiaries and herbals would have made it relatively straightforward to conceive of illustrations to accompany sections in the *Régime* that discuss foods such as plants and meat. For example, Sloane 2435 illustrates a series of twenty-one animals—including a sheep and a goat, a stag and a bear, rabbits and various birds—presented in a format quite similar to contemporary bestiaries, floating in space without any depiction of surroundings or groundlines (fig. 19). The

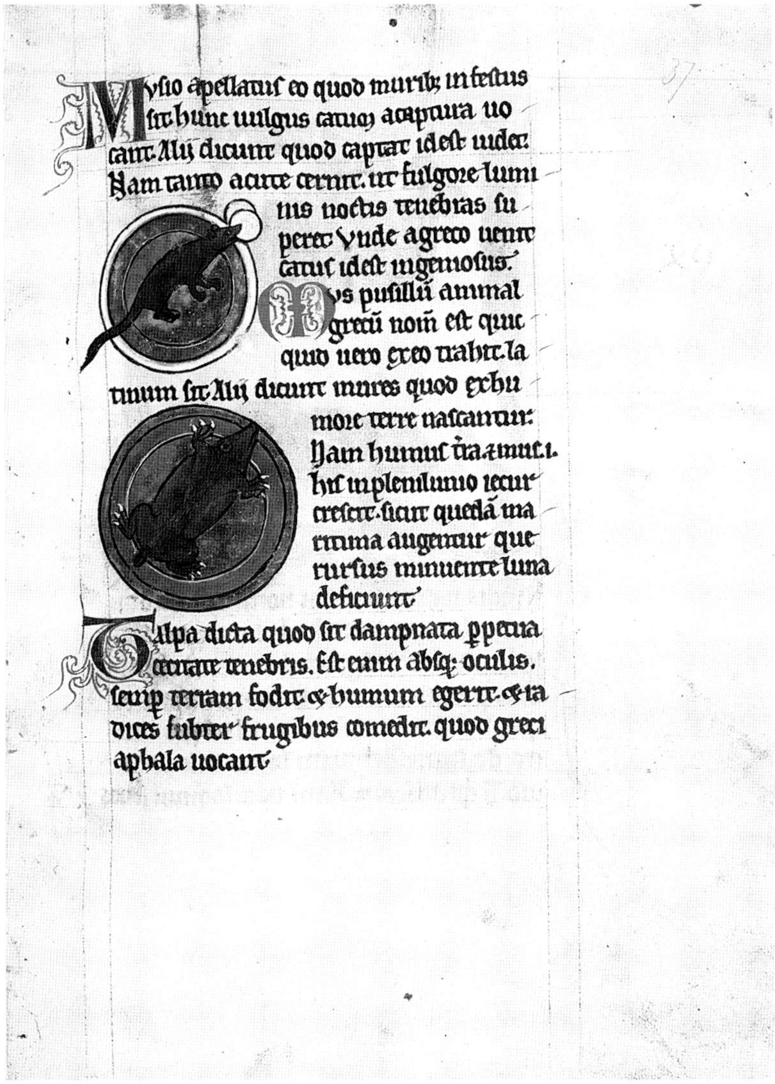

Fig. 18
Mouse, mole. Bestiary, thirteenth century. British Library, Royal MS 12 C XIX, fol. 37r. © The British Library Board.

Fig. 19 (opposite)
Stag, hare, rabbit, bear. *Le Régime du corps*, ca. 1265–70. British Library, Sloane MS 2435, fol. 48v. © The British Library Board.

shared visual language and similar topics suggest not only that these chapter-heading images worked in very similar ways for the viewer, but also that the designers of *Régime* manuscripts could have been looking at bestiaries and other encyclopedic texts as models.

As in the related manuscript genres of the herbal and bestiary, the initials in Sloane 2435 work to introduce specific chapters and visually signal the beginning of each topic. As scholars such as Minta Collins and Jean Givens have pointed out, the late medieval illustrated herbals most likely were not field guides for plant retrieval.[26] The images in such manuscripts probably served a variety of functions, not only signaling sections of the text but also contributing to the conspicuous consumption favored by the bibliophiles of this period.[27] In her discussion of an illustrated copy of the surgical text *Chirurgia*, Helen Valls likewise points out how the scenes depicted work as "visual rubrics," so that the contents of the chapter could be quickly recognized by the manuscript's users.[28] The illustrations in encyclopedic texts, which involve many images accompanying fairly short chapters, in a form that repeated over and over, were especially well-suited to the format of historiated initials, which provide their own style directives.

Historiated initials seem to have been a logical illustrative choice for compendia of all kinds, including encyclopedias, because they could be used to mark each new entry. The *Omne Bonum*, a fourteenth-century encyclopedia of universal knowledge, is one particularly extensive example that contains more than 750 initials along with full-page illuminations (fig. 20). Its historiated initials seem to be derived from a number of traditions, including legal and biblical books as well as natural history, but in some cases the accompanying text drove the image selection. Pictures often referred to themes or short passages of text. In the *Omne Bonum*, the topics for individual entries are most often nouns, which refer to objects and living things as well as concepts, but

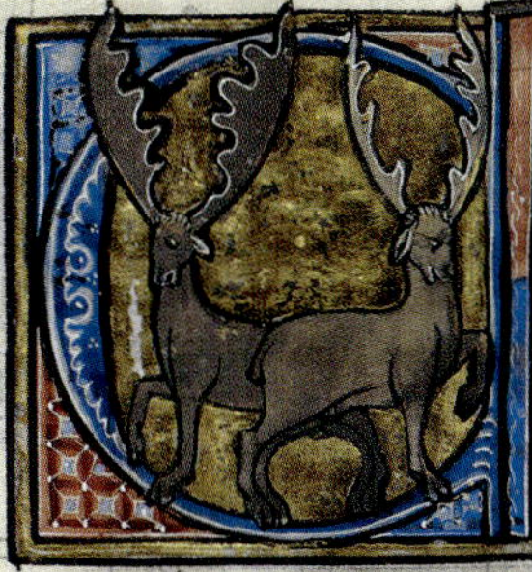

ars de
cerf ⁊
de dain
sunt
·ij· cars
froides
⁊ seces
mais
que ce
le dou
dain est ·i· po plus caude· mais
toutes voies se cuissent a[n]s
deus mauuaisement a le for
cele ⁊ engendrent gros
sanc ⁊ melancolious mais
ensi que dit vous auons des
autres cars selonc laage se di
uersefient de lor nature de do
ner bon ⁊ mauuais noussem[en]t
car chars de cerf quant il est
iones sor toutes cars sauue
gines vaut miex ⁊ li sans q[ui]
en est engendres est plus de
lies ⁊ mains a de superfluites
tout soit ce quil soit melanco
lious ⁊ quant il sunt iones il
sunt castre si vallent asses miex
⁊ est la cars plus tempree· m[ai]s
ais cars de cerf viel ⁊ de grant
eage ne doit on mie vser por
ce quele est del tout mauuai
se. de car de lieure.

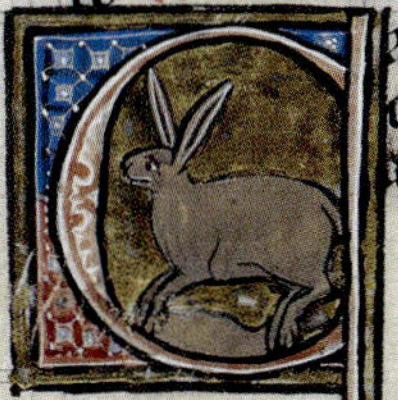

ar de lieure ⁊
sece ⁊ plus des
autres sauue
gines engendre melancolie
mais toute voie vaut ele miex
a vser que car de bouc ne de
cieure ⁊ se doiuent de tel car
garder cil qui ont la comple
xion sece ⁊ maigre porce que
le norist po ⁊ mauuaisement.
de car de conin

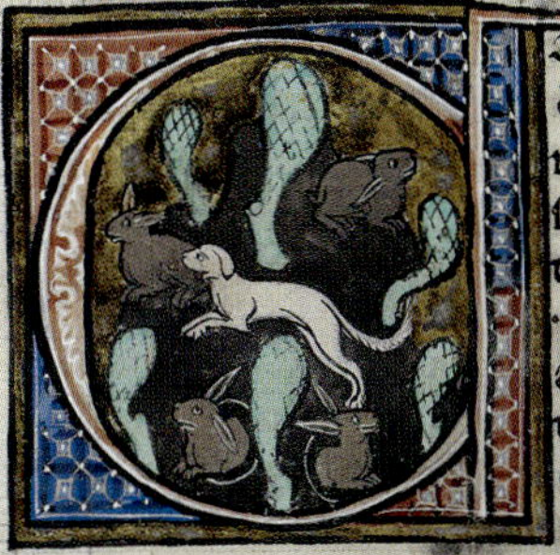

ar
de co
nin
si se
tient
·i· po
a na
ture
de lie
ure
mais ele est asses plus temp[er]ee
⁊ por con vaut miex a vser
⁊ le pueent vser cil qui de cau
de maladie sunt escape car
ele lor conforte lestomac. et
lor done appetit de mengier.
⁊ li sans qui en est engendres
est bons ⁊ sutis· mais quil est
vn po melancolious. de car
dors

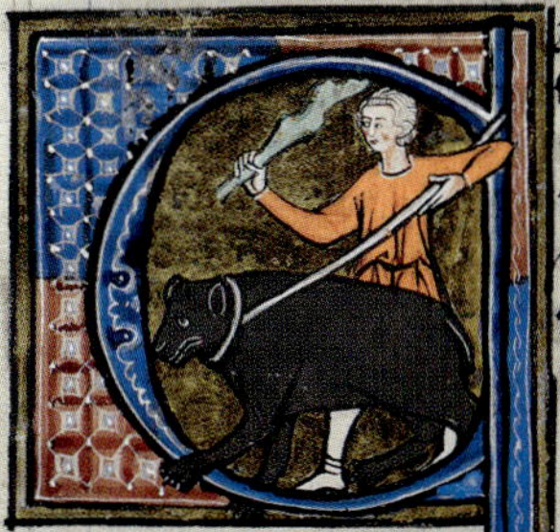

ar dors
si est
sor to
tes cars
viscou
se et
plus

dorſ

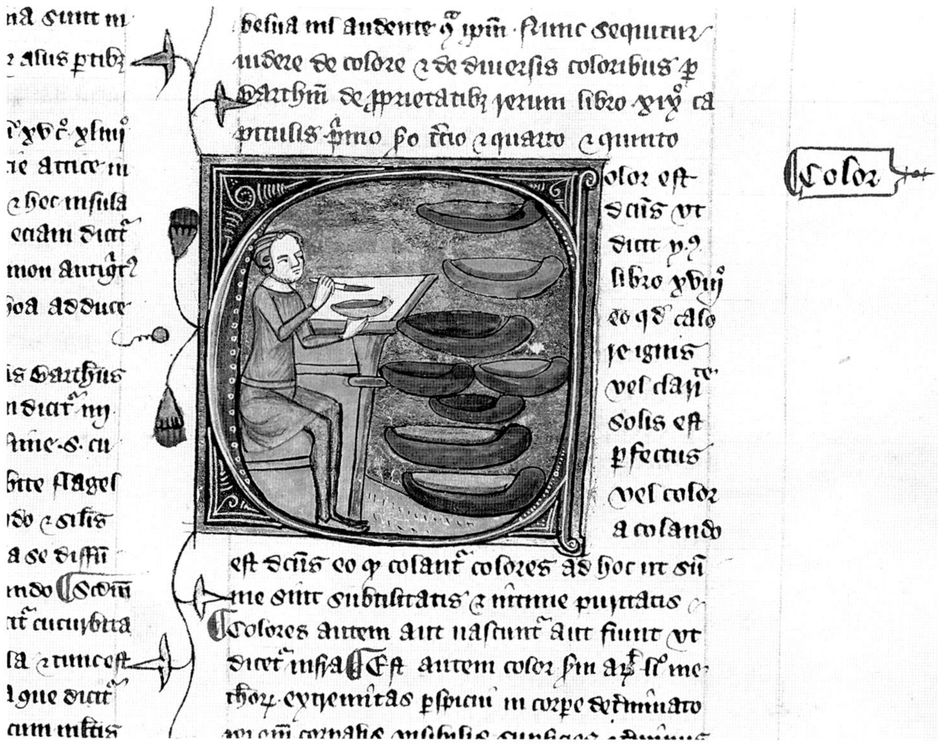

Fig. 20
Initial C(olor), with artist mixing colors. *Omne Bonum*, ca. 1360–75. British Library, Royal MS 6E VI–6E VII, fol. 329r, detail. © The British Library Board.

Fig. 21 (opposite)
Scholar lectures to students. Paneth Codex, ca. 1300. Yale Medical Library, MS 28, fol. 57r, detail. Medical Historical Library, Harvey Cushing / John Hay Whitney Medical Library, Yale University.

which are often illustrated with pictures of actions.[29] Such specificity in terms of mode of representation is also evident in the *Régime*.

When it comes to medical or scientific manuscripts that employ historiated initials, there is often a loose connection with the content of the text. Peter Murray Jones has observed that some artists were quite literal when selecting subjects, and that "taking the first or early words of the text written alongside the space left for the illuminator to fill was a very common strategy for illuminators seeking a subject for initial pictures," especially when there were many such pictures to fill.[30] When books were made as luxury items, as several of the illustrated *Régime* manuscripts were, the texts were downplayed while the images were essential for the projection of prestige and authority. For example, the Paneth Codex, a medical compendium produced in Bologna around 1300, contains fifty-seven historiated initials, primarily scenes of the physician as seated authority gesturing toward his students (fig. 21). Jones suggests that because this manuscript's artists did not have a canonical set of images to follow, they were improvising based on existing models.[31] Bologna was a center of law, and the artists were likely working in that oeuvre; the result is the frequent portrayal of the physician as scholastic authority and relatively few treatment scenes.

Despite the constricted space in which the figures of the historiated initials of the *Régime* reside, they are nevertheless involved in activities. They do things in a specific place and for a certain amount of time. Discussions of how medieval images construct narrative often involve the formulation of a relationship between images, seeing them as episodes in a larger sequence and analyzing how a series of images is understood by a viewer.[32] In his discussion of the grid-like format used in the folios of the surgical manuscript Sloane 1977, Karl Whittington argues that, although the images in the two lower registers are not actually depicting the stages of a procedure "step by step" but instead are independent scenes, they "effectively become a narrative" through their consecutive organization on the page and their position underneath a well-known narrative (fig. 22).[33] The specific effect of the arrangement in Sloane 1977 is not a given, since other illustrated copies of this surgical treatise are organized with the images spread out and integrated into the blocks of text.[34] Therefore the organization of images and their placement on the page and in relation to the text are as significant in how they can be narratively read as the content of the images themselves.

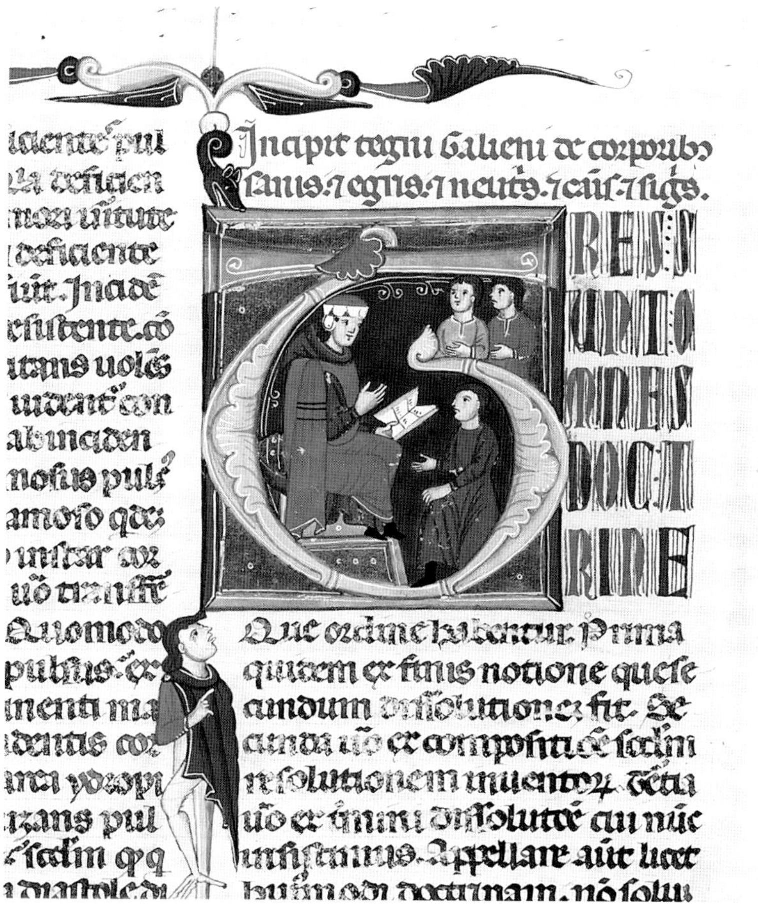

Coincidentally, many of the depictions in Sloane 1977 evoke a similar two-person structure of the *Régime*, representing both scenes of treatment and moments of consultation. In two scenes in which women consult with a surgeon regarding diseases of the breast, a woman holds out her breast to show the surgeon her disease (fig. 23). In the first scene, the woman has a dark blemish on her right breast, her left hand pointing upward; the surgeon gestures toward her, his left hand flat and raised as he holds a green jar in his right. In the second scene, the surgeon gestures with both hands, his left hand pointing upward, as the woman uses her left hand to show him the pinkish lump on her left breast, her right hand raised and open. These scenes of breast display in a medical context mirror the presentation of the breast in the *Régime* wet nurse scenes; the gestures of discussion seen here are also frequently seen in the *Régime*'s scenes of consultation between patient and practitioner.[35] Thought to have been made in northern France in the early fourteenth century, perhaps in Picardy, Sloane 1977 was likely made after the earliest illustrated versions of the *Régime*. The shared imagery of breast consultation, alongside a number of other known surgical manuscripts with similar scenes, connects the visual language of the *Régime* to another established norm of medical illustration (that medical context is further explored in chapter 3). This comparison reminds us

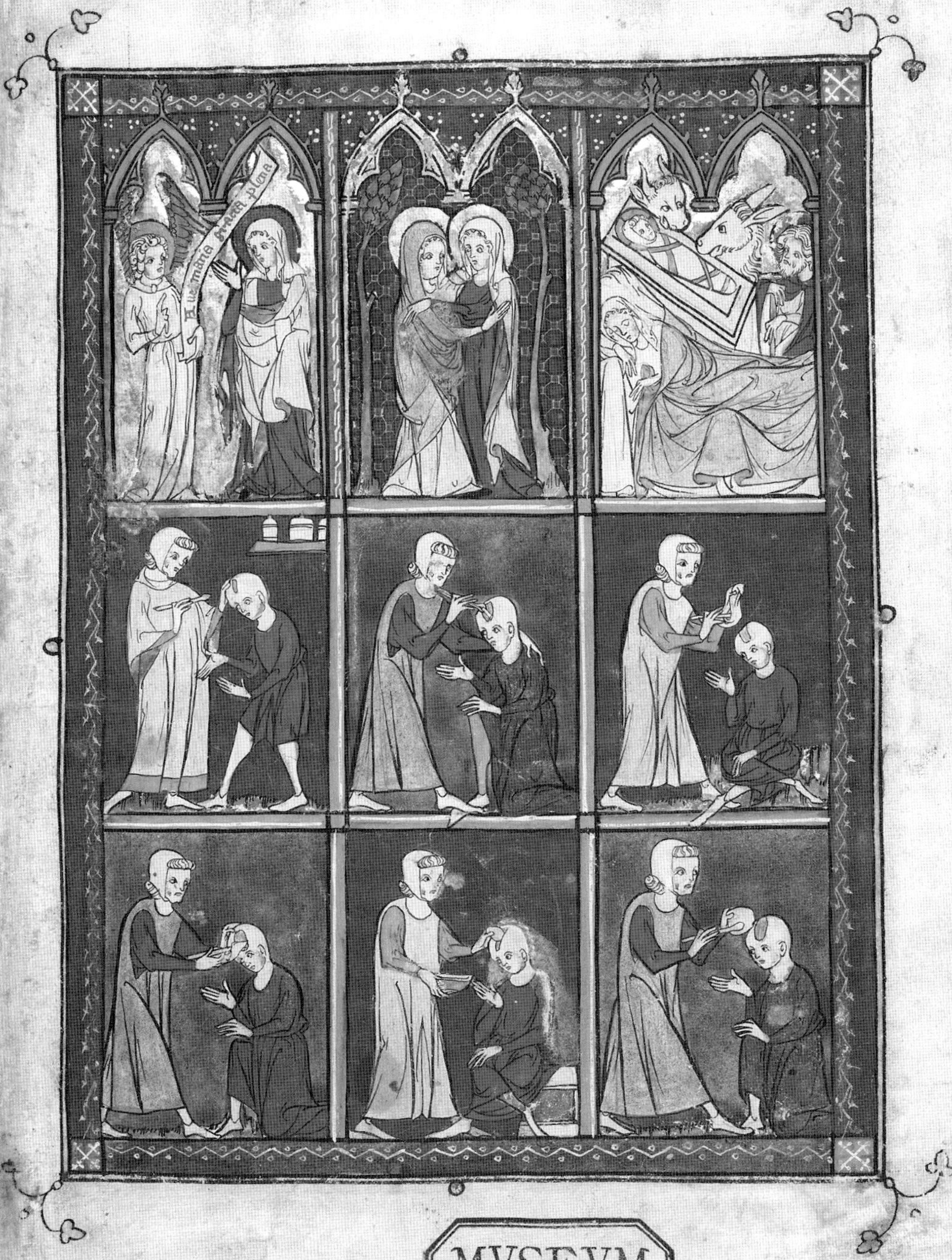

MVSEVM
BRITAN
NICVM

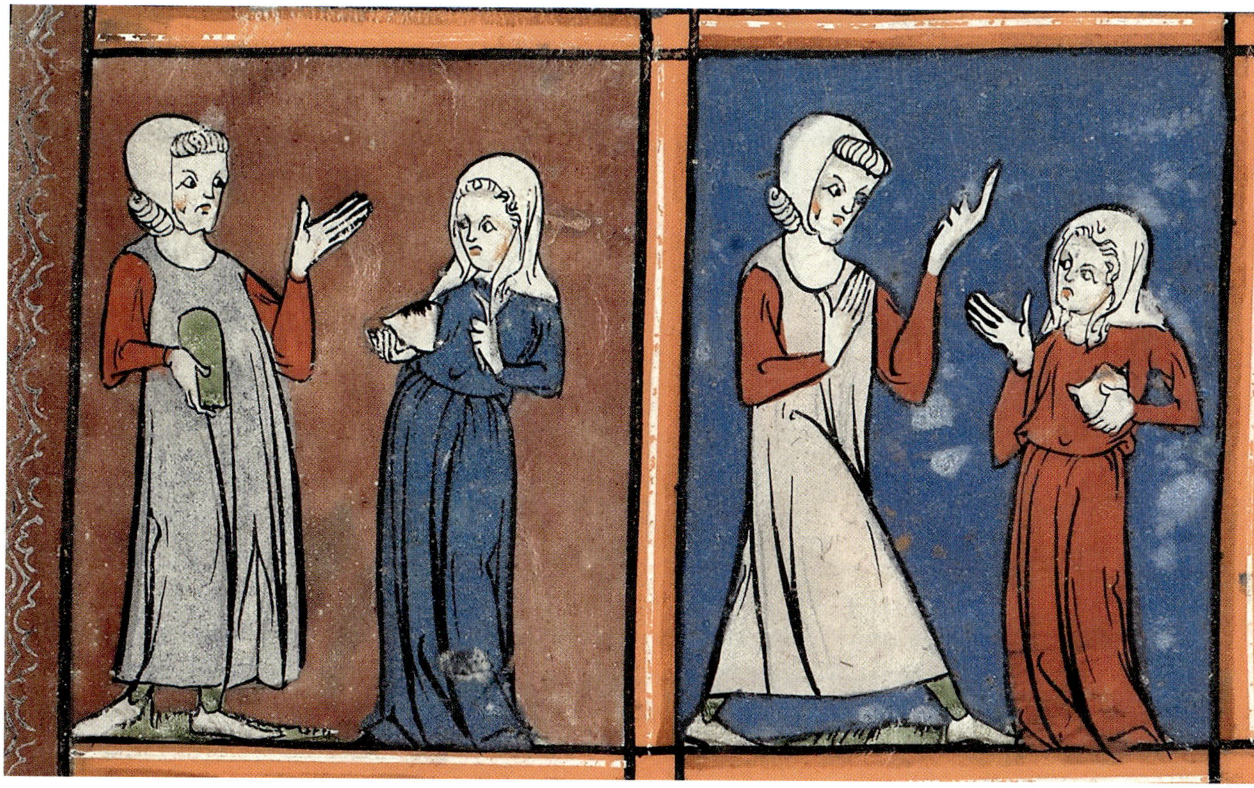

that, even when the composition of an image may not be original to the *Régime* manuscripts, frequently the subject matter was adapted and nuanced to fit this particular context and audience.

Fig. 22 (opposite)
Annunciation, Visitation, and Nativity with surgical scenes. *Chirurgia*, early fourteenth century. British Library, Sloane MS 1977, fol. 2r. © The British Library Board.

Fig. 23
Women presenting breast diseases to surgeon. *Chirurgia*, early fourteenth century. British Library, Sloane MS 1977, fol. 7v detail. © The British Library Board.

Narrative Ingenuity in Historiated Initials

Although many of the images in these manuscripts indicate the use of models from other genres, other scenes reflect artistic originality when clear models for the topic did not exist. Improvisation may be particularly necessary for manuscripts with so many images, especially for unconventional topics.[36] Indeed, numerous images throughout the *Régime* manuscripts appear to be unique and innovative, suggesting that the designers of these books were selective in their choice of which images should be based on models, and which needed to be invented outright. The *Régime du corps*, as a health guide oriented toward a domestic audience, was different from many other illuminated books, and illustrating copies of this text required initiative. The originality of the *Régime* manuscripts' visual language is bound up in the illustrative form of the manuscript: that is, the historiated initial.

As in many other late medieval manuscripts, the historiated initials in the *Régime* copies most often involve a large capital letter with a simple scene enclosed. They are

Fig. 25
Newborn care. The Bute Painter, *Le Régime du corps*, ca. 1285. Bibliothèque nationale de France, Arsenal MS 2510, fol. 25v, detail. © Bibliothèque nationale de France.

second woman on the other side of the bed, sitting on the ground washing a child in a tub to her right and our left. While the drawing styles vary, details like the headwear of the three women and the color palettes are also remarkably similar. In another fifteenth-century manuscript, Ajuda, the chapter is represented by a lone woman in the act of breastfeeding, with the infant held in her arms, a scene we also find in the earlier Leipzig manuscript.

This variety can be attributed in part to factors like date and place of production, workshop and patron idiosyncrasies, or available models. At the same time, however, each of these examples communicates something different about what is contained in this chapter, and, more significantly, what was considered by those organizing the initials as the most important thing for the reader to glean from the chapter. So often that takeaway message is a multivalent one, with the image engaging viewers to think about a range of possible narrative outcomes. A closer look at the wet nurse images from Sloane 2435 and BnF Fr. 12323 demonstrates the complexities of monoscenic narrative construction (figs. 8, 26). In both images the wet nurse displays her left hand in a gesture of greeting or acquiescence; the wet nurse's right hand falls limp in BnF Fr. 12323, while in Sloane 2435 she holds up her breast for the noblewoman. In both manuscripts, the elite figure reaches with her right hand and touches the other woman's breast. Through clothing and gesture, these scenes remind us of the inequitable power structure at play in the scene, even as we realize that the noblewomen also need something from the lower-class figures. Instead of an image that includes an infant, Sloane 2435 and BnF Fr. 12323 depict a scene in which a potential wet nurse's body undergoes physical evaluation and judgment. The isolation of the key moment in a narrative for visual depiction also engages the viewers to add what is not there, in this case, the infant. Numerous authors have pointed out the remarkable open-endedness of such a construction, suggesting that such ambiguity allows for endless possibilities, which are then repeated and multiplied each time the narrative is revisited.[42] By capturing an activity *as it is happening*, these scenes not only leave the results open and unresolved but also allow the user to participate in narrative construction.

The construction of a narrative out of these singular images might look something like this: a user of one of the illustrated *Régime* manuscripts begins by finding the section she wants, having identified the health problem for which she seeks information. This viewer sees the image, in which a scene shows the solution in progress, but with an uncertain outcome: the image offers an arrested moment with multiple potential outcomes. In a comparable scene from a bible, psalter, or book of hours, audience members would generally know how the scene's narrative was supposed to end even if the outcome was not depicted. The initials in those other textual genres explicate what will happen in the text as opposed to what the text will direct the reader to do. With the treatment or discussion scenes in the *Régime du corps*, however, that outcome is not preordained. The user might also read the description in the corresponding text, which often provides directives along with the effects or outcomes that may be achieved through practicing what the text advises.

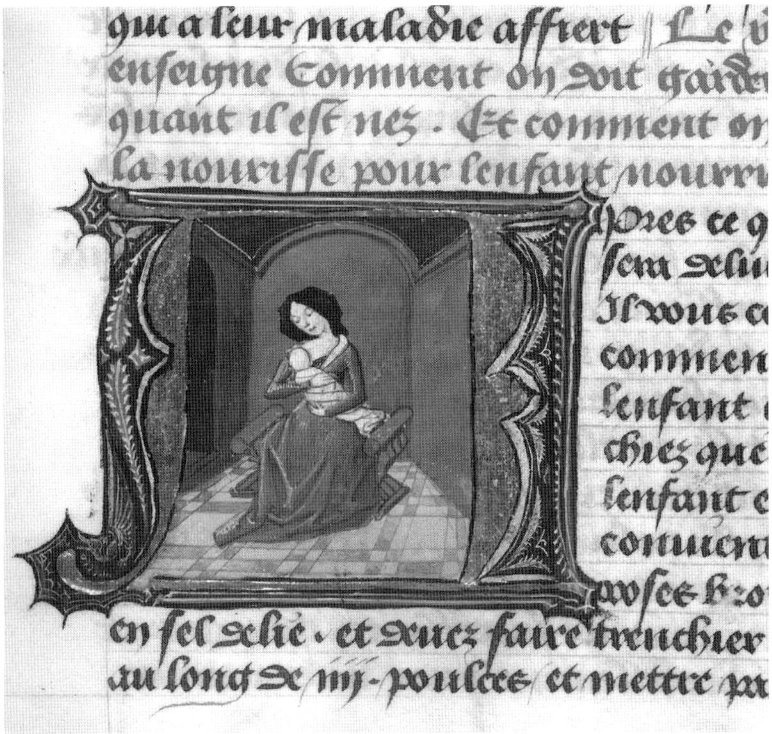

Fig. 28
Woman breastfeeding newborn.
Le Régime du corps, ca. 1470s.
Biblioteca da Ajuda, Lisbon,
Cod. 52-XIII-26, fol. 49r, detail.
Biblioteca da Ajuda.

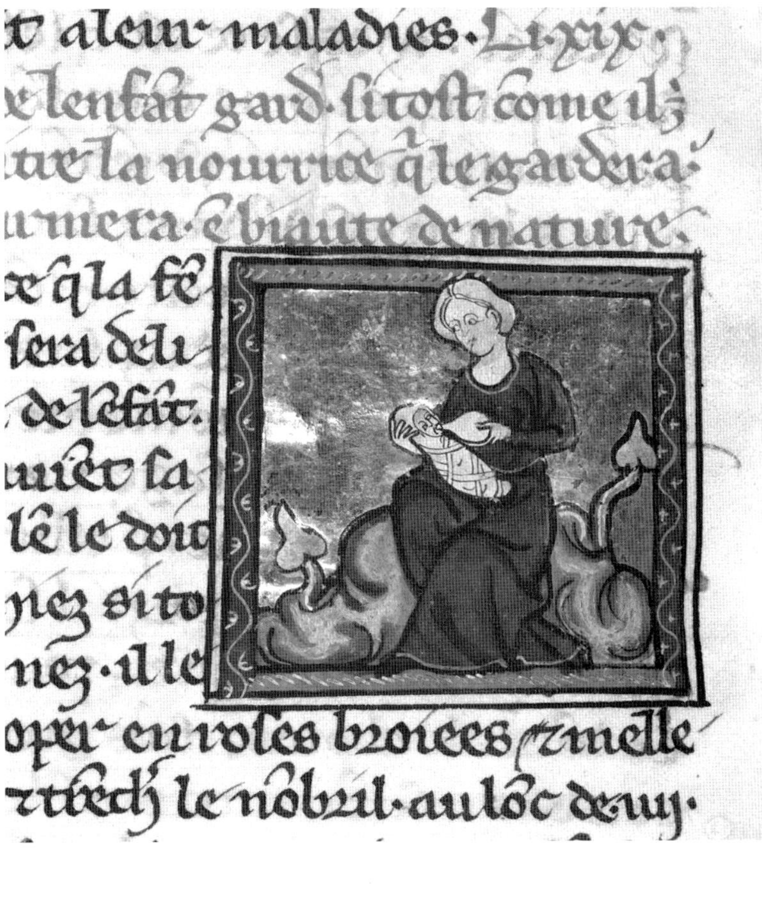

Fig. 29
Woman breastfeeding newborn.
Le Régime du corps, ca. 1270–1300.
Universitätsbibliothek Leipzig,
Cod. Haen. 3478, fol. 54v, detail.
Universitätsbibliothek Leipzig.

of the process of hiring a nurse. Klapisch-Zuber finds that in fourteenth- and fifteenth-century Florence, men almost exclusively oversaw the negotiations with the wet nurse and her husband or family, leaving their wives, the birth mothers, largely out of the process of making arrangements to send a child out to nurse.[63] In contrast, Winer has demonstrated that this was primarily the woman's responsibility in fourteenth-century Barcelona, and Debra Blumenthal does the same in relation to fifteenth-century Valencia.[64] It is all the more intriguing to see, then, the scene depicted as a physical exchange between women in these two versions of the scene, rather than as a purely financial agreement. Despite the dominance of men in other contexts, perhaps the specific circumstances of the *Régime*'s composition granted a greater role for women in this important decision. Aldobrandino was certainly aware of Beatrice of Savoy's political power and the status of her four royal daughters; perhaps these earlier illustrated copies, if indeed made within the circles of these powerful women, reflect their authority.

Fig. 27
Wet nurse scene. *Le Régime du corps*, ca. 1265–70. British Library, Sloane MS 2435, fol. 28v. © The British Library Board.

The role of the wet nurse is depicted differently in the later copies, placing either more or less focus on her role. The Ajuda manuscript, the latest of our group, contains an image of a woman breastfeeding a child for this chapter, bringing to the forefront her prominent role (fig. 28). Her status as a servant is not readily evident in the clothing she wears—female workers in the manuscript wear a variety of colored garments and head coverings—but she obviously nurses the child she holds. While the woman is dressed nearly identically to the previous chapter's depiction of the pregnant mother, her activity of breastfeeding, considering the reference to the *norrice* in the chapter heading, suggests she is a wet nurse rather than the mother. As such, this late copy veers away from the other fifteenth-century images of this chapter, but it happens to share this approach to the chapter with the earlier Leipzig manuscript (fig. 29). In depicting a breastfeeding woman who is almost certainly meant to be the wet nurse, these versions make her central to the chapter's message.

Like the scenes in Sloane 2435 and BnF Fr. 12323, these illustrations reiterate the figure's essential function in the health of the baby. But unlike those two earlier manuscripts, which depict this scene as a tense exchange between two women, these simpler scenes of nursing include the infant and potentially leave out the mother. Aldobrandino's text includes a brief statement that mother's milk is best along with some general tips for helping the baby to suckle. However, that short section is followed by a much lengthier discussion that elaborates in great detail the considerations for wet nurse selection, how she should nurse the child, and when and how the child should be introduced to solid food and weaned. In Sloane 2435, for example, this portion of text discussing the selection of a wet nurse is 118 lines over the course of three folios (29v–30v). Ostensibly modeled on one of the most common subjects in medieval art, that of the Virgin and Child, these depictions of breastfeeding offer positive scenes of a nourished infant. At the same time, however, the ambiguous identity of the nursing woman, who may represent the wet nurse instead of the mother, speaks to the persistent uneasiness that such situations must have conjured.

uiers soit fors ⁊ perillous
si con del enfant ki ne uolt
vient droitement si con deue
ntr les pies auant v les bras.
car vous deues sauoir quil doit
venir la teste avant naturel
ment ⁊ ses bras estendus sor
ses cuisses. ⁊ sil ensi ne vient
mais en si con nous auons dit
se ni a autre consel fors q̃ dauo
ir sage baille qui le remete a
point por issir en si com il doit.

Et se cest ke li enfes soit
mors si se couiend ha
ster de le feme deliurer
por ce quil ia peril trop grant.
si li dones a boire de liaue v fies
gres ⁊ dates seront cuites. ⁊ se
li dones .iij. fois v q̃tre v pl9
se mestier est .vi. de rue de sauine
v boire cannele ⁊ garance en
vin. ⁊ se le est crasse si se couce
a dens ⁊ traie ses genols dev9
se teste ⁊ ait vn coussin sous
sen ventre. car si faitement
estre fait toutes femes plus le
gierement deliurer ⁊ apres
che que le sera deliuree se doit
baignier ⁊ soi conforter de bo
nes viandes. Et se dolors et
autres maladies lor avienẽt
si facent medicine q̃ a lor ma
ladie afiert.

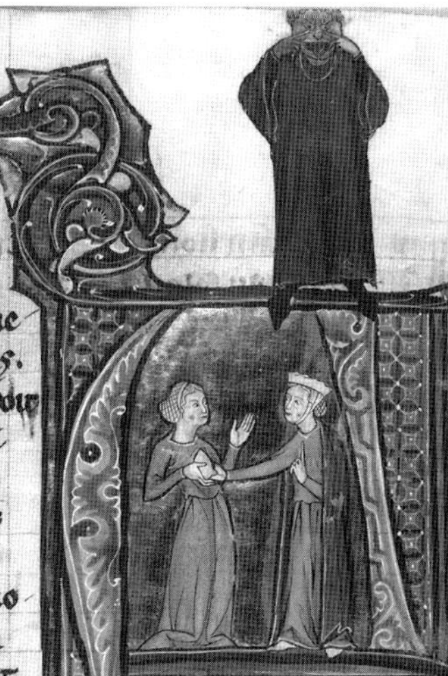

Apres
che ke
li feme
sera de
liuree
si vos
couiẽt
sauoir
coumẽt
vo9 de
ues lenfant garder. Sachies
ke si tost com il est nes le cou
ent en volepeir en roses broies
melees en sel delie ⁊ deues fai
re trenchier le bouteril au
lonc de .iiij. poces ⁊ metre par
desus poure de sandragon ⁊ de
sarquacol ⁊ de comin ⁊ de mir
re ⁊ vn drapiel de lin mollie
en oille doliue ⁊ ce est li enseg
nemens de mains filosofes.
mais il est plus seure cose de
penre .j. fil de laine retors ⁊ lie
le bouteril. ⁊ apres metre dra
piaus sus. ⁊ mollies en oille
⁊ laissier les iusq̃s a .iiij. iors ⁊
lors carra. ⁊ quant il sera cheus
si v9 deues haster dou metre sel
delie sus mele a poure de cost.
v de somac v de fiens gres v do
rigano ⁊ de ce poes saler tout
le cors fors q̃ le nes le bouce p le
bouteril ⁊ por tout le cors en

Scholarship on medieval gesture reminds us that the gestures of a scene's actors, while ostensibly directed at their scenic partners, are actually addressing the beholder of the image.[60] The upward pointing by the upper-class woman in Sloane 2435, then, is directed both to her companion and to the viewer. That gesture is not uncommon in the *Régime* manuscripts or other medical illustrations; it is usually made by a practitioner who seems to be directing or admonishing a patient (see figs. 22–23, as well as chapter 3). Such a power dynamic expressed through gesture echoes the previous chapter's image in both of these manuscripts, which depicts the pregnant woman conversing with the doctor. But in Sloane 2435, the woman's pointing gesture seems to direct the other woman, and us as viewers, to look above her as well. A peculiar mouth-pulling figure stands on the letter's upper frame, looming in a dark cloak above the noblewoman (fig. 27). At first glance one might assume the figure is an artistic doodle added later, but the thin white lines articulating edges of fabric folds and other details, the rosy cheeks, and the opacity of the paint align with the other illustrations of this manuscript. Furthermore, the gold background of the letter goes around the figure's toe, indicating it was part of the original design of the page. Although this ominous figure is perplexing and its meaning enigmatic, it boldly engages the audience by directly facing the viewer, despite its marginal status. Michael Camille has suggested that the messages of the margins are explicitly intended for the book's audience when they seem unrelated to the action of a page's main illustration, and this robed figure's orientation, facing forward and out toward the reader, certainly seems to be an unambiguously direct gesture.[61] It is true that the actions of the wet nurse and the noblewoman are directed at each other, but the latter's gesture of pointing upward at the marginal figure directs the viewer's gaze to that figure as well. The marginal figure's outward orientation, toward the viewer and parallel with the picture plane, is an unmistakable device identified in other manuscripts of this period.

Such scenes are among the most fraught in terms of the variables associated with this important decision. These two wet nurse scenes are particularly powerful depictions of monoscenic episodes that suggest multiple actions or choices that could cause different results: will the wet nurse prove adequately nourishing for the newborn, or will this important decision result in an unsatisfactory hire and an ill child? The dark figure above the scene in Sloane 2435 further reinforces the significance of this moment, while the noblewoman's anxious pointing—both to the other woman and for the viewer—also seems to provoke concern over this chapter's content. It has been suggested that narrative created through monoscenic or monophase images cannot create suspense, but these images, on the contrary, capture precisely the key "crisis" moment in the administration of health care.[62] After all, the noblewomen may have social power over the women whom they employ, but they are both responsible for the selection of and also ultimately at the mercy of those future wet nurses.

The objectification of the nurse's body is likewise furthered through the powerful role of the paying family. Although in the *Régime* images, elite women maintain the position of physical dominance, in some situations the elite mother was in fact left out

Thus, in these various European contexts, the practice of using wet nurses is clearly tied up with status and bodily control. The women who were paid to nurse tended to be lower class, sometimes slaves or other kinds of domestic servants within the household. As Rebecca Lynn Winer has demonstrated in her discussion of thirteenth-century Aragon and Majorca, the practice of using wet nurses was also explicitly linked to slavery, specifically enslaved Muslims; domestic slaves also existed in Florence in the later Middle Ages.[53] To retain their employment, they had to contractually agree to certain stipulations, the most important of which was to not become pregnant themselves while nursing, even if they were married. They also might have been required to nurse only one child at a time, and therefore would be unable to nurse their own children; this is one reason why, tragically, the "ideal" nurse would have lost her own baby.[54] Although in some contexts the child was sent out to nurse (out to the country, for example, in Florence), there are also instances in which the preferred option was to have the woman in the house, although that would also have been more expensive. If the wet nurse were living at close quarters with the family, they would be able to more closely monitor her sexual activity.[55] These circumstances inform the wet nurse assessment scenes in these two *Régime* manuscripts, in which the future nurse's body is groped, assessed, and, if hired, further exploited by wealthy elites.

In the *Régime* chapter that deals with caring for a newborn, much of the discussion is dedicated to the selection of a wet nurse based on a range of characteristics, including her age, physical condition and appearance, habits, breasts, and milk quality, as well as how to maintain her health once she is nursing. The chapter description seen in most of the illustrated copies is a version of "comment on doit garder l'enfant quant il est nés et d'eslire et connoistre la norrice pour l'enfant norrir et garder," suggesting an overt association between this chapter and the role of the wet nurse (*norrice*). Clearly, the selection of a wet nurse was an incredibly important decision, perceived to have great consequences for the infant's future. While this chapter simply states that this information is here "because mothers cannot always nurse their infants," it seems clear that the dedication of this much space in this chapter to this topic is connected to the type of elite audiences for which this text was intended.[56] Such audiences would have desired that mothers become pregnant again as quickly as possible, and using a wet nurse would allow the mother's own milk production to wane and reproductive capacities to return sooner.[57] This chapter includes numerous ominous warnings about the selection, for "sickly nurses kill children straight away"; one must be sure she does not become pregnant while nursing, "for a pregnant woman when she nurses kills and destroys children."[58] The ideal amount of time that has passed since the wet nurse has given birth to a child is one to two months, and if it has been one or two years, that is too long. Probably in many of these cases the nursing woman had lost her own baby; in other cases, a nurse's child might be weaned, or she might even hire another nurse for her own child. At any rate, it seems unlikely that a wet nurse would have been feeding more than one child at a time.[59]

Anxiety and Authority in Childcare

Fig. 26
Wet nurse scene. *Le Régime du corps*, fourteenth century. Bibliothèque nationale de France, Fr. 12323, fol. 97r, detail. © Bibliothèque nationale de France.

The wet nurse scenes provide an excellent case study for unpacking the rich and layered meanings communicated by the illustrated *Régime* manuscripts. Such images not only informed readers by expanding beyond and enriching the text but also connected to actual practices and experiences of health care in the real world. The different roles for female caregivers displayed in these representations reflect a similar diversity, while also revealing the concerns and duties of the contemporary upper-class women who were the likely owners of these books.

There is no question that status informed both the use of wet nurses as well as what kind of woman became a wet nurse. Although much of the relevant work on medieval wet nurses has been by scholars who focus on Iberia and Italy (rather than France or England), their studies remain useful for gauging general practices across Europe as well as how these images from the *Régime* might stand out.[43] Although the practice of employing wet nurses was often implicitly discouraged by the Church, it seems to have gained increasing popularity, with those who could afford it, by the thirteenth century.[44] Despite the existence of an idealized notion of the mother suckling her own child, which was further supported by medical texts and in literature, more and more elites were inclined to use wet nurses; one reason, of course, was lineage. As Christiane Klapisch-Zuber puts it, "they must have been governed by infinitely stronger and more dynamic values than medico-moral literary heritage."[45] Numerous sources at the time suggested that breast milk could be tainted by intercourse, so much so that it could poison the child.[46] Aldobrandino was one of these, stating that a nursing woman "should not sleep with a man, since it is the thing which most corrupts milk . . . because a pregnant woman kills and destroys the child when she breastfeeds."[47] Furthermore, for wealthy families interested in having more children closer together to increase the likelihood of surviving sons, waiting two years until a child was weaned for the next pregnancy was simply too long; without such limitations, children might be only a year apart in age.[48] Klapisch-Zuber even suggests that this would have been preferable to an elite woman, as it "permitted her to enjoy complete liberty" from the burden of suckling between births.[49] Paid breastfeeding was also a clear sign of status for these urban elites, bolstering the prestige of wealthy husbands and indicating the pronounced fertility of the wives. There is plenty of evidence that the four royal daughters of Beatrice of Savoy, for instance, would have been keenly aware of the importance of their procreation. For example, Eleanor of Provence was considered fortunate to get pregnant early and have a son when she was just sixteen; she also had three daughters and another son (although the youngest daughter died at age three).[50] In contrast, it took her sister Margaret nearly ten years before she gave birth to a male heir (she eventually gave birth to eleven children).[51] The popularity of the *Régime* with female or mixed audiences has been tied to obvious concerns about fertility with such readers, and in several unillustrated copies the text accompanies a range of additional works associated with fertility.[52]

autres maladies leur auienēt
si facent medicine qui a leur
maladie affiere. Li .xix. chapistre
cōment on doit lenfant garder
puis quil est ne. ⁊ cōment on
doit cognoistre ⁊ eslire la nourrice
pour garder ⁊ nourrir lenfant.

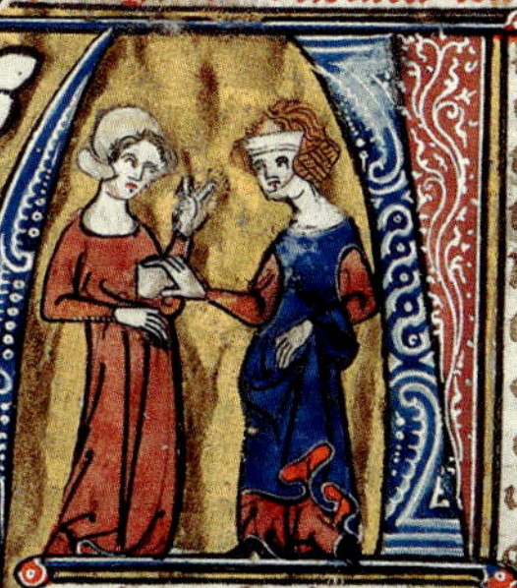

Apres ce
que la
feme
sera de
liuree.
si vous
couu
ent sa
uoir
cōment
vous deues lenfant garder. Sa
chies que si tost cōme il est ne
le couuient enuolepper en roses
broiees mellees en sel delie. et
deues faire couper le nombril
au lonc de .iiij. pouces ⁊ mettre
par dessus pourre de sandragon
⁊ de sarquacol ⁊ de cōmin ⁊ de
mirre ⁊ vn drapel de lin moullie
en oile doliue. ⁊ cest li enseigne
nemens de mains philosophes.
mais il est plus seure chose de
prendre .i. fil de laine retors ⁊
lier le nombril ⁊ apres mettre
drapiaus sus moullies en oile
⁊ laissier les iusques ~~au matin~~
a .iiij. iours ⁊ lors cherra. ⁊ quāt
il sera cheus si vous deues haster

de mettre sel delie sus melle a
pourre de cost ou de soumac ou de
fiens grec ou dorgano. ⁊ de ce
poes saler tout le corps fors q̄
le nes ⁊ la bouche. pour le nom
bril ⁊ pour tout le corps endurcir.
pour ce que si tost que li enfes
est nes tout le corps est tendre ⁊
delie si sent legierement choses
chaudes ⁊ froides apres. qui trop
legierement le grieuent ⁊ pour
roient sa naturel forme chāgier.
et le puet on faire dune fois
se mestier est. especialment ceuls
qui auront asses de superfluites.

Apres le doit on lauer
diaue tiede ⁊ doit la
nourrice ses oreilles
⁊ ses narines espraindre ⁊ es
purgier. ⁊ se garde bien que ele
ait tousiours les ongles roeig
nies que elle ne puisse lenfant
greuer. ⁊ mette as ieux .i. pou
duile doliue. apres le doit lauer
⁊ li mettre son petit doit dedens
le fundement ⁊ tout belement
ouurir pour les superfluites .
mielx espurgier. ⁊ sa verge es
praindre belement pour mielx
orner. ⁊ le garir de froit tant
cōme elle pourra. Et quāt elle
le voudra lender. si doit les
membres souef touchier ⁊ estē
dre ⁊ drecier ⁊ le mettre a point.
⁊ li donner bele forme car cest

Pour cou quil ia gñt
peril. Et li doit on do
ner a boire augue ou
fiens grec ⁊ dates se
iour cuites. ⁊ se li do
nes trois fois ou qñte
se mestiers est. ou pl'
Ou vous li dounes ui
de rue .ii. dragmes. en
uin tiede. ou ius de
sauine. ou boire cha
mele ⁊ waranche en
uin. Et se ele est cras
se si se couche a dens.
⁊ tiraies les ienous ui
ers la teste. ⁊ ait .i.
cousin souz le uentre
Car si faitement demo
rer. fait toutes femes
plus legierement deli
urer. Et qñt ele se
ra deliuree. si le doit
on baignier. ⁊ recon
forter de boines via
des. Et se dolours ⁊ au
tres maladies lor a

uienent. si facent me
decines qui a lor ma
ladies fasierent. Li .xx.
chapitres. coment vos
deves lenfant warder
puis quil est ne de mere.

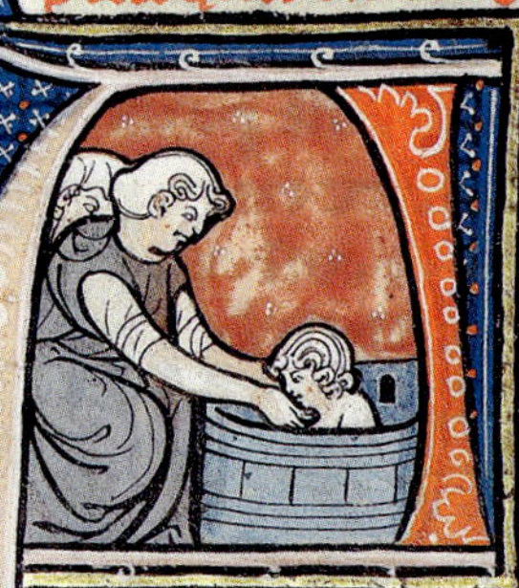

Apries
cou q̃
li en
fes se
ra nes.
⁊ la fe
me de
liure
e. Si vous estuet sauo
ir coment vous le de
ueres garder. Si tost
com il iert nes le co
uient envoleper en
roses broies. meslees
a sel delie. Et deuestr
enchier le bouteril
au res de quatre paus
Et metre sus poudre
de sanc de dragon. ⁊
sarcacol. ⁊ de comin.

Three other fifteenth-century copies depict this chapter with a different focus, showing a lying-in scene instead (figs. 30–32). In all three manuscripts, the woman is unclothed except for her bedclothes and a headwrap and has bare shoulders or even bare breasts. In each manuscript, the two attendants are dressed essentially identically, suggesting they have similar status; across the manuscripts these figures are dressed alike, especially notable in their headdresses. Although we can only speculate on the reasons for this change in iconography, the visual tone of this chapter notably shifts in light of this change. In contrast to the somewhat aggressive display of bodily exploitation that we see in the two wet nurse scenes, or the isolation of a lone nursing woman, here the emphasis is on intimacy, motherhood, community, and the central role of attendant caregivers. Lying-in, the practice of secluding women for four to six weeks after childbirth, was fairly common by the later Middle Ages, especially in elite households.[65] Although lying-in and its conclusion with the rite of churching (the purification rite that signaled a woman's reentry into the community) are complex practices that could be both limiting and empowering for new mothers and their female caregivers and attendants, Elizabeth L'Estrange points out that "it is possible that aristocratic women positively interpreted and received those practices that were designed especially for them as mothers, especially if those practices were intended to give them care and respite and to emphasize their social standing."[66] These women may have welcomed the suspension of usual duties, including pregnancy and sex, along with the recognition of a successful birth. Furthermore, "the refocusing of the household and the family's interests, spaces, and finances on the mother placed the woman 'on top' in a way that upset the usual routine."[67]

The depiction of lying-in was an international iconography, especially common in biblical scenes, and appeared in a wide range of media, including manuscripts, frescos, birthing trays, and panel painting. The authority of the upper-class woman in the *Régime* lying-in scenes is subdued in comparison with the wet nurse scenes, but it is not absent; her status is suggested by her privileged treatment and her surroundings. At least in late medieval France, the canopied bed was linked to wealth, power, respect, and distinction, with the royal woman's bed "not just used for confinement and childbirth," but also seen as "a place of political authority."[68] Canopy beds are clearly articulated in the lying-in scenes from the Cambridge and Sloane 2401 manuscripts, but not in the image from the Morgan manuscript. L'Estrange explores the extensive preparations of the lying-in space, especially by the aristocracy. Special attention was paid to bed linens and other luxurious fabrics, which can often be seen in depictions of lying-in scenes.[69] In the primarily Northern European manuscripts from the fifteenth century that are the focus of her study, the births of holy figures such as the Virgin Mary or John the Baptist were commonly portrayed in contemporary spaces that reflected the birthing environment of the manuscripts' readers.[70]

In reflecting on the reasons for the shift from wet nurse to lying-in in the illustrative tradition for this chapter of the *Régime*, we might begin with the ambiguity and even anxiety inherent in the wet nurse scenes. The ominous creature in the upper

Fig. 30
Newborn care. *Le Régime du corps*, ca. 1450. Cambridge University Library, MS Ii.V.11, fol. 34v, detail. Reproduced by kind permission of the Syndics of Cambridge University Library.

Fig. 31
Newborn care. *Le Régime du corps*, fifteenth century. British Library, Sloane MS 2401, fol. 37v, detail. © The British Library Board.

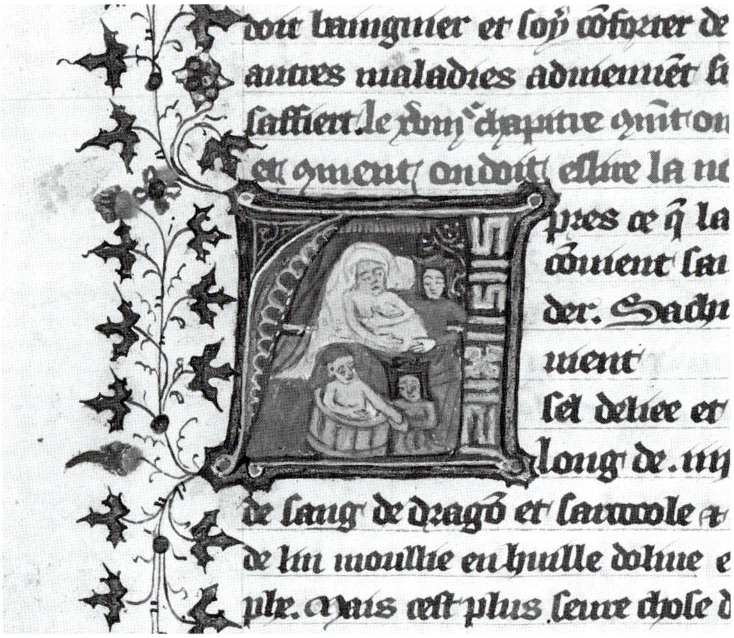

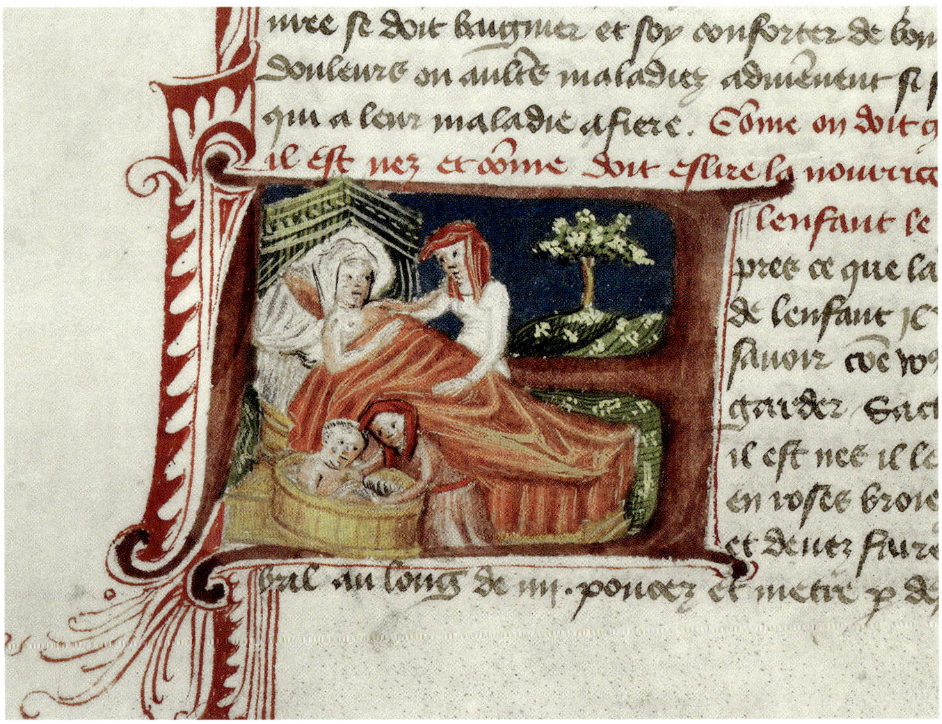

margin of Sloane 2435 to which the elite woman points emphasizes the dire consequences of making a poor choice of nurse. Furthermore, it is not clear in these two depictions of the wet nurse scene whether the exchange is happening before or after the child is born; in the images that accompany the preceding chapter in these two copies, the pregnant woman's condition is not especially visible. At any rate, there is little in the images to indicate whether a successful childbirth has taken place; that ambiguity is key to the tension and poignancy of the earlier wet nurse scenes. In contrast, the lying-in scenes depict overtly *successful* childbirth; the baby is included in the image, cared for alongside the new mother. As the lying-in iconography gained traction in the later Middle Ages, especially so in books of hours aimed at an audience similar to the audience for the illustrated *Régime* manuscripts, it is easy to imagine why this image became a more popular one.

Touch and Status

In the scenes explored above, a wide range of nuanced messages are conveyed to viewers. Complicated relationships are alluded to through the use of clothing, positioning, and gesture. These indicators of status are enriched further through the employment of touch—who is touched, who does the touching, who avoids touch, and what kind of touch occurs. These visual connections between people in the *Régime* images inform real-world encounters between people with different social roles and unequal authority in relation to one another. The childbirth scenes present compelling examples of intimacy at work.

In the lying-in scenes from the *Régime* manuscripts, the women with the most status are rarely the figures who actively touch others. One exception is in the Morgan version, where the mother leans toward the tub and actually places her hand on the edge of it, as if to reach out toward her new baby (fig. 32). For the most part, the power of touch returns to the caregivers, as is the case in many of the other scenes of medical treatment throughout these manuscripts. These birth scenes are dominated by women who provide care and touch the newborn in the absence of men.[71]

In part because the scene illustrating the chapter on newborn care changes over time, we are witness to the varied nuances with which this material was depicted. The wet nurse scenes found in two of the earlier copies, Sloane 2435 and BnF Fr. 12323, are case studies in how touch connects to status. The exposure of the breast by the lower-class woman signifies a kind of submission, an acquiescence, or at least tolerance, of the touch; the noblewoman accepts this offer apparently without hesitation. In Sloane 2435, the wet nurse's right hand literally offers the breast to the other woman; while that woman touches the breast with her right hand, her left hand points and gestures up at the creepy figure in the margin, an almost scolding gesture that mimics what we see the physician do in some other images (see fig. 27). In most of the other scenes of touch in the *Régime* manuscripts, the persons being touched are receiving treatment,

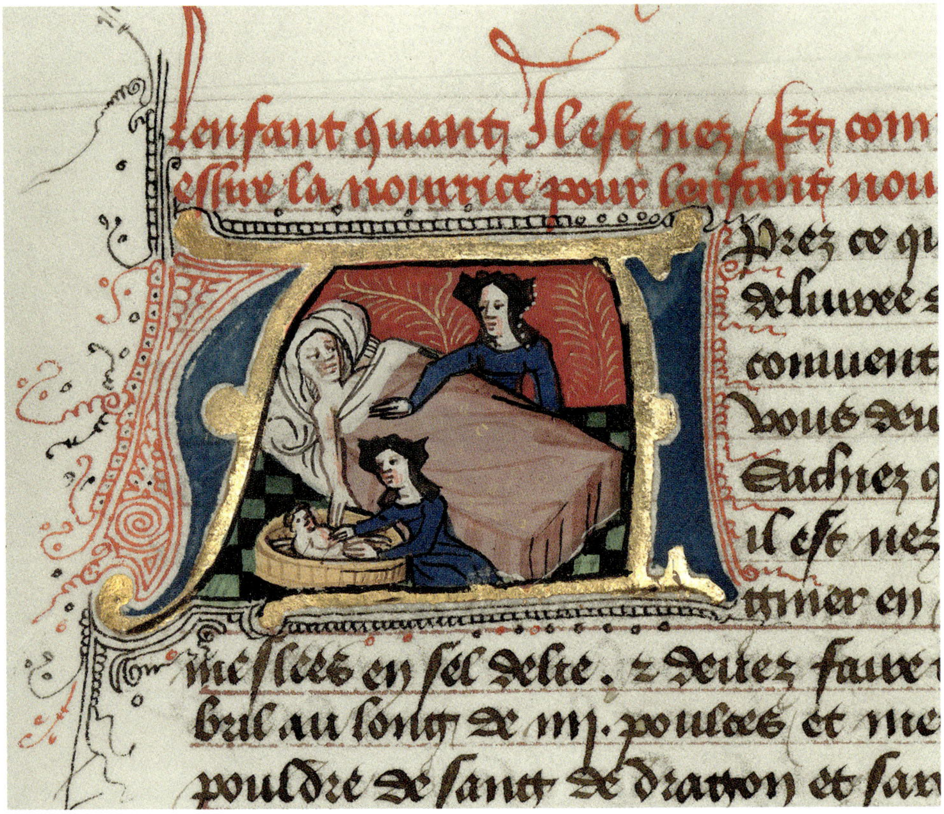

Fig. 32
Newborn care. *Le Régime du corps*, ca. 1440–50. The Morgan Library & Museum, MS M.165, fol. 44r, detail. The Morgan Library & Museum, New York. Purchased by J. Pierpont Morgan (1837–1913) in 1902.

and so they may be more inclined to respectfully submit, hoping for improvement of their own health. But the touch in the wet nurse scene is connected to the health benefit of a third party, the infant, who is not depicted. That changes the tone of the exchange, in which the authority of the wealthier woman is asserted. These encounters may evoke the more clinical breast examination scenes from surgical texts, in which the physician's authority is represented by his avoidance of touching. In the wet nurse exchange scenes, however, touch *is* power, while it also demonstrates the method by which women acquired the knowledge they needed to make a judgment call about the nurse. In the intimate space of the home, a woman can gain power in terms of both physical dominance and empirical knowledge that a physician cannot attain without touch.

Other forms of touch also take place in the *Régime* illuminations. In the scenes of copulation, for example, skin-to-skin touching, and thus a certain level of intimacy, is over time removed from the scene completely. While those scenes may seem peripherally related to health care, they certainly engage with notions of power and authority as they relate to physical contact. In Sloane 2435, the heads of the man and woman are visible, along with a portion of their upper bodies, but otherwise the details of their activities are left to the imagination (see fig. 14). In a brief but witty discussion on images of copulation, Camille argues that the image metonymically references those parts we are not allowed to see, through the man's arm. Considering the curtains of the bed canopy, he states they represent "the opening that cannot be represented, the part of the female body being penetrated."[72] This image reflects a long tradition of authors who assert the procreative dominance of men; Aldobrandino follows this thinking, presenting conception as a phenomenon in which the male provides the primary generative material, while the woman is viewed much like a vessel.[73]

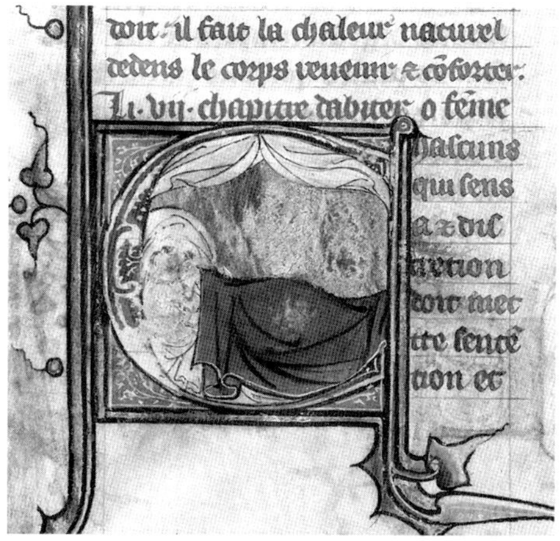

Fig. 33
Copulation. *Le Régime du corps*, fourteenth century. Bibliothèque nationale de France, Fr. 12323, fol. 78r, detail. © Bibliothèque nationale de France.

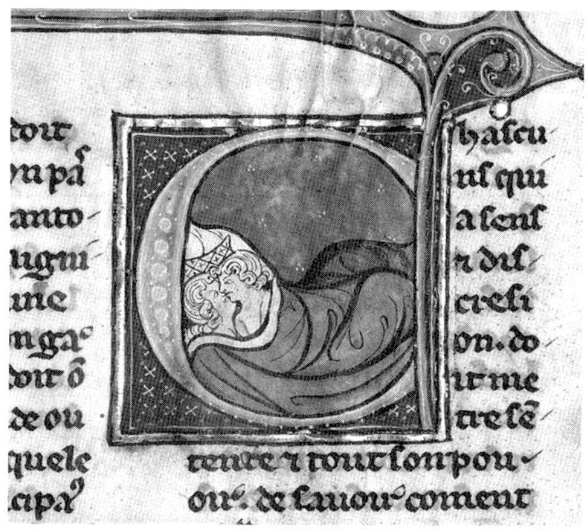

Fig. 34
Copulation. The Bute Painter, *Le Régime du corps*, ca. 1285. Bibliothèque nationale de France, Arsenal MS 2510, fol. 9r, detail. © Bibliothèque nationale de France.

While the curtain of the bed is also a component of the image that appears in BnF Fr. 12323 (fig. 33), the positions of the figures in the bed are no longer accessible because of the defacement that has occurred sometime between the image's creation and our viewing today.[74] Although the erased details make it difficult to discern this image clearly, it does not appear as though the erect arm of the man is part of this image's composition. Other marginal illumination on the page, possibly a hybrid or fantastical beast, has also been rubbed out, suggesting a later puritan motivation to rid this folio of what was deemed unnatural or inappropriate. In the version of this image in the third manuscript from the early group, Arsenal 2510, male domination or authority is deemphasized further (fig. 34). There is no assertive arm or parting curtain, nor do the figures wear caps to clearly distinguish their gender. In fact, with the absence of clear attributes, these two figures look almost identical, preventing us from determining absolutely whether the man or the woman is on top.

The toning down of this chapter's initial continues with the fifteenth-century copies, in which the couples move outside of the bed entirely. In the Morgan manuscript, the couple embraces amorously but are shown on top of the bedcovers and fully clothed (fig. 35). The dominance of the man, who is clearly positioned on top, is still very pronounced in this image. In contrast, both the Cambridge manuscript and Sloane 2401 display a scene in which the two are not only completely clothed, but also stand up in their embrace (fig. 36). There is no bed in the scene, and the couple could be in any number of public or private spaces—in fact, in Sloane 2401 they stand outdoors. In the Ajuda manuscript, the couple is also fully dressed and upright. Although they are seated on the edge of a huge canopied bed, its deeply skewed perspective pushes them forward into nearly standing positions (fig. 37). The vertical orientation of the figures in these copies not only takes them one step further away from the suggestiveness of the bedroom but also puts them on an equal footing, for neither figure is on top of the other. As the depiction of intimacy decreases throughout the series, the sense of male domination diminishes as well. The absence of touch here suggests a reduction in male authority or an equalizing of power, while in other *Régime* images, authority is tied to who has the control over the denial as well as the initiation of physical contact.

Similar notions of authority are tied to the abundant depictions of physicians in the illustrated *Régime*, informing how we think about the management of health care within the context of the household. Although I consider the representations of the physician in these *Régime* manuscripts more fully in chapter 3, it is worth noting here that the physician appears eight times in Sloane 2435, for example, and has similar representation in most of the other manuscripts. Regardless of the fact that the authority of the physician is largely absent in the text of the *Régime du corps*, his role in health care is pronounced in the initials of all the illustrated copies except for the Arsenal manuscript. That should not be particularly surprising, considering the upper-class, and at times aristocratic or royal, audiences for these books; these were exactly the same audiences that could afford consultations with professional physicians.[75] Aldobrandino himself was apparently the physician of Beatrice of Savoy, after all. The physician's status is established in part through the clothing he wears, which distinguishes him from both the patients and the other attendants or workers in the manuscripts. However, clothing is not the only visual signifier of the physician's authority; it is also suggested with gesture and touch.

The physicians in the *Régime* images have quite specific gestures, often ones that imply authority and the giving of directions.[76] For instance, in the BnF Fr. 12323 image associated with the chapter on pregnancy, a woman stands across from a physician, but her condition is not pronounced (fig. 38). Instead, primarily through the use of dress and gesture, such depictions highlight the physician's authority, the status of the patient, and the relationship between them. In the parallel scene from Sloane 2435, the physician makes a similar gesture toward the notably elite woman, while his left hand is being used expressively (see chapter 3). Elsewhere in that manuscript, the gesture he makes with his right hand is open and oriented toward the other figure, while the left points upward to make his point. Occasionally the doctor holds up a urine flask or hands a cup containing a purgative to the patient, but direct physical contact is largely absent. The physician in BnF Fr. 12323 points his right hand assertively toward the pregnant woman while his left hand holds a glove. In this manuscript, he is often shown holding gloves that have been removed; sometimes the patients also have their gloves removed (see chapter 4). The Leipzig manuscript also depicts several scenes in which the physician has his gloves removed. It is logical to assume that the physician took off his gloves for a reason; however, there is still usually no physical contact made with the bare hands. Was the removal of gloves done to keep the gloves clean? Or did this action have to do with formalities or social practices? Perhaps it was only polite to take off your gloves during such a consultation.

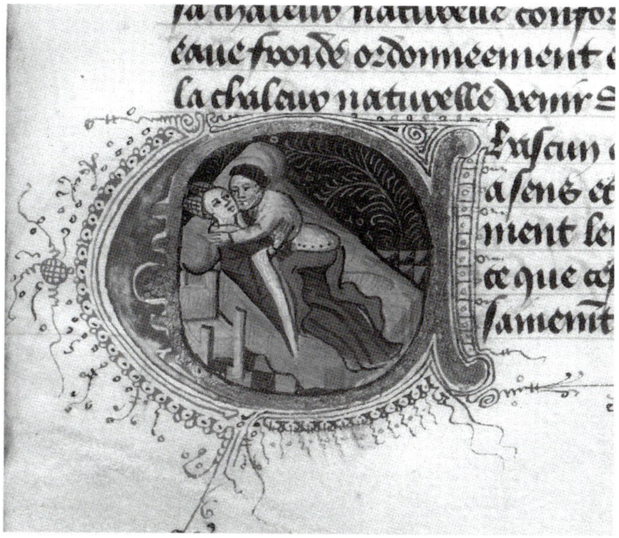

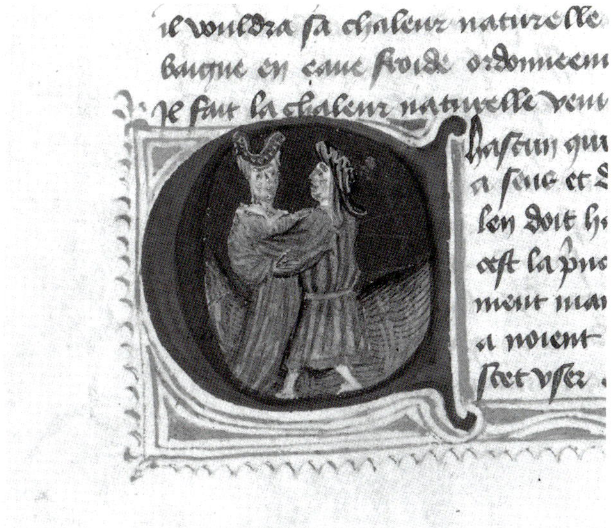

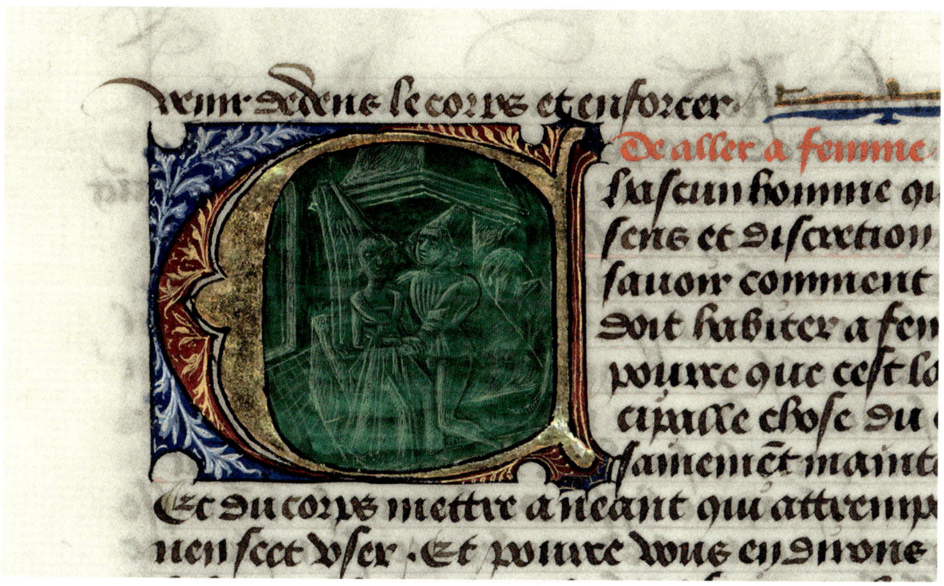

Fig. 35 (above left)
Copulation. *Le Régime du corps*, ca. 1440–50. The Morgan Library & Museum, MS M.165, fol. 17r, detail. The Morgan Library & Museum, New York. Purchased by J. Pierpont Morgan (1837–1913) in 1902.

Fig. 36 (above right)
Copulation. *Le Régime du corps*, fifteenth century. British Library, Sloane MS 2401, fol. 16v, detail. © The British Library Board.

Fig. 37
Copulation. *Le Régime du corps*, ca. 1470s. Biblioteca da Ajuda, Lisbon, Cod. 52-XIII-26, fol. 16v, detail. Biblioteca da Ajuda.

Can we read the removal of gloves as a sign of touch, even though the touch itself is left unrepresented? On the one hand, the removal of gloves suggests a need to touch directly with the fingers; on the other hand, that touch is rarely shown in the same image with the gloves. As is often recommended with texts that focus on the pulse as an important diagnostic tool, taking the patient's pulse presumably required the removal of gloves—for the physician as well as for the patient.[77] Yet the images that depict a physician holding gloves rarely show a demonstration of such pulse-taking. In her assessment of several images from another surgical manuscript, Montpellier Bibliothèque interuniversitaire, MS H 089, Helen Valls suggests that such gloves added to the seriousness of the scene, one in which a notable spatial distance exists between

encore qui faire le pourroit vin
droit il nuche a ceuls qui che
minent porter nete voe de leur
pais ⁊ meller en yaue qui est
mauvaise que boire couvient ⁊
faire boulir ⁊ faire la clere en
la maniere que nous vꝰ avons
dit ⁊ user. se de ces choses na loi
sir du faire. si puet user vin ai
gre ⁊ oignons ⁊ laitues a vin
aigre. ⁊ se ainsi est que elle soit
amere. si la boive avec chucre.
Et pour plus briement dire. oi
gnons ⁊ vin aigre ⁊ põmes gre
nates ⁊ toutes choses aigres de
struisent la mauvaistie de tou
tes mauvaises yaues quil cou
vient user.

Et sil avient chose quil
couviegne nagier par
mer. devant que li hõs
entre en mer. ij. iours ou. iij.
menguisse mains quil ne seult.
⁊ le premier iour quil entrera
en la mer ne doit nule viande re
garder. anchois li couvient flai
rier choses de bonne odour ⁊ mẽ
gier fruit qui conforte la cervele.
sicõme cooins. põmes grenates ⁊
autres põmes aigres. Et sa soi
ce quil couviegne boivre nest il
pas mauvais se ce nest a outra
ge. ⁊ le trop boivre ⁊ la grant
abhominacion si est le remede
de boire. i. pou de semence dache

en vin ⁊ en ius daloisne. ⁊ mẽ
gier roisins qui ne sunt mie me
urs. ⁊ faire ce que dit vꝰ avons
v chapitre de boivre. **Li. xviij. cha
pitres cõment la feme se puet
garder puis que elle est enchain
te. ⁊ cõment elle se puet aidier
a delivrer.**

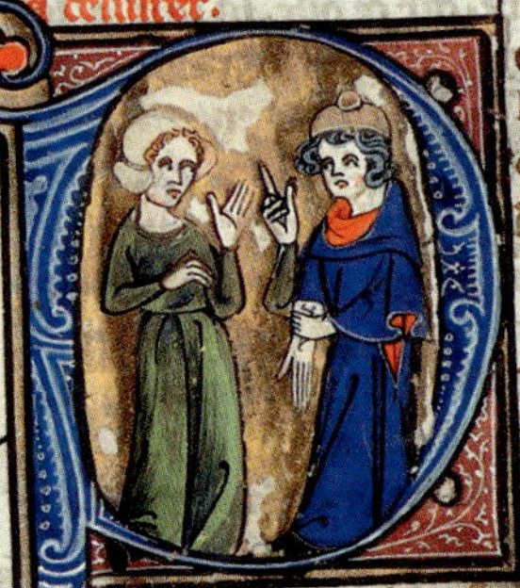

Pour
bien
entendre ce
que
nous
vous
dirons
vous
devez
savoir que li enfes v cors
de la feme si est ausi cõ
me le fruis es arbres.
car vous vees premiere
ment que la fleur ou le
fruit vient qui se tient
foiblement a larbre et
par pou de vent ⁊ de pluie
chiet. ⁊ apres quant le
fruit engroisse si se tient
fort ⁊ ne chiet pas volen
tiers. ⁊ quãt il vient quil
est meur si chiet ausi cõ
me la fleur legierement.
Tout ainsi devez vous
entendre de la fame que
v premier mois ⁊ v secont

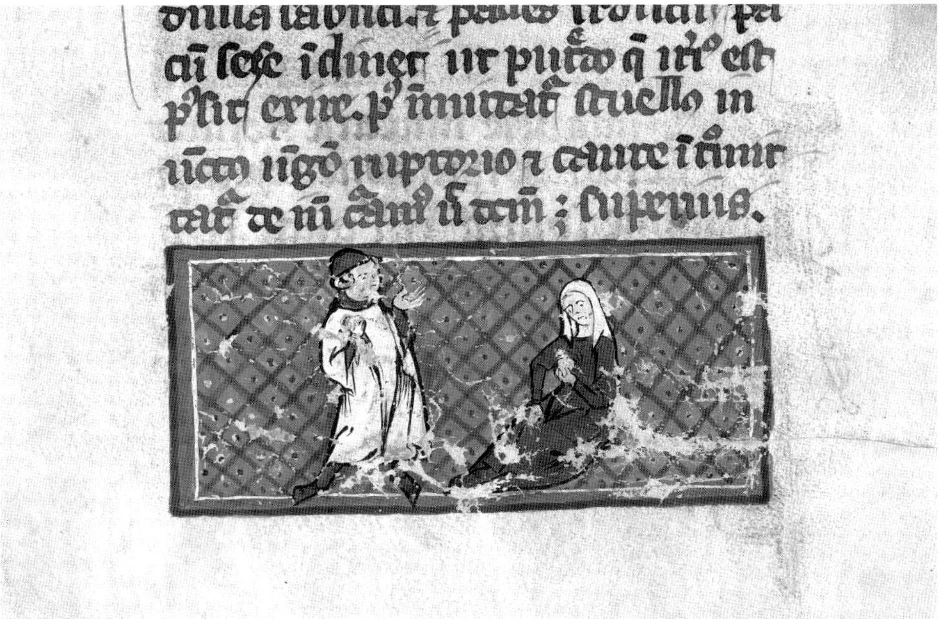

Fig. 38 (opposite)
Pregnancy. *Le Régime du corps*, fourteenth century. Bibliothèque nationale de France, Fr. 12323, fol. 95v, detail. © Bibliothèque nationale de France.

Fig. 39
Woman presenting breast disease to surgeon. *Chirurgia*, fourteenth century. Montpellier, Bibliothèque interuniversitaire, MS H 089, fol. 22r, detail. © BIU Montpellier / IRHT (CNRS).

practitioner and patient (fig. 39). She suggests that these images mirror the warning in the accompanying text that the pictured ailment is not one the surgeon should take on.[78] The surgeon's particular gesture and gloves are read in this case as an articulation of the gravity of the situation and his reluctance to intervene. The surgeon's touch is otherwise prevalent in this manuscript, making the four instances with gloves, more formal clothing, and distant proximity particularly notable.

The lack of touch may then be as much about the patient as it is about the practitioner, serving as a way to demonstrate gravity. It may have been a sign of respect not to touch, since these patients had status themselves. According to Michael McVaugh in his discussion of medieval writing regarding physicians' behavior with patients, doctors are advised to "examine the patient yourself as much as modesty allows."[79] Several authors writing in the thirteenth century talk about the right tone in which to speak to patients: William of Saliceto warns, "you should not get too friendly with your patients, should maintain a certain aloofness; looking thoughtfully at the ground, saying little, lets them see that you are thinking hard and builds up their faith in you."[80] Coincidentally, another text, an Anglo-Norman treatise on visiting and treating patients that also discusses proper behavior in such exchanges, exists in copies, including British Library Sloane MS 3525, an unillustrated manuscript that also includes the *Régime*.[81] The lack of touch in the scenes with physicians may have to do with both the assertion of objective authority and the maintenance of an appropriate tone to garner respect from the patient, while respecting the status of the patient as well.

The prevalent lack of touch in the *Régime* illustrations also correlates with established taboos in the medical field regarding touch, especially when dealing with female patients. As Monica H. Green has explored in relation to the areas of gynecology and obstetrics, there was persistent anxiety about male physicians touching women, especially during childbirth or for genital examinations. Even as academic medicine became more involved in women's health care, male practitioners avoided the impropriety of touching women, often enlisting female assistants to carry out their directions.[82] Although the treatments in the *Régime* manuscripts are of a much less fraught nature, usually involving clothed patients and men as well as women, the absence of the physician's touch clearly reflects these broader concerns.

Conclusion: The Intimate Household

Across the board, when patients are actually touched by practitioners, those practitioners are dressed differently, more modestly or humbly, implying they are surgeons, barbers, or assistants; some of them are also women. This can be seen in scenes of bloodletting, cupping, vomiting, and purging, and even in some specific consultations in the "parts of the body" section, as will be further explored over the course of this book. The figures engaging in treatment do not necessarily represent poverty or low status, but they are illustrated in a distinctly different fashion from the professional physicians. In the cupping scene from Sloane 2435, for example, a woman who wears a hairnet around her bundled, braided hair and a simple chemise holds the cups over a fire, applying one to the bare back of a male patient, his head covered in a coif (fig. 40). Her body is bent to better reach the man receiving treatment, who appears seated on the ground with a blanket over his lap. The patients are often sitting in such scenes; they have acquiesced to being touched. A different kind of authority is presented here; clearly the patients are allowing the practitioners to touch them in the course of treatment, whether that is holding out their arm to cut the vein for bleeding or turning their bare back toward the practitioner so that she may apply the glass bells for cupping. It is even possible that some of these people are household servants or employees of the patient; they were familiar people, following the directions of the physician. As scenes like the cupping treatment above demonstrate, a certain comfortableness is evident in the willingness of the patients to submit to the intimacy required by their care. In addition to the level of intimacy required for administering treatment, with some of these remedies, the patient will be put into a particularly vulnerable position as the treatment runs its course (purging or vomiting, for instance). These treatments most certainly took place in the home, and many would have resulted in excess bodily fluids. Who would have been responsible for disposing of blood or vomit? No doubt it was often the household servants.[83]

As the images related to childbirth epitomize—the wet nurse exchange, as well as the nursing and lying-in scenes—most of the treatments and other forms of care represented in the *Régime* required touching and intimacy in which the physician was not at all involved. The physician is represented several times in most of the *Régime* manuscripts, but these are not situations that require close contact or bodily engagement.

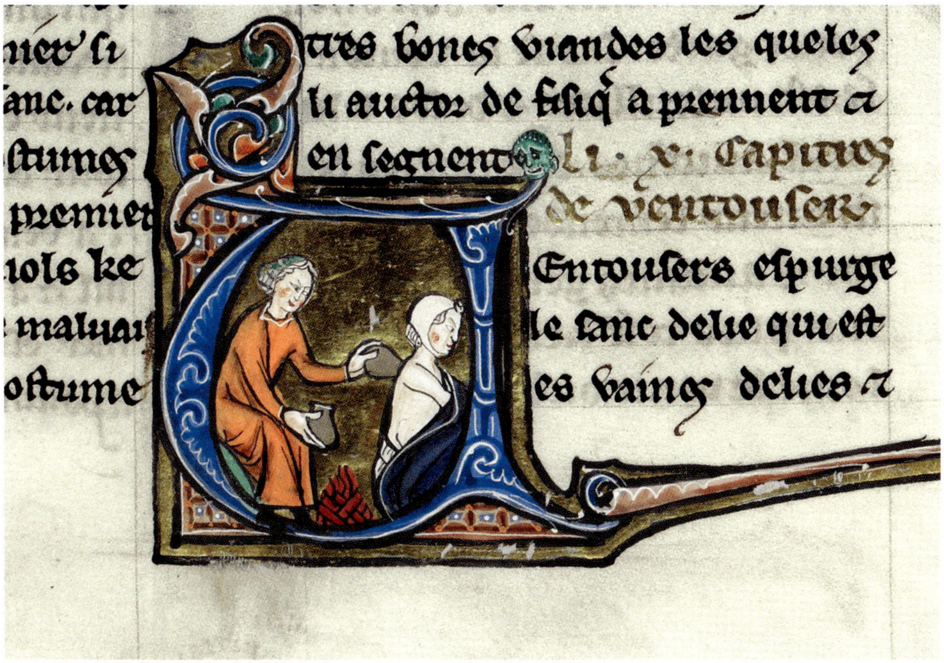

Fig. 40
Cupping. *Le Régime du corps*, ca. 1265–70. British Library, Sloane MS 2435, fol. 14r, detail. © The British Library Board.

On the contrary, touching is done by other practitioners: attendants, nurses, and caregivers of all kinds. The well-dressed physician enters the space of the household, potentially bringing with him the canonical medicine represented by the *Régime* text itself; at the same time, his knowledge and authority represent just one kind of knowledge, and that expertise must yield to the larger household networks of people and practices. These illustrated manuscripts guide the book users' expectations of these different types of interactions, potentially preparing those readers for how they should behave when consulting with physicians and how to anticipate different norms of behavior when there are changes in status, as when dealing with other types of practitioners, assistants, and household members.

The intimacy of everyday household care is suggested by the nature of the touching we see in these scenes, in which patients' bodies are cut, disrobed, positioned, handled, consoled, caressed. These people are weak and exposed, their bodies are messy, and, in the intimate space of treatment, people are present to guide them through these vulnerable moments. Those moments took place within the household, a place where nearly everyone was preoccupied with activities that facilitated the sustenance and maintenance of all the bodies that lived within that sphere (that household context is further explored in chapter 4). A disrobed patient, after all, has removed many of their signifiers of status, and allowing someone to cut your arm for bleeding necessitates submission. Everyone's bodies create the same kinds of waste, which must be dealt with by someone. While these lavish illustrated copies are clearly communicating status, they simultaneously evoke a context in which household networks wove together multiple knowledges, at times transforming public knowledges into more personal, immediate, and intimate ones. It is precisely that heightened intimacy of these interactions that is evident when these copies of the *Régime* are illuminated.

The *Régime* images also unsettle authority through their creation of ambiguous narrative resolution that moves into the real space of the medieval household. The many players within a scene—the practitioner and patient, but also the book user—enact the narrative beyond the space of the image, not unlike the way medieval plays and other forms of performance moved devotion or narrative action into the space of the viewer.[84] Nonsequential historiated initials foster unresolved narratives that suggest even more potentiality than images that are part of a series, and they do so by engaging the viewer in imagining multiple conclusions simultaneously. The viewer of the *Régime* images becomes the composer of the narrative, specifically a health-related one, initiating action in a way analogous to enacting health care itself. This involvement of the viewer moves the activity into the spaces of living, and nothing was more real than the realities of caring for children, family, and other household members. The open-ended narrative form of the historiated initials ultimately created a situation in which many images in these books provided the reader with the simultaneous possibilities of survival and succumbing, comfort and pain, heartbreak and celebration, indeed, a multiplicity of imaginable futures at once.

THE ILLUSTRATED MANUSCRIPTS AND THEIR AUDIENCES

2

In BnF Fr. 12323, the initial for the chapter on *fromages* consists of a large "F" with twenty-one rounds of cheese, depicted as simple white circles fanned out in three rows between the two arms of the letter (fig. 41). The abundance suggests that this scene shows the moment right after the cheese has been made, the large batch laid out to age. A parallel image appears in Sloane 2435, in which fourteen similarly colored cheeses are shaped and piled in three levels (fig. 42). In contrast with these two earlier illustrated copies, the fifteenth-century manuscripts show the cheese in a slightly larger spatial context. Rather than engaging the letter to serve as shelves for the newly crafted cheese, the artist depicts it as it might have been stored within a household: laid out on a table, with an airy basket for storage hanging above.

The similarities between the cheese images in Sloane 2435 and BnF Fr. 12323 indicate a close relationship between these two manuscripts, even if we are unable to articulate precisely what that relationship is. The different layout of the cheese images in the later copies of the *Régime* likewise reflects connections that are most evident in visual terms. The existence of such parallels, despite the different styles of the manuscripts, makes a strong case for their interconnectedness. The shared characteristics evident across this later group of manuscripts imply strong connections among them; these connections are further strengthened by the clear familial networks across Europe, but especially across the English Channel, that they represent.[1]

It may not seem that a lot is riding on what the designers decided about how to represent cheese. But the curious abstraction from the chapter on cheese in Sloane 2435 and BnF Fr. 12323 encourages us to ask what choices an artist or designer might have had, and why they made the selections they did. Were there pattern books or other models to use for images of food? If not, did the cheese's painter create this image from scratch? We might also wonder how a medieval viewer might have approached or understood such a scene. Perhaps it was determined that multiple rounds of cheese conjure

user que nuls de ces deux. Cil q
sunt cuis en l'eaue conforteut la
chaleur naturel. & especialment
quant il sunt si cuis quil ne sunt
ne mols ne durs. car pour l'eaue
il samendent & perdent leur
mauuaistie. & valent miels &
miels nourrissent son les men
gue en tel maniere que en tou
tes les autres manieres con les
puist cuire ne user.
Les oefs fris sur toutes
les autres manieres
valent pis. car il se
conuertissent en mauuaises
humeurs. et engendrent fume
es & abhominations. & pour ce
les fait il mal user. Cil que on
mengue auec char ou en autre
maniere on les doit blasmer &
loer selonc la compaignie des
autres choses ou il sunt melles.
car ceuls qui sunt mengies a
uec bonnes espices sicome auec
poiure. canele. gengibre & auec
char. si se cuisent miels en lesto
mac & donnent meillour nour
rissement & acroissent plus le
talent de gesir o feme que cil
que on mengue auecques four
mage qui namendent pas ain
chois acroissent leur malice.

De toutes manieres de four
mages.

Fourm
ages
sicome
dit y
saac
sunt
gene
ralment
du tout
mau
uais. car li formages est
pesans & engroisse la for
cele. & de ce uous proues a
perceuoir. car qui lusse lon
guement il couuient quil
ait douleur de flans. mau
uaise teste & gros encende
ment & pierre es rains
~~es rains~~ & en la uessie. mais
il est mauuais plus et
mains selonc la diuersite
de luser con en fait. Car
qui le mengue quant il est
fres & nouuel si a nature
de remondier la fourcele pour ce
quil est froit & moiste u premier
degre & s'il se cuist bien a lesto
mac. si encrassie & nourrist mie.
S'il est mengie quant il est uiel
selonc ce quil est plus uiel si est
plus chaut & uaut pis a user
car il engendre mauuaises fu
mees & mauuaises humeurs &
chaudes & seches & fait sur
toutes autres manieres de four

the food better than one circle would; that said, fourteen or twenty-one does seem a bit excessive. It is true that when cheese is made, many rounds are created from one batch, so perhaps this approach is also meant bring to mind many rounds stacked on shelves. As an object that may have been seen most often in multiples, the number could be less significant here than the simple suggestion of abundance.

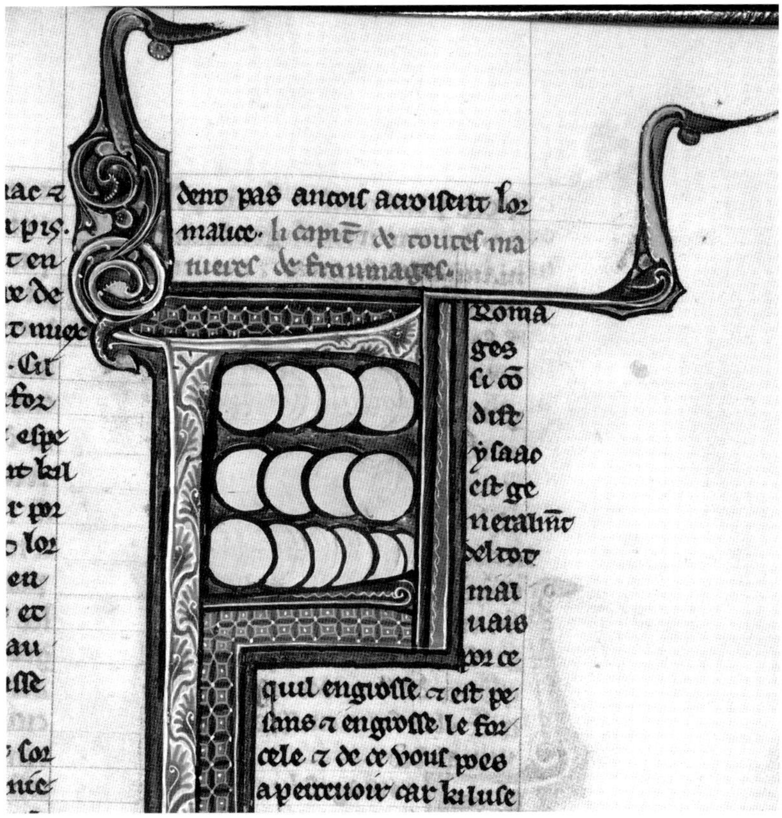

Cheese was a food created in the household context; it was given value and discussed in the *Régime*'s text, but that assessment also took place via the accompanying images. As a result, cheese, like all the substances or activities depicted in the illustrated *Régime* manuscripts, was infused with associations: nutritional value and other health benefits or risks, circumstances of production within the household, and cultural or social connotations, including those tied to status. Although we might assume that cheese was understood to have healthful benefits because it is included in a health text, this chapter's accompanying text describes cheese as being rather unhealthy: "As Isaac says, cheese is generally completely bad because it swells the belly, making it heavy and inflated," and "people who have used it for a long time . . . have pains in their side, a bad head, dullness of wit, kidney and bladder stones."[2] If the reader must consume it, fresh cheese is more nourishing, while older cheese is best for therapeutic uses, such as comforting the stomach.[3] Furthermore, at various historical moments, it seems cheese was seen as a lower-class food, associated with peasants and laborers.[4] Whether or not this was an association prevalent when Sloane 2435 was made in the late thirteenth century, it does seem surprising that a food not seen as particularly beneficial to one's health would receive the special recognition offered by the historiated initial. When the abstraction we see in the two earlier manuscripts gives way to the later scenes with a table, some of these ideas about the chapter's content may have changed (fig. 43). With no people in either type of image, we might be inclined to read them as static, inert scenes, but with the expanded space in the later initials, the invisible presence of the human as cheese maker is more pronounced.

Fig. 41 (opposite)
Cheese. *Le Régime du corps*, fourteenth century. Bibliothèque nationale de France, Fr. 12323, fol. 128r. © Bibliothèque nationale de France.

Fig. 42
Cheese. *Le Régime du corps*, ca. 1265–70. British Library, Sloane MS 2435, fol. 69r, detail. © The British Library Board.

The prologue of the *Régime* tells us that the text was composed by Aldobrandino for Beatrice of Savoy, and apparently this new vernacular and domestically oriented collection of medical material moved quickly throughout Europe, possibly as each of

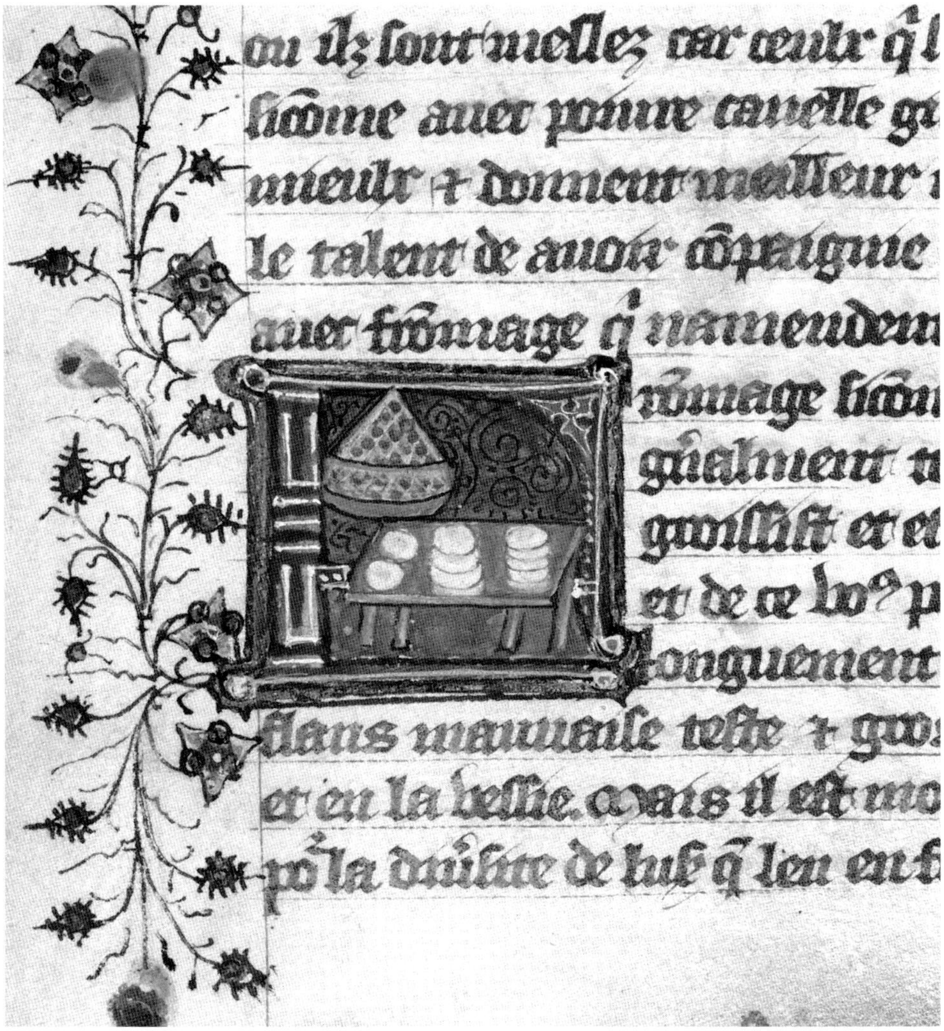

Fig. 43
Cheese. *Le Régime du corps*, ca. 1450. Cambridge University Library, MS Ii.V.11, fol. 77r, detail. Reproduced by kind permission of the Syndics of Cambridge University Library.

her daughters brought the text into her home and introduced it to a new audience. As Monica H. Green points out, even though Beatrice's copy does not appear to have survived, if she was the first female owner of the text, "given the content of its genesis it would not be improbable to imagine that she had copies made for her four daughters."[5] Although the earliest illustrated copies of the *Régime du corps* were created within just a few decades of the text's composition in 1256, they cannot be tied directly to Beatrice or her daughters, and it remains unclear whether the "original" copy presumably made for Beatrice was illustrated or not. Individual commissioners have not been identified for these illustrated copies, but it is often possible to narrow down their patronage or ownership to a small group of men and women, or at least to make a case for the social group in which the manuscript was made. Understanding these less precise audiences remains productive, especially for establishing the types of late medieval audiences that may have been interested in the *Régime* and similar texts.

The dissemination made possible by the movement of Beatrice and her daughters, which is supported by the narrative in the text's prologue, provides a structure for approaching these illustrated manuscripts with more specific questions about how they came to be, what role women and their households might have had in their production, and what kinds of audiences might have had access to them. Who were these women, Beatrice and her daughters, and why might they have been interested in manuscripts with images of things like cheese? As the chapters on cheese, game, spices, newborn care, and many other topics suggest, the intersections between health care, household activity, and social status remain central to understanding this group of manuscripts and their audiences.

A Royal Context for the *Régime*: A Powerful Family

According to the prologue that accompanies many versions of the *Régime du corps*, in the year 1256 Aldobrandino of Siena (d. 1287), physician to Beatrice of Savoy (1207–1265), countess of Provence (married to Raymond Berengar V, count of Provence), was asked by Beatrice to compile the text for her in anticipation of traveling to visit her daughters.[6] All four of these daughters were or would become queens: of England, France, Germany, and Sicily.[7] While some scholars have suggested that this prologue presents an apocryphal story, in part because there is no documentary evidence of the commission, others have taken the prologue, which accompanies a number of the earliest copies of the text, as a likely scenario.[8] In this context, it is probable that copies were made for the daughters themselves: Margaret of Provence (1221–1295) married Louis IX, king of France (1214–1270), in 1234; Eleanor of Provence (1223–1291) married Henry III, king of England (1207–1272), in 1236; Sanchia of Provence (1228–1261) married Richard, earl of Cornwall (1209–1272), in 1243 (Richard became king of Germany in 1256); and Beatrice of Provence (1231–1267) married Charles, count of Anjou (1227–1285), in 1246 (Charles became king of Sicily in 1266).[9] Henry III and Richard of Cornwall were brothers, as were Louis IX and Charles. Sanchia and Beatrice of Provence, the two youngest daughters, died in the 1260s, but Margaret and Eleanor both lived into the 1290s.[10] This family of women remained close and connected well beyond the time of their marriages, suggesting continued dialogue in political, literary, and artistic realms.

Although there has been some debate about the date of Aldobrandino's text, most scholars seem to have settled on 1256.[11] With this in mind, the two earliest surviving illustrated copies, Sloane 2435 and Arsenal 2510, dated to around 1265–70 and 1285, respectively, were made quite soon after the text was first composed. The sororal link between the courts of England and France in this period, fostered by the particularly close relationship between Eleanor and Margaret, offers a probable context in which the earlier group of books may have been moved back and forth across the English Channel as the result of events like inheritance or gift exchange.[12]

Ample evidence suggests that these women—especially Margaret, queen of France, and Eleanor, queen of England—were involved in commissioning other lavish manuscripts in this period. Queen Margaret, Beatrice's daughter and the wife of King Louis IX, was a prolific patron of the arts, as was her husband, and Queen Eleanor has been linked to the collecting of a wide range of manuscripts, including chivalrous romances, poetry, and devotional books.[13] Margaret gave a three-volume moralized Bible to either her sister Eleanor or her brother-in-law Henry III, possibly to celebrate the latter couple's visit to Paris in 1254 (now divided across several libraries, this *Bible moralisée* is usually referred to as the Oxford-Paris-London version).[14] The *Bibles moralisées* are among the most luxurious and extravagant manuscript productions of the thirteenth and fourteenth centuries. Seven copies were made over the course of the fourteenth century, intended for kings and queens of France and their closest relatives.

That meeting in Paris in December 1254 involved all four sisters, their spouses, and the dowager countess Beatrice of Savoy; it is the only documented case of such a reunion. John Lowden describes this trip as "extraordinary"; Louis IX and Margaret had just returned from six years of crusading and, according to chronicler Matthew Paris, demonstrated great warmth and hospitality toward the visitors.[15] The connections fostered through these marriages and relationships were celebrated and provided optimism for a new period of friendship between France and England. Matthew Paris wrote that Louis IX told Henry III, "Have we not married two sisters, and our brothers the other two? All that shall be born of them, both sons and daughters, shall be like brothers and sisters."[16] Eleanor and Margaret seem to have had a particularly strong relationship, which they maintained over decades and great distances, including during the years that Margaret was on crusade in the Levant (primarily in Damietta, Acre, and Jaffa) with Louis IX from 1248 to 1254.[17] There were clearly significant political implications in commissioning and bequeathing manuscripts in a wide range of genres.[18]

In addition to these women who are linked to the practices of book production, collection, and giving, there are also important book patrons both earlier and later in the genealogies of these families. Earlier female supporters of (in some cases very luxurious) manuscript production include Blanche of Castile (1188–1252), Louis IX's powerful mother, and Eleanor of Aquitaine, Henry III's controversial grandmother (ca. 1122–1204). In fact, Blanche of Castile probably commissioned the earliest copy of the *Bible moralisée*, possibly for her daughter-in-law Margaret in celebration of Margaret's marriage to Louis around 1234, or for herself (Vienna, Österreichische Nationalbibliothek Cod. 2554).[19] Several children and grandchildren of both Margaret and Eleanor are associated with manuscript patronage; one pronounced example is Isabella of France (ca. 1295–1358), who was queen of England and the likely patron of many books, including the Queen Mary Psalter.[20] Isabella has connections to two of Beatrice of Savoy's daughters: she was the granddaughter of Margaret *and* she was married to Eleanor's grandson, Edward II (1284–1327). One of Margaret's daughters-in-law, Marie de Brabant (1260–1321), commissioned many manuscripts as well.[21] Indeed,

Marie may have commissioned Bibliothèque municipale de Rennes MS 593, a copy of the *Image du monde* (a text often associated with the *Régime*), which may have eventually passed into the inventory of Queen Clémence of Hungary.[22] Cambridge Ii.V.11 includes the coat of arms of Eleanor's sixth great-grandson Henry VII, king of England (1457–1509), and his queen, Elizabeth of York (1466–1503), demonstrating that descendants of these women have been linked to illustrated copies of the *Régime* as well.

Although the specific trajectories of these illustrated copies are quite different, they collectively indicate exchanges of various forms across the "border region" between Paris and England over the course of two hundred years.[23] Several of the illustrated *Régime* manuscripts are now located outside of France; three of those are in collections in England, and the other two were likely in England for part of their lives. These manuscripts reflect the complex, multifaceted nature of book production and dissemination in France and England in this period, which grew over time to adjust to greater demand from a wide range of lay readers and collectors. These relatively luxurious copies of the *Régime* were clearly created in contexts similar to those of other types of books intended for royal patrons, and they were communicating the important values of luxury, literacy, and cosmopolitanism. The movement of these books, linked with the activities and spheres of Beatrice and her daughters, suggests a female-focused network that, over centuries and across lands, made a profound impact on the communication of various knowledges and ideals.

Initial Circulation: The Earlier Group

The known copies of the *Régime du corps* illuminated with historiated initials are divided into an earlier group of Sloane 2435 (ca. 1265–70), Arsenal 2510 (ca. 1285), and BnF Fr. 12323 (ca. 1350), and a later group of Cambridge Ii.V.11 (ca. 1450), Morgan M.165 (ca. 1440–50), Sloane 2401 (ca. 1450–1500), and Ajuda 52-XIII-26 (1470s). Overall, they were created over a period of approximately two hundred years, and this is reflected in their pronounced stylistic diversity. Despite this, and the fact that the number of initials each manuscript contains varies greatly—ranging from thirty-seven to 149—these manuscripts still display striking similarities in subject and form. The existence of such parallels, regardless of the different styles of these manuscripts, makes a strong case for their interconnectedness. By considering these books as two distinct groups, it is possible to see different trends in the copying and dissemination of the illustrated *Régime*. The manuscripts in the earlier group, including one created just a few years after Beatrice's possible commission, can be seen as developing within circles very similar to hers, primarily among the nobility, if not royalty. The later manuscripts reflect a broadening audience that included wealthy, but not necessarily royal or noble, elites. For both groups, there is compelling evidence that these manuscripts were desirable for both their particular content and their luxurious display, and that the collecting of these books was tied to expressions of prestige and household wealth.

Fig. 44
Bathing. *Le Régime du corps*, ca. 1265–70. British Library, Sloane MS 2435, fol. 8v. © The British Library Board.

Produced about a decade after the text was composed, Sloane 2435 was made in northern France, probably soon after 1265, making it the earliest of the illustrated copies.[24] Sloane 2435 includes just two texts, the *Régime* (Redaction B) and Gossuin de Metz's *Image du monde*, and both texts include illuminations by the same artist (*Régime du corps*, fols. 1r–75v; *Image du monde*, fols. 77r–133v). The latter is an encyclopedic poem covering theological, geographical, and astronomical topics. It was the first such encyclopedic work written in French, and Sloane 2435 contains one of the earliest surviving copies of the text.[25] The manuscript's dating is partially based on the 1265 recension of the *Image du monde* included with the manuscript, and the date is also written at the end of the text. Coincidentally, two other early illustrated copies of the *Image du monde* were produced in the same region; one contains the 1265 recension (Bibliothèque nationale de France MS Fr. 14964), and the other (Bibliothèque nationale de France MS Fr. 14970) was illustrated by the Bute Painter, the artist of Arsenal 2510, another illustrated copy of the *Régime* discussed below.[26] Alison Stones has identified the artist of Sloane 2435, whom she calls the "Aldebrandin Master," as the artist of several other manuscripts as well. They were likely made in Cambrai in the 1270s and 1280s for either ecclesiastical or noble patrons.[27]

Sloane 2435 is an incredibly luxurious production, its embellishment among the more elaborate illustrated *Régime* copies (fig. 44). Seventy-two historiated initials illustrate the *Régime*, while the *Image du monde* is accompanied by forty images, including thirteen historiated initials and twenty-seven diagrams in rectangular frames. Additionally, several initials contain animated borders that extend from the initials, and many smaller, decorative initials are also finely realized in gold and multiple colors. The artist's figure drawing is remarkably delicate, precise, and legible despite the small size of the figures. The artist employed gold leaf not just for the background in many scenes contained in the initials; many folios in the manuscript have gold in multiple places on the page, including in the ascenders and descenders, as well as gold script in place of rubrication in some chapters. The book literally sparkles as one turns the pages, creating a dazzling effect. Such characteristics suggest a very elite patron with abundant resources to produce a manuscript of somewhat unusual content.

The only textual indication of a possible patron, however, is in this manuscript's prologue, which is written in gold and states that the text was "made for" (*fist por*) a mysterious "Benoit de Florenche." Scholars have not been able to identify this individual, nor is he found elsewhere in the historical record. Stones hypothesizes that, if this manuscript were made for a Florentine living in northern France in this period, he might have been part of the ecclesiastical community or a wealthy merchant.[28] Because we cannot identify Benoit, the name prevents a more specific argument for the manuscript's connection to French or English royalty, although the richness of this book suggests that Benoit would have had to have been extremely wealthy indeed. One possible scenario could be that the book was commissioned by a royal or noble individual as a gift to Benoit. There also remains the question of how the manuscript eventually came to England. It is tempting to link this early copy to the Savoy sisters, especially

complexion. Car cil ki est
caus ⁊ se des nature ⁊ sue vo
lentiers nest mie si bons li
travaus come a celui ki a
nature contraire a cestuy. a
cels ki sunt foible ⁊ relie
vent de maladies doit estre
plus tempres li travaus que
a ceus ki sunt fort ⁊ viste
⁊ por che est bone cose a gar
der que lom face toutes coses
selonc che ke se nature pu
et porter. Car selonc che ke
li philosophes dist toutes
les oeuvres confait outre ce
ke li nature ne puet compor
ter covient que les metent le
cors anient. Dou travillier
ne vous dirons or plus fors
ke ki se sent pesant par tra
vail quil ait fait li repos si
est se medichine si con dist
ypocras. ⁊ ki set le maniere
dou travillier. doit savoir
le maniere dou reposer.

Li .vi. capitres dou bagnier.

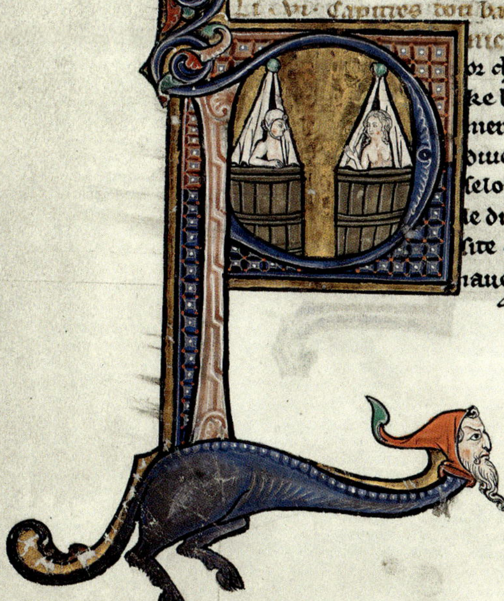

Por che ke bagniers est divers selonc le diversite des iaues.

Si vos dirons premierement le
diversite des iaues. ki sont bones
por baignier ⁊ a coi eles font
bien ⁊ mal. Apres vos dirai co
ment on doit user le baignier.
Toutes les iaues en
coi on se baigne ou
eles sunt douces ou
eles sunt dautre maniere. Ce
les ki ne sunt douces sunt de
maintes manieres si con sunt
iaues ki ont nature de souffre.
autres ki ont nature dalum.
autres ki sont salees. autres
ki sunt ameres autres ki ont
nature de salnitre. autres ki sunt
gissees autres ki ont nature
de fier. autres ki ont nature da
rain. autres iaues sunt de mer
⁊ toutes ces iaues ki par lor
nature sunt douces premierement
prendent autre nature par les
conduis u elles passent. si com
celes ki ont nature de souffre.
⁊ por le passer kele fait illuec
si cange se nature. ⁊ escauffe. ⁊
ensi poes entendre des autres ⁊
toutes ces iaues ki sunt teles.
naturelment si les puet on fai
re par artifice. Si con de faire bol
lir soffre en iaue douce. ⁊ ensi
des autres. Mais por che que li bag
niers en ces iaues nest mie co
vegnables a celui ki molt se
sante garder. ⁊ ki a le cors sain

Fig. 45
Grain. The Bute Painter, *Le Régime du corps*, ca. 1285. Bibliothèque nationale de France, Arsenal MS 2510, fol. 39v. © Bibliothèque nationale de France.

because Sloane 2435 was likely made only about a decade after the text was supposedly composed at Beatrice's request, and a parallel scenario exists in the *Bible moralisée* given to Eleanor by Margaret.[29] Lowden has proposed that British Library Add. MS 18719, the London-made (and final) copy of the *Bible moralisée*, was created in the 1280s or early 1290s on behalf of a French royal—likely Margaret of Provence herself—thus creating another path of exchange from England to France in the later thirteenth century. He also persuasively argues that Margaret and Louis IX were the intended recipients of what is now known as the Toledo *Bible moralisée*, an earlier copy completed in 1234 or 1235 in connection with their marriage; this manuscript was eventually given by Louis IX to Alfonso X of Castile in the 1250s or 1260s, to recognize the union created by the marriage of their children Blanche of France and Ferdinand de la Cerda (Cathedral of Toledo, *Bible of St. Louis*, vols. 1–3, and Morgan Library MS M.240).[30] Unfortunately, there is no concrete evidence for such a link in the case of Sloane 2435.

Arsenal 2510 (housed at the Arsenal branch of the BnF) is dated a decade or two later, around 1285.[31] The manuscript includes the abridged Redaction B of the *Régime* and is accompanied by a few folios of recipes (*Régime*, fols. 1r–57r; other medical texts on the last few folios, 57v–59r). The manuscript includes an explicit that names Aldobrandino, Beatrice, and her daughters, as some copies do with a prologue, and calls the text "the flower of the rose of all books of medicine," suggesting it was understood as an essential tool for maintaining good health.[32] The explicit also refers to Beatrice of Provence, the daughter of Beatrice of Savoy, as "de roine de Sezile," implying that Beatrice was queen of Sicily at the time it was made (thus placing it after 1266).[33] There is also an inserted bifolio (fols. 33 and 34) by Jehan Neriot, who apparently had possession of the manuscript and took it to Bruges and Flanders in the sixteenth century; on an interleaf, a statement suggests he was lent the book from the House of Madame of Vendôme.[34] While no patron or original owner is tied to the manuscript, this suggests that the manuscript stayed in the northern regions of France through that period, and possibly in the hands of women from the nobility. With thirty-seven images, Arsenal 2510 has the fewest initials of any illustrated copy of the *Régime* (fig. 45). Many of the scenes themselves diverge from the norm, depicting an unusual perspective, spatial organization, or grouping of figures. The style of the illustrations is unusual, too, with a pronounced linearity to the drawing of the figures, as well as a prominent "sense of dramatic expression, movement, and gesture."[35] Stones describes this artist's style further as "aimed at commanding and directing the attention of the viewer to the activities of the figures represented," expressed through the use of "frontal faces with flattened-out ears, profiles surrounded with curling locks, and dramatic backturned poses."[36] The recognizable style seen in Arsenal 2510 has been convincingly ascribed to an artist known as the Bute Painter, who is tied to at least sixty extant manuscripts.

The attribution of this book's illustration to the Bute Painter comes out of Stones's work on the artist of the Bute Psalter, Getty Museum MS 46 (fig. 46).[37] The various projects associated with the Bute Painter link the artist to production in several northern, French-speaking provinces—such as Artois, Flanders, and Hainaut—in the 1260s,

se. basilicō. Choses
au chaudes au cuer
froit. si sont zidoare.
musch aumbre soie sa
frans girofes siloes
cubebes fueille ynde
enula. Choses froides
au cuer caut. sont pie
lle margerites sandles
coral blanc. Tou sont
choses pour maitenir
le cuer en sante. Et si
meterons fin a ceste p̄
tie. Ichi endroit fine
la seconde partie de la
perautique. apries por
reson de tous leuus.

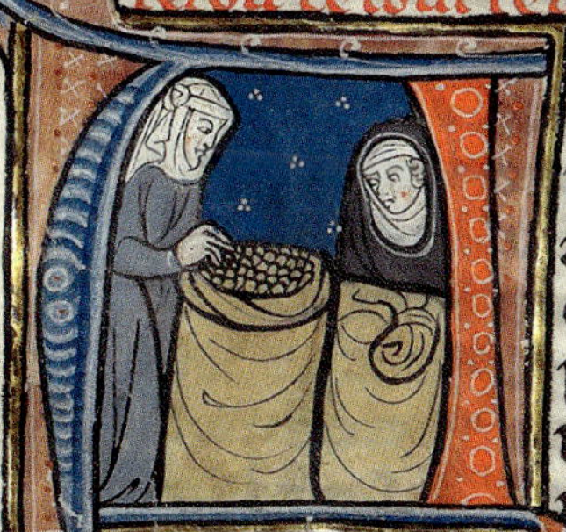

pries
cou q̄
dit v̄
avōs
en le
premi
re par
tie. ⁊
en le seconde. Si vous
aprenderons a conoi
stre en le tierche par
tie. q̄ū q̄l couenra u
ser. Et i aura diuers
chapitres. Li chapitre.
Li p̄miers chapit̄s
sera de toutes ma
nieres de bles.
Li secons de tous be
urages.
Li tiers de toutes char̄.
Li quars de tous trem
ois.
Li cuins de tos fruis.
Li .vi. de tous poisson.
Li sietismes de toute
manieres dierbes.
Li witismes de toute
manieres dues. ⁊ de
froumages ⁊ de lais.
Li nueuismes chapi
tres si parole de tou
tes espisses. Et est li
daerains chapitres
de ceste tierche par
tie. Ichi endroit po

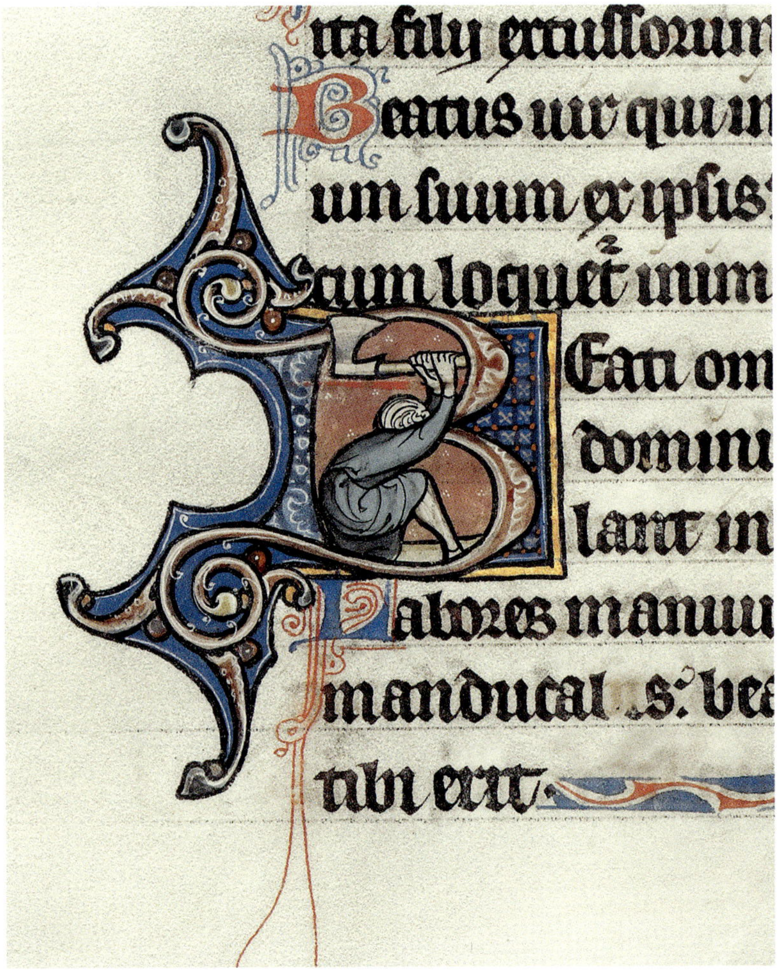

Fig. 46
A man holding an axe above his head. The Bute Painter, The Bute Psalter, ca. 1285. The J. Paul Getty Museum, MS 46 (92.MK.92), fol. 188v, detail. Digital image courtesy of the Getty's Open Content Program.

1270s, and 1280s. The area in which the Bute Painter worked included the cities of Cambrai (Hainaut), Tournai and Lille (Flanders), and Saint-Omer (Artois), all significant centers of civic and ecclesiastical activity and well known for book-making and manuscript illumination.[38] Several illustrated copies of the *Régime* have been tied to prominent production centers in precisely this region of northern France (Sloane 2435, Morgan MS M.165, and Cambridge Ii.V.11). The manuscripts that display the Bute Painter's work are tied to wealthy, primarily clerical patrons; particularly sophisticated manuscripts have been linked to the patronage of an important ecclesiastical figure, a prelate in the diocese of Cambrai and county of Hainaut, and another to the Dominicans of Lille. Simpler secular texts produced later in his career are linked more frequently to lay audiences.[39] While Arsenal 2510 is among the simpler and more cheaply made manuscripts worked on by the Bute Painter, displaying a relatively limited palette of pinks and blues, gold leaf is not completely absent, if somewhat minimally used. The strong visual affinities between Arsenal 2510 and other work by the artist support this attribution.

Stones argues that a woman was likely the patron or recipient of the Bute Psalter, probably one within the larger social circle of Sanchia's husband Richard of Cornwall or the Hainaut court. Richard of Cornwall was also the brother of Henry III (husband of Eleanor). Alternatively, if the book came to the Hainaut court through Jeanne of Hainaut, daughter of the count of Hainaut and sister of Philippa, wife of Edward III of England, it also links the production of the Bute Painter to the Savoy circle: Edward III (1312–1377) was the great-grandson of Henry III and Eleanor of Provence.[40] In either scenario, the Bute Psalter would be circulating in a royal context. The Bute Painter is also associated with at least two copies of the *Image du monde*, although Arsenal 2510 does not include that text.[41] Arsenal 2510 has not been tied to a specific patron or owner, but the identification of the manuscript's artist as the Bute Painter helps pinpoint a date in the 1280s and Cambrai as a location for its creation. Moreover, the broader network of both book producers and commissioners reflected in the Bute Painter's body of work supports the idea that the illustrated *Régime* manuscripts come out of an elite, royal context, one clearly tied to Beatrice's daughters and their families or descendants.

The final manuscript of this early set, BnF Fr. 12323 (fig. 47), appears to have been made several decades after the other two but retains much in common with the earlier Sloane 2435. Fifty-two historiated initials accompany the *Régime* text in this manuscript, several of which display damage or possibly intentional defacement. Nineteen total images accompany the *Image du monde:* twelve historiated initials (primarily depicting natural materials and phenomena), as well as seven rectangular-framed images of diagrams. BnF Fr. 12323 begins with several medical recipes (by Jean Pitart, Jean de Chalon, Jean d'Aunoy, and others), then a version of the *Image du monde*, followed by the *Régime du corps*, and concludes with a tract by Paris medical faculty on the plague of 1348, commissioned by King Philip VI (medical notes, fols. 1r–27r; *Image du monde*, fols. 28r–70v; *Régime du corps*, fols. 71r–135r; treatise on the plague, fols. 135v–144r).[42] The manuscript contains the mixed redaction of the *Régime* text.

The first folio of the manuscript contains a prologue that states: "Very noble and powerful Monseigneur Charles, Count of Valois, Chartres, of Alençon and Anjou, ordered this book be made, which is good and profitable for healing all manner of old and new wounds, and for countless other diseases as well."[43] This statement references Charles of Valois (1270–1325), who was Margaret of Provence's grandson, but it is unlikely that this manuscript was actually made for him. To have been made on Charles's behalf, the manuscript would need to have been at least begun before 1325; however, the final text included in the manuscript is the 1348 report on the plague by the Paris medical faculty to the king of France, Philip VI (Charles's son).[44] The reference to Charles of Valois is more likely related to the particular texts included in the manuscript, specifically to legitimize the section of the text that has been attributed to Jean Pitart (or Pitard, or Picart). Charles was a patron and supporter of Pitart, a surgeon working in France during the late thirteenth and early fourteenth centuries.[45] It is now thought that the medical text associated with Pitart (and found in BnF Fr. 12323) was actually a later compilation by another author, perhaps one of Pitart's students, who knew of the connection to Charles and used that reference to legitimize the text.[46] Thus the references to Charles of Valois, the royal surgeon Jean Pitart, and Philip VI have to do with the original patronage of the texts included here, rather than the patronage of this specific manuscript. Although the reference to Charles de Valois in the text does not speak directly to the commissioning of this specific manuscript, the reference, along with the inclusion of the 1348 plague text commissioned by Charles's son Philip VI (1293–1350), supports a royal context for the book's creation. The courtly and Parisian connections are indicated in the manuscript's inclusion of texts by Pitart, who spent part of his career in Paris, as well as in the reference to his royal patron. It thus seems likely that it was made in Paris, rather than a northern French city, around the mid-fourteenth century.

These details of BnF Fr. 12323 do not fully explain its similarities to Sloane 2435; Sloane 2435 could have been in Paris in the decades following its creation. The strong

courrant & ou vaines sunt. & qui
ont couleur rouge obscure & sa-
mees de coleur rouge. & ont la
teste petite & sunt semblans a
coues de sons. Mais qui mielx va-
lent sunt celes qui ont le ventre
rouge & sunt verdes dessus le dos
mais q̃ elles soient en yaue cou-
rant ce sunt les meilleurs. Et
puis que vous saues le queles sont
bonnes. or vous dirons nous a
quoi elles valent.

Elles valent a ceuls q̃
sunt lentilleus & qui
ont goute rose. et a
maniaule couleur rouge & boutõ-
nee. & a plaies de lonc temps fai-
tes qui ne se pueent souder. Mais
que on se doit auant saignier de
vaine. car si cõme dit auicenes le
sanc que elles espurgent vient
plus de parfont que ne fait celui
des ventouses. Encor couuient q̃
nous vous apreignons que deuãt
ce que vous mettes les sansues
que vous les gardes .i. iour puis
que elles seront prises & les me-
tes en yaue clere froide pour es-
purgier ce que elles ont u ventre.
& seroit bon de les nourrir de sanc
daignel ou dautre chose deuant
ce q̃ on les meist. & apres estuet
que la ou on les doit mettre con
i soit bien frote & con i mette .i. pou
de sanc de buc por plus tost prēdre.

Et quant eles seront plai-
nes & vous les voudres
oster. prenes .i. pou de cen-
dre ou .i. pou de sel ou verlaurac
ou verde soie arse ou lin ars ou
esponge arse ou laine arse & le
getes sus si cherra maintenant.
& puis que elle sera cheue si couuient
con leue le liu de bonne yaue chau-
de & que li remanans du sanc soit
espurgies par ventouse. Et se li
sans ist plus quil ne deust & vous
le voules estanchier. si mettes
par dessus .i. drapel moillie en vin
aigre. se ce vault. bon est. & se nõ
si faites ce qui plus restraint. pre-
nes une pieche de toile & la fai-
tes ardoir & en faites poure de
liee & la mettes par dessus. autãt
fait poure de galles arses & pou-
re de balaustes arses & poure
de terre rouge. & poure de cendres
bien deliee. car merueilleusemēt
toutes ces poures restraignent
le sanc. Li .xii. chap. du purgier.

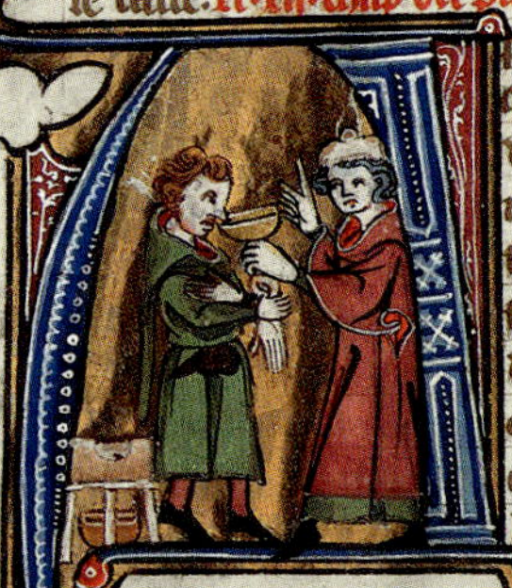

Apres ce
que dit
vous a-
uons du
saignier
si vous
dirons
cõment
on doit
le corps

similarities between the Sloane 2435 and BnF Fr. 12323 manuscripts allow for at least the possibility that Sloane 2435 (or a similar illustrated copy) was in mind when BnF Fr. 12323 was made. Both Sloane 2435 and Arsenal 2510 have been tied to production around the northern city of Cambrai and were probably made within twenty years of each other. Despite this, their images differ considerably in terms of both style and content. In contrast, the content and number of images in Sloane 2435 are much closer to BnF Fr. 12323 than the Arsenal manuscript, and Sloane 2435 and BnF Fr. 12323 both include the *Image du monde* alongside the *Régime*. While specific commissioners or first owners have not been identified for the manuscripts, all three—Sloane 2435, Arsenal 2510, and BnF Fr. 12323—can be tied to the temporal and regional trends of secular and vernacular book production aimed at wealthy elite audiences, even the nobility.[47] It is clear that the *Régime du corps* became a popular text among royal families (especially France and England), and the argument that the *Régime* was handed down and copied within the spheres of Beatrice's royal daughters and their immediate descendants can be supported.

Fig. 47
Purging. *Le Régime du corps*, fourteenth century. Bibliothèque nationale de France, Fr. 12323, fol. 84v. © Bibliothèque nationale de France.

The Companion Text of *L'image du monde*

Several manuscripts that include the *Régime du corps* also contain the *Image du monde*, an encyclopedic poem containing significant astronomical as well as theological and geographic content. Copies with these two texts include the earliest *Régime* manuscript, the unillustrated BnF Fr. 2021, as well as the illustrated copies Sloane 2435 and BnF Fr. 12323, and continue to appear in some copies well into the fifteenth century.[48] The pairing suggests that medicine itself was quite broadly defined, associated not just with health care but with other practices, including astrological learning, that facilitated well-being through encyclopedic knowledge. Another copy, the unillustrated University of Pennsylvania LJS 55, includes the *Image du monde* and a *Régime* fragment alongside other encyclopedic works, supporting this characterization as well.[49] In the illustrated copies, the juxtaposition of the *Régime* images with the celestial diagrams of the *Image du monde* puts the *Régime* in dialogue with the broader visual language of scientific diagrams and encyclopedic knowledge. The *Image du monde* is often illustrated, and, as such, the pairing of these two texts in the deluxe copies seems rooted in the types of audiences for whom these copies were likely made.

Written by Gossuin (or Gossouin, or Gautier) de Metz around 1245, the *Image du monde* is not exactly medical and it does not provide astrological tables for the reader to navigate, but it does contain discussions of eclipses and other astronomical phenomena.[50] The *Image du monde* covered theological, geographical, and astronomical topics and is illustrated with planetary diagrams, lunar and solar eclipses, and depictions of the elements. These might include a diagram of the planets, with Earth at the center and seven concentric rings labeled with the planet's names, or illustrations of solar and lunar eclipses in which a large triangle is used to represent the affected zone between

la plus hautaine
Est li cieus que len voit si plains
Des estoiles com fait serains
Com cil qui tous en est veles
Cil cieus qui est si esteles
Est li firmamens qui tornoie
Deau tour il est si grant ioie
Et si tresdouce melodie
Qu'il nest nus sil lavoit oie
Qui iamais voulsist chose faire
Qu'a dieu venist a contraire
Tant lavroit a parfair
La ou il repeust oir
Tousiours & avoir lonc sore
Si tres ioieuse melodie
Sont aucun furent q̃ disoient
Que li petit enfant looient
Com il tient en lor dormant
Qu'il disoient quil oient chantant
Les angles dieu en paradis
Qu'il les ont en tel ioie mis
Mais de ce ne scet nus le voir
Fors dieu qui tout a savoir
Que les estoiles ou ciel mist
Tel pooir avoir lor emprist
Qu'en terre na chose diverse
Ne dedens mer tant soit perilse
Qu'ou ciel ne soit figuree
Par estoiles & compassee
Sont nus ne puet savoir le nombre
Fors dieu q̃ par lui seul les nombre
Et de chascune scet le non
Com cil q̃ tout fist par raison
Des estoilles con puet veoir
Puet on bien le nombre savoir

Et quierre par astronomie
Mais cest une bele mestrie
Na en terre chose petite
Qu'ou ciel nait sa vertu cinte
En herbe ou en fruit ou en flour
Soit de faiture ou de coulour
Ou de q̃l chose que ce soit
Na riens en terre questre doit
Ne qui en lui prenge naissance
Qu'estoile ni ait sa puissance
Par nature soit male ou bone
Itele come dieu li donne
Pour planetes & firmament
Ceste figure vous present

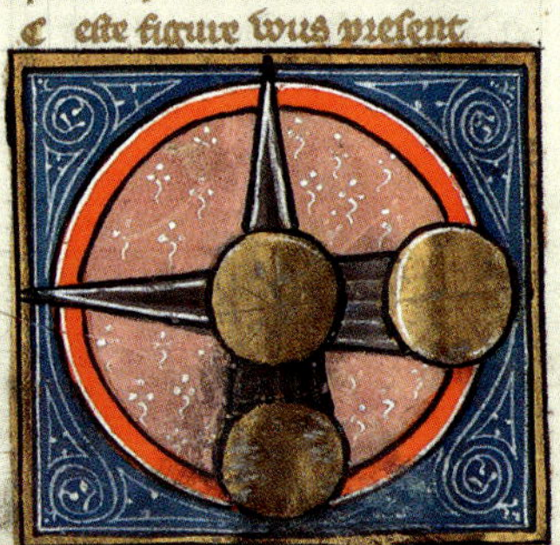

Mais plus quencores scot escrit
Avons le firmament descrit
Puis vous en dirons la mesure
Pour miex entendre la faiture
De ce quest sus le firmament
Et de paradis ensement

Ci fenist la seconde partie de cest livre. Et comence la tierce.

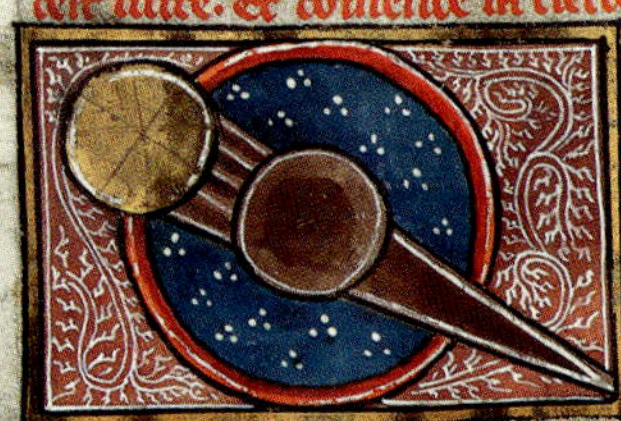

celestial bodies. Forty images are included with the *Image du monde* in Sloane 2435, and BnF Fr. 12323 contains nineteen (fig. 48). It appears that in both cases, these two texts, the *Régime* and the *Image du monde,* were conceptualized together, their illustrations likely overseen by the same designers and artists. The color palettes and general aesthetics within each manuscript support this assumption. The illustrations in the *Image du monde* are, more often than not, contained in rectangular frames instead of initials, creating a visual distinction between the two texts within the manuscript through the format of the images on the page.[51]

Numerous illustrated copies of the *Image du monde* exist without the *Régime.* In addition to BnF Fr. 14964 and BnF Fr. 14970, Rennes 593, a particularly deluxe manuscript of the *Image,* was made around 1300 in Paris (fig. 49). This particular manuscript was illustrated by the Master of Thomas de Maubeuge, an artist tied to around twenty-nine manuscripts made in Paris in the first half of the fourteenth century, and was partially written by the scribe named Robin Boutemont; this information helps date the manuscript to 1303. Sophie Cassagnes-Brouquet has proposed that an aristocratic audience was intended for this rich manuscript, as were many of this artist's works.[52]

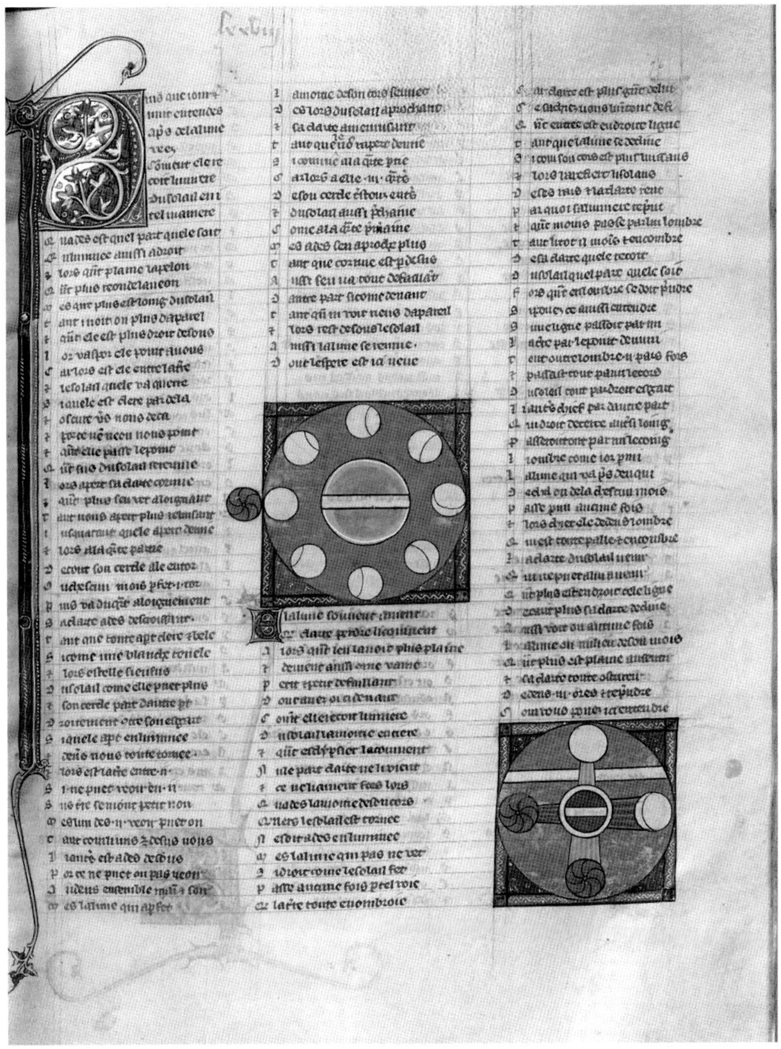

Fig. 48
Diagrams of the influence of the moon on the Earth. *L'image du monde*, fourteenth century. Bibliothèque nationale de France, Fr. 12323, fol. 55v. © Bibliothèque nationale de France.

Fig. 49
Phases of the moon and the influence of the sun and moon on the Earth. Master of Thomas de Maubeuge, *L'image du monde*, 1303–4. Bibliothèque municipale de Rennes, MS 593, fol. 76r. Bibliothèque des Champs Libres, Rennes, France, Les Tablettes rennaises.

There are strong suggestions that, in the case of Rennes 593, the aristocratic audience was also female. In her book exploring the inventory of French Queen Clémence of Hungary (1293–1328), Mariah Proctor-Tiffany explores the likelihood that a certain manuscript listed in the inventory is Rennes 593.[53] Clémence was a later owner of this manuscript rather than the original patron, but she probably inherited it from another female member of her family. According to Tracy Chapman Hamilton, the original patron was likely Marie de Brabant (1255/1260–1321), Clémence's mother, or Jeanne of Navarre and Champagne (1273–1305).[54] That Marie de Brabant's mother-in-law was none other than Margaret de Provence, one of the four queenly sisters, suggests that, indeed, the *Régime du corps* and the *Image du monde* were circulating among very similar audiences in the thirteenth and fourteenth centuries. The female ownership and readership for Rennes 593, a lavishly illustrated copy of the *Image du monde*, supports the possibilities of female audiences for the illustrative tradition of the *Image* more broadly, and thus for other manuscripts that also include the *Image*.

The Rennes manuscript also includes Brunetto Latini's *Livres dou Trésor*. The *Image du monde* and Brunetto's *Trésor* are often discussed alongside the *Régime* as evidence of the popularization of encyclopedic and scientific information in the thirteenth century.[55] Although none of the illustrated manuscripts of the *Régime* includes the *Livres dou Trésor*, the *Trésor* does accompany an unillustrated copy of the *Régime*, Bibliothèque nationale de France Fr. 1109, which includes a wide range of encyclopedic and moralizing texts.[56] Although analyses of all such comparative manuscripts are beyond the scope of my study, examples like these provide useful documented parallel scenarios for the creation of similar manuscripts. Texts often associated with the *Régime*, including the *Image du monde* and *Livres dou Trésor*, were copied and lavishly illustrated at the same time as several of the illustrated *Régime du corps*; it is reasonable to presume that these comparable productions were intended for similar audiences.

Further Expansion: The Later Group

The political and commercial connections between France and England in the thirteenth and early fourteenth centuries persisted into the later fourteenth and fifteenth centuries, though admittedly in a different form as a result of the Hundred Years War (1337–1453), the context out of which several of the later manuscripts came: Cambridge Ii.V.11, Morgan MS M.165, Sloane 2401, and eventually Ajuda 52-XIII-26. The Hundred Years War was an extended series of conflicts that involved periodic English occupation of parts of France.[57] The city of Rouen, for example, where the Morgan and Cambridge manuscripts were likely made, was in English hands from 1419 to 1449. Several key English magnates were present in Normandy during this period; some have connections to manuscript production as well. John, Duke of Bedford, famous for his artistic commissions and collecting of books, was French Regent between 1422 and 1435 (after Henry V gained control of Normandy in 1420). And Richard, Duke of York, was in France between 1440 and 1445; three of his children were born in Rouen in that period. He was the father of Edward IV, king of England, and the grandfather of Elizabeth of York, queen to King Henry VII (whose arms appear in the Cambridge manuscript; see below). Earlier, French manuscript production centers like Cambrai or Paris had connections to England in part fostered by the strong ties of sororal relationships across the courts of England and France. Over the fourteenth and fifteenth centuries, the making of books, and specifically of illustrated manuscripts of the *Régime du corps*, continued despite pandemics and political conflict. The precise combination of people in cities like Rouen created the right environment for artistic entrepreneurship and cultural exchange that propelled continued dissemination of the *Régime du corps*.

Cambridge Ii.V.11 contains the *Régime du corps* as well as a short selection of French and Middle English recipes (*Régime*: 71r–85r; recipes: 85v and 86r). On the last folio after the recipes there is also a couplet and a reference to a later owner; scholarly consensus is that the manuscript was made in France in the mid-fifteenth century, likely in the Rouen region.[58] It includes 143 historiated initials, reflecting the increased illustration program of the later copies (fig. 50). The manuscript also includes likely evidence of later, royal owners. The arms of Henry VII, king of England (1457–1509) and Queen Elizabeth of York (1465–1503) are found on folio 6v. This was likely added after 1486, when the couple was married; based on this date, Henry was a later, probably second owner of the manuscript, who may have purchased it or received it as a gift.[59] The determination of royal, English ownership by the late fifteenth century raises questions about where and for whom the Cambridge manuscript was originally produced. The English presence in the area around Rouen in the mid-fifteenth century was prominent; Elizabeth of York's grandfather Richard, Duke of York (1411–60) was in residence in that area, and her father, Edward IV, was born in Rouen in 1442. Edward was a pronounced collector of Continental, specifically Burgundian, manuscripts; another, later illustrated copy of the *Régime,* Ajuda 52-XIII-26, may have been produced for him in Bruges. That the Cambridge manuscript took such a path to the collection of Henry VII seems quite plausible.

While inheritance is certainly one way manuscripts might have come into the hands of Henry VII and Elizabeth of York, Henry was also an avid book collector in his own right. Emphasizing Henry's move away from the type of books that characterized his predecessor Edward IV's patronage, Kathleen Scott considers the Cambridge *Régime* manuscript to be representative of the type of books Henry VII collected: smaller, more modest manuscripts, often secondhand and intended for personal use rather than display.[60] Indeed, the collection reflects Henry VII's interest in French manuscripts: his collection was primarily made up of French secular texts, and his library probably also led to the establishment of a Flemish school of painting at the English court. He employed a royal librarian to acquire books for him abroad, the first of whom was Quentin Poulet, a native of Lille who was well connected with French manuscript ateliers.[61] Furthermore, Henry went to the trouble of putting elaborate ownership pages into such manuscripts, including the Cambridge illustrated *Régime;* such actions by a collector suggest personal attachment or interest.[62] While we might be disinclined to consider the Cambridge *Régime* truly modest, considering its abundant illumination, the personal subject matter and the intimate scale of the images position this book as among those Henry acquired through interest rather than for display. Another health-related manuscript associated with Henry's family, Fitzwilliam Museum MS 261, contains the arms of Margaret Beaufort, Henry's mother; the book may represent their shared interest in matters of health and well-being.[63] This narrative also reminds us that, while some of the earlier *Régime* manuscripts—Sloane 2435, for instance—point to a royal pedigree through their deluxe execution, the more modest appearance of later copies does not rule out a similar audience.

garder cestadire de user le enfieures sicome faire eaue dorge et autres chos
que les auteurs de plusieurs apruuent. Et sachiez que le pain qui est fait
dorge a comparaison de cellui de fourment est plus froit et donne moins nour
rissement et fait ventositez et douleur de flans et acroist toutes
froides maladies et restraint le ventre et tient la nature de toutes
choses de lorge dont il est fait. Du milet.

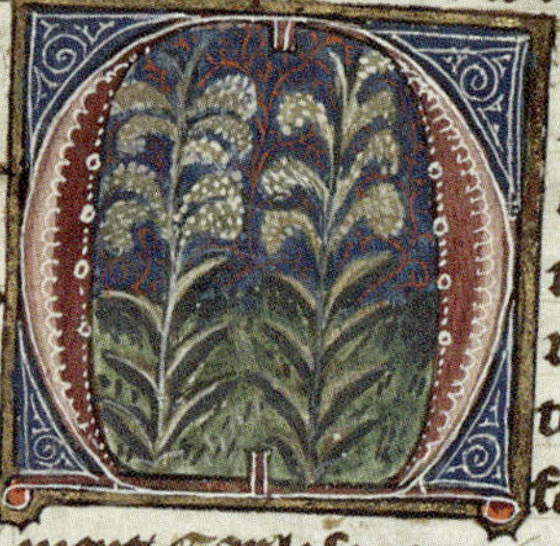

ilet et paniz sont froiz ou premier degre et
secz ou second et vous disons ensamble de
ces deux pource quilz ont une mesmes na
ture ia soit ce que le pain donne moins de nour
rissement que le ~~pain~~ milet. Sachiez que sur
toutes graines que lomme use et dont len
fait pain donnent ces .ij. moins de nourrisse
ment. Car le sang qui en est engendre est petit et mauvais. Et pource
ceulx qui en veulent engressier et avoir habondance de bon sang ne
le doivent user car ilz restraignent le ventre et font enfler la four
celle cestadire lestomac. Mais a cellui a qui il le convient user il le peut
user a lait et a huille damandes et a char grasse car char grasse luy
fait perdre sa malice. Et sachiez que milet et paniz valent plus a ma
ladies oster quelles ne font a sante garder comme len le vueille user
comme de le mettre rosti et chault aux torcions et a toutes douleurs
qui par ventositez sont engendrees et en autres pluseurs maladies.

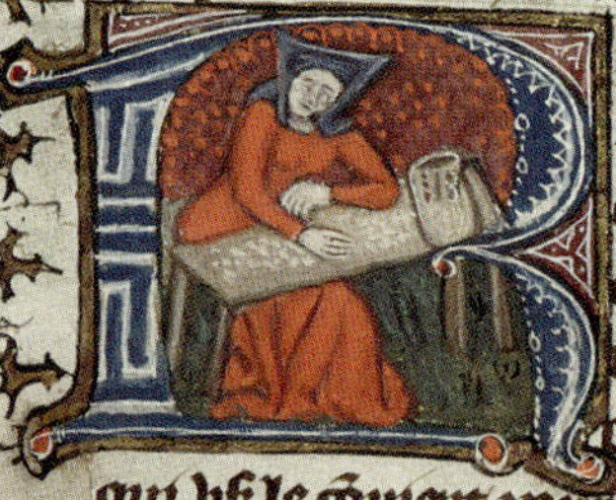

is est chault ou premier degre et sec Du ris.
ou second et sa chaleur est attrempee mais il
est de sa nature pesant et demeure moult
en lestomac et restraint le ventre et pource
ne le doivent user ceulx qui ont ventosite et qui
ont foible estomac a cuire les viandes mais
qui user le convient pour sa malice oster et pour donner assez de nourris

Fig. 50
Millet, rice. *Le Régime du corps*, ca. 1450. Cambridge University Library, MS Ii.V.11, fol. 49r. Reproduced by kind permission of the Syndics of Cambridge University Library.

The Cambridge manuscript closely resembles another copy in the late group, Morgan Library MS M.165 (fig. 51). The Morgan manuscript has been dated to between 1440 and 1450 and is also attributed to French production in Rouen.[64] It contains 149 images total; in addition to the 147 historiated initials in the *Régime*, there is a scene of creation on folio 5r and an astrological diagram on 125r. The close mirroring of these two manuscripts suggests that the Cambridge manuscript, about which less specific details on place or date have been established, may also have been created in similar circles. Morgan MS M.165 includes the *Régime du corps*, followed by the letter to Caesar by Pseudo-Hippocrates (*Lettre d'Hippocrate à César*), the book of Galen, zodiac and planetary tables, and excerpts from the *Flos medicinae Scholae Salerni* (*Regimen sanitatis*), or medical aphorisms (*Régime du corps*: fols. 5r–113r; other texts: fols. 113v–125r).[65] Several of these texts are included in both manuscripts and contain the same *Régime* redaction, known as the "roger male branche" version of Redaction B.

The Morgan manuscript in particular embodies the cross-channel market for manuscripts that existed during the Hundred Years War; Rouen's increased prominence as a book-producing center was driven in part by English patronage.[66] The artistic environment and book trade in Rouen between 1420 and the 1440s was remarkably robust, the result, at least in part, of the fall of Paris in 1420, after which some artists relocated to Normandy for its increased security and prosperity. The early sixteenth-century rebinding of the Morgan manuscript has the initials "P.P." of "a Rouen binder who worked for the English trade in 1517."[67] And later in the sixteenth century, the manuscript was owned by a Thwayte, perhaps the Englishman John Thwayte who was chaplain to the archbishop of Canterbury in the early sixteenth century. A John Thwayte was also a later owner of the section of a *Bible moralisée* now at the British Library (Harley MS 1526 and 1527); this is the copy of the *Bible moralisée* that exchanged hands between Eleanor of Provence/Henry III and Margaret of Provence/Louis IX.[68] Thus, like the Cambridge volume, the Morgan manuscript also provides evidence of a later English owner less than a century after the construction of the book. Furthermore, it appears the book was still in Rouen in the earlier sixteenth century, being prepared in such a way that would put it in the stream of books intended for England. In contrast with the Cambridge manuscript, however, the references to the binder P.P. and possible owner John Thwayte indicate this book did not end up in a royal collection. Although this book was likely produced in the context of the English royalty in France, a wide range of classes were present as part of the court entourage or with the military.

Rouen was clearly a site of important cultural and artistic exchange during the war and especially under English rule in the 1420s through the 1440s, and the manuscripts produced under these circumstances reflect that change.[69] That complicated context is well demonstrated in both the Cambridge and Morgan copies, which point to a widening group of individuals commissioning and collecting illustrated manuscripts. A number of specific English individuals have been identified as clients of the artists working in Rouen, to the point where many of the identifiable artists working in the Rouen style are named after those patrons.[70] Many of these figures were associated

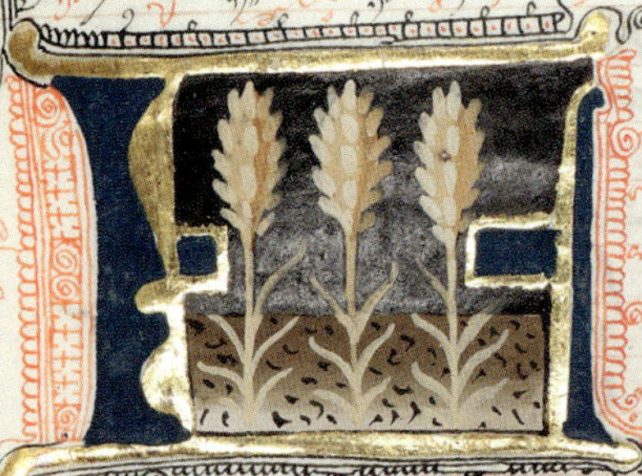

ar est une maniere de ble q
est semble a fourment mais
il est plus gros et est froit et
sec attempreement et a vertu
de donner grant nourrisse
ment au corps quant il est
bien cuit mais il enfle vent pou
le ventrail et vault plus a
maladie oster que a sante garder especiaulment aux ma
ladies chauldes. De bren de fourment.

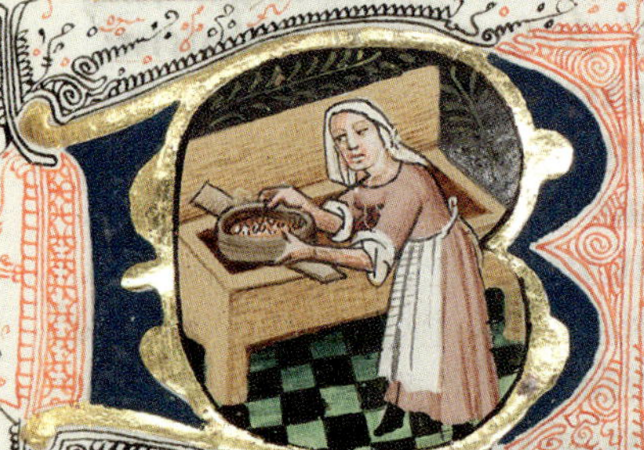

ren de fourment est chault
et sec et le nourrissement
quil donne est petit et mau
vais mais sa couleure a ver
tu de nettoyer les boyaulx
et quant il est mis en eaue
chaulde et frotez et coulez &
apres bien mariez soit cuit
a maniere de gruyau il a vertu de purifier la poittrine
de grosses et mauvaises humeurs et si ne fait point
enfler la fourcelle et y demeure pou. Et pource le
peult len donner en fievres et aultres maladies
chauldes avec le sucre attourne en tele maniere co
dit est. Mais bren dorge vault mieulx pource ql
nourrist plus que celui de fourment et refroidist
Et encore faire boullir bren de fourment en eaue
et en vin et de ce faire emplastre chault dessus
les mameles qui sont enflees et dures pour
habondance de lait. les desenfle et les met attan

with the war effort or the civil administration that followed; the commissioning of art was one way to project permanence and stability. The households of Henry VI or of his lieutenants "needed to appear plausible as the representatives of the legitimate king of France and duke of Normandy"; an illuminated manuscript also would have been a logical souvenir.[71] The fifteenth-century movement of clients, owners, artists, and books between France and England highlights the permeability of the English Channel as a border region, representing a later phase of exchange that built on and grew out of earlier interactions between the Provençal sisters. And of course, the existence of later *Régime* copies seems unlikely without the earlier circulation generated by women like Beatrice and her daughters, especially the illustrated copies.

The third in the fifteenth-century group, Sloane 2401, contains 137 historiated initials and shares much with the other two late copies, despite their different styles (fig. 52). The *Régime* is the longest text in the manuscript; in addition to the *Régime*, there are a number of other shorter texts and recipes, primarily medical in nature (*Régime du corps*: fols. 1r–88v; various medical texts: fols. 3, 88v–136r). These include several texts that have appeared with the *Régime* in other copies (including Morgan MS M.165 and Ajuda 52-XIII-26), such as the Pseudo-Hippocrates letter to Caesar and the book of Galen.[72] Sloane 2401 also contains the same redaction as the others, Redaction B "roger male branche." Additionally, Theresa Tyers argues that the specific remedies included in this compilation suggest the manuscript was aimed at a female audience responsible for health care in the home.[73] While a specific location of production has not been identified, it seems likely that it was created in a similar milieu to the other copies with which it shares so much. The similarities between Sloane 2401 and the other copies in terms of subject matter and form are pronounced.

The Cambridge and Morgan copies both appear to have made their way to England by their second or third owners, and Sloane 2401 also has a reference to a sixteenth-century owner. The manuscript includes a conjoined coat of arms, suggesting it was owned by Margaret, wife of Richard Brydges of Ley, Weobley, Herefordshire.[74] Richard seems to have been related to Rowland Brydges of Ley, Weobley (1472/73–1540), who was in the law profession, an MP during Henry VIII's reign.[75] Elizabeth Brydges (1510–1568), daughter of Rowland Brydges and Margaret Kelom, was a literary patron and translator, and may have been Richard's cousin.[76] If Richard's wife, Margaret Brydges, jointly owned Sloane 2401, she and her family represent an upper-class and elite, but not royal, audience, generally fitting in with the types of owners seen for several of the later group of illustrated *Régime* manuscripts—and in this case, a specifically female audience as well.

An additional copy with historiated initials, Ajuda 52-XIII-26, shares much with this group of later manuscripts in terms of the *Régime* chapters it illustrates yet also stands out as a manuscript attributed to two artists working in Bruges at the end of the fifteenth century (fig. 53). The manuscript, now located in the Biblioteca da Ajuda in Lisbon, Portugal, contains a frontispiece and 147 historiated initials with the *Régime* text and several additional texts. These include the letter to Caesar by Pseudo-Hippocrates

Fig. 51
Farro, bran. *Le Régime du corps*, ca. 1440–50. The Morgan Library & Museum, MS M.165, fol. 65r. The Morgan Library & Museum, New York. Purchased by J. Pierpont Morgan (1837–1913) in 1902.

chosez de bonne odour et megier fruit de bone odour q̃ cofort la fourcelle si come sont coingz pomes grenatez et aultrez pomez aigres Et ja soit ce quil le conuiengne vomir nest pas mauvaiz se nest a oultrage et le trop vomir amet grant abhominacion oster est de boire vn pou de semence dache en et en me dalicne et mengier voisine qui ne sont pas meurez et faire ce q̃ dit vous auons en chapit de vomir

Comme la feme grosse se doit garder

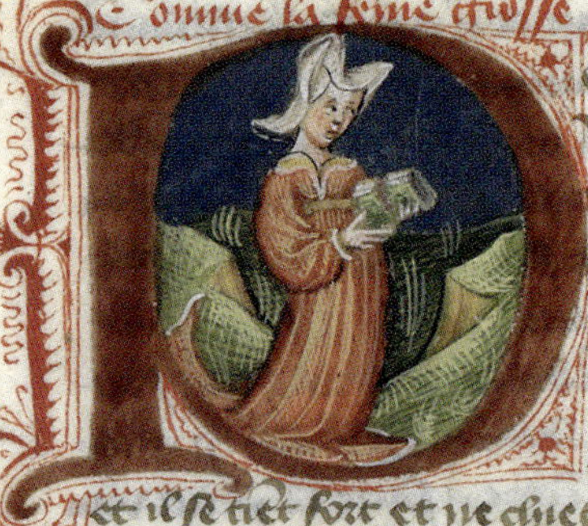

Pour bien entendre ce que no⁹ duions vous deuez savoir que lenfat en corps de la feme est ausi come le fruit des arbres q̃ vous voiez premierement q̃ la fleur ou le fruit vient qui se tient fieblemet a labre et pour pou de vent et de pluie chiet et apˀe que le fruit engroissist et il se tiet fort et ne chiet pas voulentiers Et quat il est meur il chiet come la flour ainsi legierement tout ainsi deuez entendre de la feme Car en premier moiz et en second et en tiers peult aneantir sa grossesse se elle ne se set garder en quart ne en v^e^. nest mie si grant peril et la peult len saingnier et purgier en cel teps et ouurer en lui se mestier est si come dit ypocrate pour ce q̃ lenfant se tient fort si come le fruit qui nest pas meur Mais au temps quelle est preste de deliurer il ya peril si come deuant Et pour le peril eschiuer no⁹ aprendrons come chascune feme grosse se doit garder. Premierement se doit garder de toutez chosez amerez et des chosez trop salees Car si coe dit le philosophe pour ces chosez mengier pourroit lenfat sans onglez et sans genoulx naistre. et toutes chosez qui facent bien ormer et qui leur puissent maladie puissent faire venir si come chiches fasolez vice et lupis et ne doit pas trop mengier a vne foiz ne diuses viandes (fols. 138r–52r), the Book of Galen (fols. 152v–154v), and a Latin text, *De mundo* (fols. 155r–65v).[77] The first two French texts are ones we see in other manuscripts alongside the *Régime*. *De mundo* is a short astrological text in Latin, made up of excerpts from the *Imago mundi* by the twelfth-century author Honorius Augustodunensis. Although it has a similar title, apparently this text is different from the later French work by Gossuin de Metz, *L'image du monde*, which appears in a number of other *Régime* manuscripts.[78]

The Ajuda manuscript mirrors Cambridge, Morgan, and Sloane 2401 through both images and some textual content; it also contains the same redaction, Redaction B "roger male branche."[79] Its dating by various scholars to the 1470s is based on numerous factors, including artistic attribution and style, and it may have been produced for the English king Edward IV.[80] The book includes signs of its sixteenth-century ownership, including the inscription "No. 1291," which has been identified as a number from Henry VIII's library, and a frontispiece with the arms of Thomas Boleyn KG (ca. 1477–1539), suggesting that, after its original commission, the book entered the royal library before being gifted to Boleyn, an important figure in Henry's court. At a later point in the manuscript's history, it entered the collection of Portugal, where it remains today.[81]

In the 1470s and 1480s, there was a robust production of manuscripts for Edward IV in Bruges. Edward fled to Flanders and Burgundy when he was removed from the throne in 1470, and this exile may have prompted his interest in manuscripts in the coming years. The large 1479 commission by Edward IV from Philippe de Mazerolles demonstrates the extent of his later manuscript patronage, and the Ajuda *Régime* manuscript could be part of that production.[82] It is likely that the Ajuda manuscript was among those produced in the workshop overseen by the Master of the Harley Froissart, who is thought to be the same person as the artist Philippe de Mazerolles. Scot McKendrick and Luís Campos Ribeiro both attribute the bulk of the manuscript's images to this artist, whose work is relatively well documented through a variety of other extant works; the manuscript also displays the work of a second artist whose identity is less assured but could be the Master of the London Wavrin.[83] Campos Ribeiro describes the book as a combination of styles that bring together an "older French style" (Mazerolles) and a more "innovative Flemish approach" offered by the second artist, indicating the results of the rich artistic environment created in Bruges in the last quarter of the fifteenth century.[84] The Ajuda manuscript is therefore the latest known copy to include an extensive program of historiated initials. Moreover, the Ajuda manuscript is a reminder that extravagant illustrated copies of the *Régime* remained of interest to the most elite of patrons, including royalty, even as the group of fifteenth-century copies generally reflects a widening audience.

The similarities among these later copies indicate close relationships; these relationships could mean that one of these manuscripts served as a model for the others, or that there were other copies influencing the group that do not survive. The similarities are not only formal and artistic but also textual: the manuscripts contain the same redaction of the *Régime* and often similar accompanying texts. Although both

Fig. 52
Pregnancy. *Le Régime du corps*, fifteenth century. British Library, Sloane MS 2401, fol. 36v. © The British Library Board.

iii. iours ou .iiii. si mengusse moins quil ne
souloit Et le premier iour quil y entrera ne
doit pas seaux regarder ancois lui convient
flairer choses de bonne odeur et mengier fruis
de bonne odeur qui confortent la fourcelle. si
comme sont coins pommes grenates et autres
choses aigres. Et ia soit ce quil le conviengne
dormir. Il nest pas mauvais se ce nest a oul
traige. Et le trop dormir avec grant abhomi
nacion oster est de bonne vigne pou de semence
seiche en vin ou en ius dalume et mengier rai
sins qui ne sont pas meurs. Et faire ce que dit
vous avons ou chapitre de dormir. Comment
la femme grosse se
doit garder.

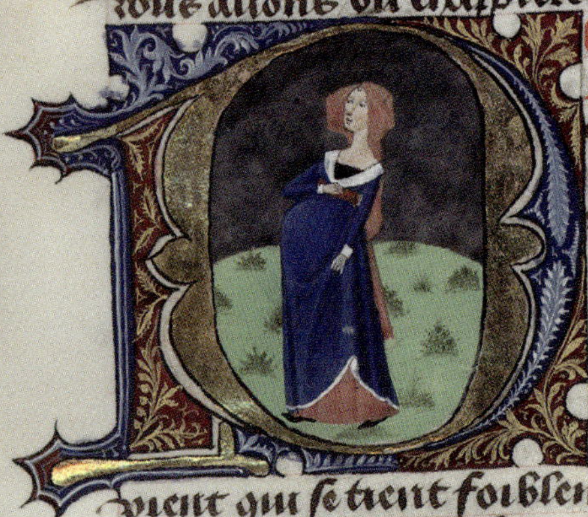

Pour bien entendre ce
que nous dirons vous
devez savoir que lenfant
ou corps de la femme
est ainsi comme le fruit
des arbres que vous
veez premierement
que la fleur ou le fruit
vient qui se tient foiblement a larbre. Et pour
pou de vent ou de pluye chiet. Et apres que le
fruit engrossist il se tient fort et ne chiet pas
volentiers. Et quant il est meur il chiet ainsi

the Cambridge and Morgan manuscripts were likely made in France, both eventually wound up in English collections. While a definitive place of creation for Sloane 2401 remains out of reach, it seems likely that it is difficult to place precisely because of the inherently complicated nature of cross-channel manuscript production in northern France and England in the fifteenth century. The Ajuda manuscript also represents Continental production for an English patron several decades later, suggesting the lasting interest in the *Régime du corps* in this iteration with extensive historiated initials.

Fig. 53
Pregnancy. *Le Régime du corps*, ca. 1470s. Biblioteca da Ajuda, Lisbon, Cod. 52-XIII-26, fol. 47r. Biblioteca da Ajuda.

Regional Manuscript Production

The three earlier copies appear to have all been made in France, at least two of them in northern French cities such as Cambrai; the four later copies, while still written in French, seem to be primarily products of Continental production for English patrons, some in English-dominated northern French cities such as Rouen. Before the Hundred Years War began, French manuscript production centers like Cambrai or Paris had important connections to England, fostered in part by the strong ties of familial relationships across the courts of England and France. Moving into the fourteenth century, the northern counties of Hainaut and Flanders developed strong ties with England and the English court. Lucy Freeman Sandler points out that the continued use of French in English-made books throughout the fourteenth century demonstrates how closely tied to each other these nations were.[85]

Although the temporal gap between the latest copy in the early group of illustrated *Régime* manuscripts and the first copy in the fifteenth-century group is substantial, it is likely that widespread pandemics and political turbulence affected manuscript production.[86] Indeed, the inclusion of the 1348 plague report of the Paris medical faculty in BnF Fr. 12323 suggests the impact of the plague as well as the connection that compilers made between that text and the practices recommended in the *Régime*. Nevertheless, over the fourteenth and fifteenth centuries, the making of books, and specifically of illustrated manuscripts of the *Régime du corps*, continued, and in some contexts flourished unabated. Royal collectors were active over the course of the fourteenth century. It is perhaps initially surprising that much of that production also took place in northern France in regions like Normandy, one of the centers of the conflict between England and France during this period. But in actuality, the unique entrepreneurial circumstances in such cities fostered continued dissemination of the *Régime du corps* in manuscript form.

At the time that Aldobrandino constructed the text, and over the next century or so, Paris was a major center of manuscript production that served both royal patrons based in the city and a wide range of other types of clients. Grounding their research in a wide range of records, Richard H. Rouse and Mary A. Rouse demonstrate that hundreds if not thousands of people—including scribes, illuminators, bookbinders, parchment-sellers, and *libraires*—participated in commercial book production in Paris between 1200 and 1500 to feed the demand for manuscripts.[87] The *libraire* was a particularly important figure in the production of manuscripts in this period; this person served as book-seller and book-contractor, organizing the materials and managing the various craftspeople involved in a commission. Commercial book production in Paris was concentrated in two particular neighborhoods, along the rue Neuve Notre-Dame and in the area around the church of St. Séverin.[88] As Rouse and Rouse point out in their extensive study, it was not simply the presence of the University of Paris that drove the city's book trade; Paris's role as royal capital also led to a market of wealthy clients including "crown, court, royal servants, prelates, and cathedral canons."[89] The output of this production center was varied, depending on the type of client, but included the king, queen, and their families, all the way down to university students. The same network of producers made extremely luxurious books commissioned by royalty, less ostentatious books for others, and even exemplar *pecias* (or quires) that were rented out to students and scholars to copy on their own—creating a relatively wide accessibility because of this diversity and increasing affordability.[90]

Alongside the major book-production city of Paris, centers of book production existed in a variety of smaller provincial cities, including northern cities like Cambrai, Lille, and Rouen, and indeed, cities throughout France.[91] The artists associated with two illustrated copies of the *Régime*, the Aldobrandin Master and the Bute Painter, have been tied to manuscript production in a variety of these northern French regions, including Artois, Flanders, and Hainaut. In the specific case of the Bute Painter, the artist, described by Stones as an "itinerant craftsman," has been tied to work produced in Cambrai, Tournai, Lille, and Saint-Omer.[92] The artists associated with the Ajuda manuscript, Philippe de Mazerolles and the Master of the London Wavrin, are tied to production in the Flemish city of Bruges.[93]

Manuscripts did not necessarily stay where they were produced, however; especially in cosmopolitan royal circles like that of Eleanor and Margaret, books were often used as gifts and traveled across Europe. As demonstrated by the *Bibles moralisées*, illustrated manuscripts were often copied with the intention of being used as gifts to foster diplomatic relationships or to celebrate marriages and other familial alliances. In her discussion of Clémence of Hungary's collections as evidenced by the surviving inventory of 1328, Proctor-Tiffany has demonstrated that her collections were developed through inheritance as well as through purchase. Clémence's library included numerous books inherited from her ancestors, but the inventory also reflects the fact that her collection was disseminated not only through some gift-giving and bequests but also through the sale of her books—often purchased by other individuals (some of whom were royal, but not all).[94] Indeed, manuscripts made on the Continent in cities like Paris, especially those intended for elite audiences, easily made their way to England. This is not to suggest that manuscripts were not being made in England; on the contrary, England had an equally robust tradition, and the production of illustrated books in particular was centered in London and Norwich.[95] English book production enjoyed the patronage not only of courtly clients but also of newly wealthy country families, such as the Luttrells or the St. Omers; monastic audiences continued to be patrons of illustrated manuscripts in England as well.[96]

The dominance of Paris changed as a result of the Hundred Years War and the Black Death. After the fall of the city to the English in 1420, several other cities in France filled in the gap. For example, Rouen's artistic and book-making cultures, geared toward both domestic and foreign markets, took off between the 1420s and 1440s, with artists relocating to the region of Normandy in search of job security.[97] Rouen bookmakers were producing for both the French and the English. Some artists even traveled across the Channel, setting up shop in England to better serve the patrons they had been working for in Rouen.

Rouen was clearly a site of important cultural and artistic exchange during the war, especially under English rule in the 1420s through the 1440s, and the manuscripts produced under these circumstances reflect that exchange. That complicated context is well demonstrated in both the Cambridge and Morgan copies, which point to a widening group of individuals commissioning and collecting illustrated manuscripts. This cross-cultural environment for creation and dissemination continued throughout the fifteenth century, as seen in the robust manuscript production in Bruges in the 1470s and early 1480s that is indicated by the Ajuda manuscript. Earlier, the network created by Beatrice's daughters likely contributed to the circulation of the *Régime du corps*. The fifteenth-century manuscripts represent a later iteration of that exchange, as books, clients, and even artists moved back and forth across the English Channel. These manuscripts represent the links between those five women, certainly, but their trajectories also potentially initiated connections across cultural divides for several centuries.

Artists working in cities like Rouen may have found a good number of English patrons; for some artists, the patronage of the English was pronounced enough that it was worth relocating to England at the end of the war. Numerous scholars have pointed out the diversity of patrons for such artists; as Catherine Reynolds explains, "English, English French, and French French patrons turned to the same artists and the artists accepted the available jobs."[98] The English market remained important, although after 1450 French artists had to export their work across the Channel to reach those audiences.[99] The economic products created by these artists and booksellers benefited from the conditions created by the war. The clear interconnectedness between France and England, even during conflict, is reflected in the objects themselves. Indeed, the particular circumstances of book production and consumption in northern cities like Rouen are precisely what make it difficult to parse the distinctions between English versus French or Franco-Flemish production. This robust cultural exchange contributes to the difficulties of determining whether a fifteenth-century manuscript should be considered English. According to Martha Driver, the books of this period were "quite often copied by multilingual scribes and illuminated by peripatetic artists for patrons of different nationalities . . . the question of what it might mean to say that a manuscript is 'English' or 'French' is a complicated one."[100] The challenges of distinguishing between English and French production in this period are obviously not limited to the

Régime du corps. Other illuminated medical manuscripts have also been connected to English patrons in Rouen.[101] Although the texts would not necessarily be intended for the same kind of clientele as the *Régime du corps*, they are a reminder that the market for manuscripts of this kind of didactic material, even illustrated copies, was not insignificant. These books moved across geographies and over time, introducing new ideas and fostering existing relationships, demonstrating the potential impact of objects on the complex and intertwined culture that audiences were negotiating in this period.

Conclusion: Female Networks

This group of illustrated manuscripts demonstrates a similar version of the text, associations with France or England or both, and a generally similar artistic attitude toward illumination that employs the historiated initial as a chapter marker. By considering the two groups independently, however, we see trends that change between the earlier and later periods of illustrated *Régime* production. The first group represents French production within primarily royal or noble circles and can be tied more readily to the descendants of the possibly original textual patron, Beatrice of Savoy, and her daughters. All four manuscripts of the latter group share remarkable similarities in terms of both the number of images included and the content of those images, so much so that it is hard to believe they were not created in conjunction with one another. In contrast with the earlier group, the later manuscripts reflect a shift away from France and toward England, not necessarily through exclusive English production of the manuscripts but in part through their collection and then travel from France and Flanders to England. All four were in England fairly soon after their production, and, while royal circles still played a role in their movement and collection, a different kind of audience is involved: the households, including the wives, of wealthy men who were lawyers, chaplains, and merchants. The provenances for these books are often speculative, but we can nevertheless ascertain much about class and gender in relation to their possible owners and users.

The *Régime du corps* text was a domestic health guide, one that might have been commissioned for a countess to give to her four royal daughters. As such, this text, as well as the illustrated copies of it that are the focus of my study, seem most likely to have circulated in a similar context. While we can tie these manuscripts to general groups of people, and we have some references to male and female owners, we cannot attach any of these illustrated copies directly to Beatrice's female descendants or their immediate circles. Yet both the circumstances of production and the later male owners of these manuscripts more often than not link them to the networks created through the legacies of these women. Green has suggested that a kind of "medical reading community" of aristocratic women existed in France, of which these women were likely a part.[102] At the same time, these illustrated *Régime* manuscripts were never exclusively "women's books"; they suggest instead the complex dynamics within upper-class and noble households during the thirteenth, fourteenth, and fifteenth centuries. Sloane 2401, for example, displays a joint coat of arms, speaking to the shared relevance of the *Régime*'s content for both men and women concerned with fertility and household management. A man's coat of arms or his name appearing in a manuscript does not necessarily mean that he used the book much, nor does it rule out other users in his household, including women. The immediate and extensive copying and dissemination of this text—in either illustrated or unillustrated copies—may not have happened at all without Beatrice and her daughters. Daughters, who moved widely across medieval Europe and became members of new households when they married, could potentially do this more efficiently than sons; *four* daughters, even more so. This expanding female network would have made quick work of spreading the various ideals and knowledges that were inherent in the illustrated *Régime* manuscripts. The changing circumstances for these books over time—through relocation and through the creation of new copies—led to a shifting in audiences and a greater reach for the text that will be explored further in the next chapter.

As the possible female patronage of the original text indicates, and as many of the images in these illustrated copies demonstrate, the topics covered in the *Régime* would have largely fallen under the purview of women within such households. Those households also contained tens if not hundreds of additional people who contributed to the ongoing activity of a court or household; certainly many people were more intimately involved with the activities depicted in the manuscripts than either the man or woman who was the ostensible "head" of such a family. I investigate this particularly complex context further in chapter 4, looking at the range of household members and workers who were also potential readers or users of these manuscripts.

In considering these manuscripts as two groups, we see an extension beyond royal or noble circles to those of wealthy professional elites, a shift that can be seen more broadly in book collecting and patronage in the fifteenth century. Taken alongside evidence that books were just one of the many materials used by newly moneyed groups to emulate nobility, it hardly seems surprising that these manuscripts participated in that phenomenon. With their pictorial emphasis on clothing, food, and access to physicians and other forms of health care, the illustrated *Régime* manuscripts depict much within household life that reflected status. They explicate how life was lived within such households, where the seemingly routine was always also a powerful expression of status or ambition for that status. If we recall the discussion about cheese at the beginning of this chapter, these manuscripts simultaneously encapsulate the mundane and the luxurious.

By establishing the kinds of elite households in which these manuscripts likely circulated, this chapter has built upon the conclusions of chapter 1—that is, the notion that the images of these illustrated copies provide a unique opportunity for book users to engage with the narrative ambiguity of health management that would have also been a reality in their daily lives. Such illustrations did not simply entertain but also contributed to the experience of using these books, guiding the reader's expectations and demonstrating a range of behaviors appropriate for those in such households. Those audiences may also have been empowered by the manuscripts' images, which provided a context for how to navigate different encounters and intervene on behalf of themselves and their household members.

Access to learned knowledge was another commodity that symbolized status, and interest in this commodity was hardly limited to men. As the next chapter will demonstrate, the likely audiences for the illustrated *Régime* copies parallel the types of audiences intended for a variety of medical and other scientific texts. Regimen texts, in particular, were aimed at audiences who desired access to privileged knowledge and sometimes gained it through books. Women were rarely the intended audiences for many types of medical texts, but, as the *Régime* demonstrates, exceptions exist. The *Régime du corps* was likely commissioned and then disseminated by women, and the topics it covers suggest a robust interest in the maintenance of health within the households of a wide range of audiences. With the illustrated copies in particular, the encounters depicted bring attention to the negotiation of various types of relationships, a prominent one being with the authoritative medicine of the physician.

THE MEDICAL CONTEXT FOR THE *RÉGIME DU CORPS*

3

Physicians are depicted frequently in the illustrated copies of the *Régime du corps*. In a representative consultation scene from Sloane 2435, a well-dressed woman and a physician stand facing each other (fig. 54). Dressed in a red bliaut and wearing on her head the popular fillet and barbette over hair bundled in a net, the woman tilts her head slightly downward as she makes an inquiring gesture with her hands. Her right hand seems to indicate her belly, while her left hand is held up to the doctor in acceptance. The man—wearing a bright blue robe with slit sleeves, a rounded cap, and a fashionable hairstyle—points at the woman in a gesture of advice or direction. Although the man is not shown actively treating the woman, we know he is a physician because of his clothing and gesture in relation to her. This illustration accompanies the chapter on pregnancy, and, despite the ambiguity of the woman's pregnant state, the physician's authority is still evident through the nature of their interactions.

The prevalence of physicians depicted across the illustrated copies of the *Régime* cannot be attributed to chance, but rather to the intentional inclusion of a variety of associations made with these figures. They invite further consideration of what such images would have represented for viewers, for book owners, and for those who might have been patients. Naturally, these representations of well-dressed doctors would have signaled status: the status of the physician as well as the status of his patients. And that status would have extended to these books' audiences, as individuals who would have had the resources to own books as well as the privilege to consult and retain elite doctors. The depicted physician also serves as a prompt to consider the type of medicine he represents; that is, learned medicine. Aldobrandino was himself a physician to elite patrons; moreover, the sources upon which he based his text demonstrate his access to and mastery of learned medical traditions. Indeed, the genre of regimen literature, of which the *Régime* is a prime example, ties the established medical tradition to the status of wealthy lay patrons who commissioned such works.

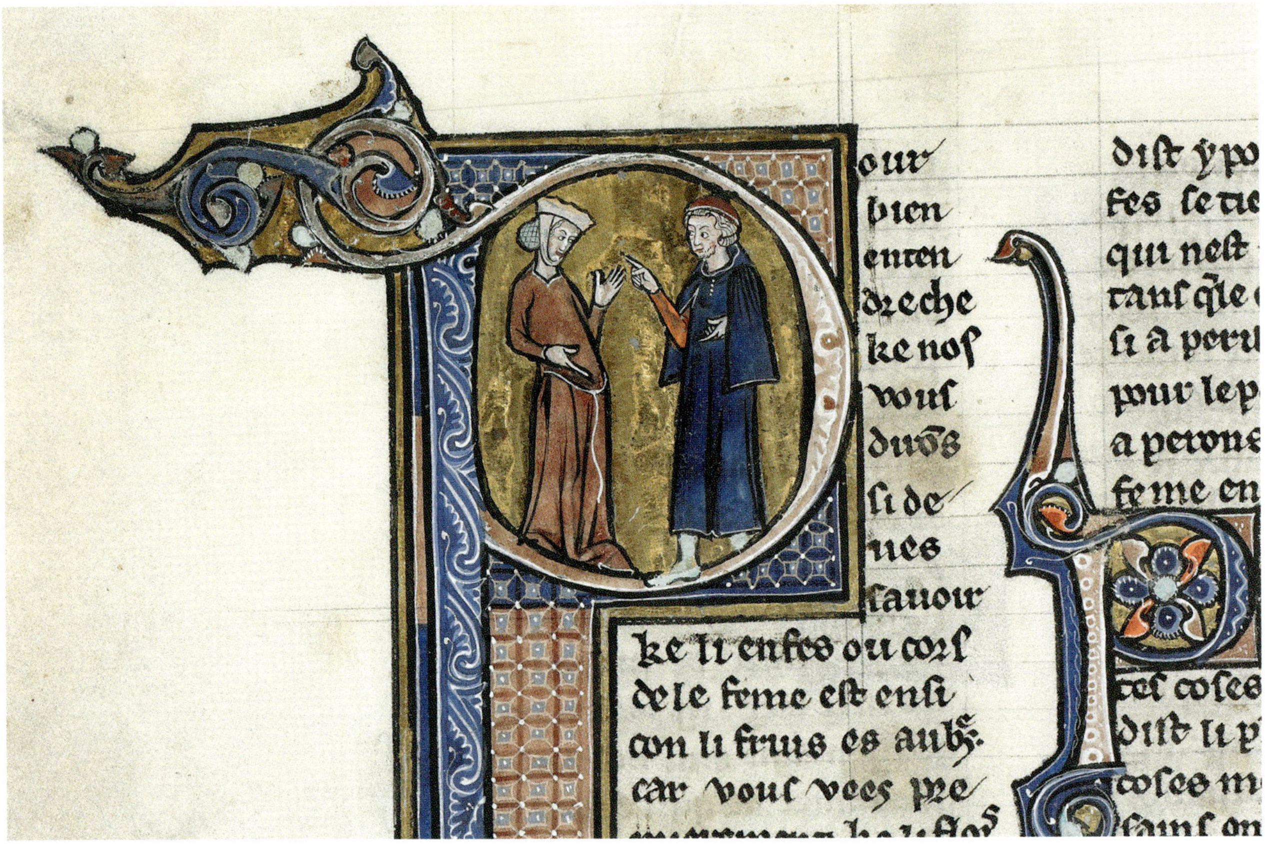

Fig. 54
Pregnancy. *Le Régime du corps*, ca. 1265–70. British Library, Sloane MS 2435, fol. 27v, detail. © The British Library Board.

The illustrated copies of the *Régime* undoubtedly reflect prominent medical traditions of the period in which they were made. This chapter offers a discussion of the role of the physician in late medieval health-care practice, prompted by the numerous depictions of physicians and other practitioners in the *Régime* illustrations. As illustrated copies of Aldobrandino's text, the manuscripts under consideration are informed by textual traditions as well as pictorial ones. Therefore, I not only place Aldobrandino's text within the broader network of late medieval medicine but also consider how the *Régime* images are in dialogue with other medical imagery circulating at this time. The contexts of these medical traditions and practices do not, however, provide a complete picture of medieval health care, nor do they fully reflect the complexities evident in the images of the illustrated *Régime* manuscripts.

Physicians may have been among the possible readers of the *Régime du corps*, but, as a closer look at the accompanying texts in various copies demonstrates, the text maintained a diverse audience that was frequently domestic lay readers, akin to the users for illustrated copies that I proposed in chapter 2. This chapter concludes that, while learned medicine was central to the development and popularity of the *Régime*, such medicine as represented by the physician's expertise was just one of many modes of health care available to the *Régime*'s audiences. The domestically oriented readership of the *Régime* then leads me back to the images of the illustrated copies; their representation of the household becomes the focus of extensive consideration in chapter 4.

The professional physician described above is but one of a wide range of practitioner types that appear throughout the illustrated copies of the *Régime*. Barbers or surgeons, physician's assistants, and women are also seen administering medical treatments. And we might recall the wet nurse and childbirth depictions discussed in chapter 1, health-care scenes dominated by female caregiving communities. Such images remind us of the diversity of late medieval health care and suggest that even as university-trained physicians were gaining prominence and power, more humble methods of treatment, often inside the home and under the supervision of household members, remained significant. The illustrated *Régime du corps* manuscripts make evident the dialogue between these different modes of health care through their various paths of dissemination.

Physicians and Perceptions of Expertise

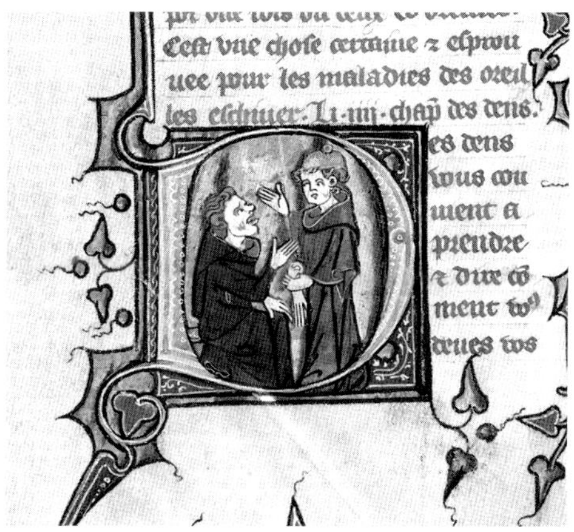

Fig. 55
Teeth. *Le Régime du corps*, fourteenth century. Bibliothèque nationale de France, Fr. 12323, fol. 104v, detail. © Bibliothèque nationale de France.

The scenes depicting practitioners distinguish the *Régime* manuscripts as a tradition preoccupied not just with asserting the presumed authority in the actions of these figures but also, and more importantly, with the interactions those individuals have with their patients. Such treatment scenes, in addition to highlighting the role of physicians in late medieval society, also illuminate the encounters such providers had with those who took advantage of their expertise. While physicians are relatively prevalent in the *Régime* images, reflecting their primary engagement with elite patients like Beatrice and her family, the profession itself was in a continuous state of flux and negotiation throughout the later Middle Ages. As doctors became a more defined group, they had to navigate changing demands for their skills and competition from other types of caregivers. The diversity of health-care methods meant that neither physicians nor their patients relied exclusively on learned medicine. Elite patients and established physicians existed within a health-care landscape that consisted of a wide range of practices across social classes. Rather than signifying an academic readership, images of physicians reinforce the status of manuscript owners and users. Furthermore, the illustrations include a wider range of practitioners of different classes and genders, highlighting the diversity of choices available for those managing household health.

Fig. 56
Frontispiece of master with students. *Le Régime du corps*, ca. 1270–1300. Universitätsbibliothek Leipzig, Cod. Haen. 3478, fol. 2r, detail. Universitätsbibliothek Leipzig.

Fig. 57
Liver. *Le Régime du corps*, ca. 1440–50. The Morgan Library & Museum, MS M.165, fol. 59v, detail. The Morgan Library & Museum, New York. Purchased by J. Pierpont Morgan (1837–1913) in 1902.

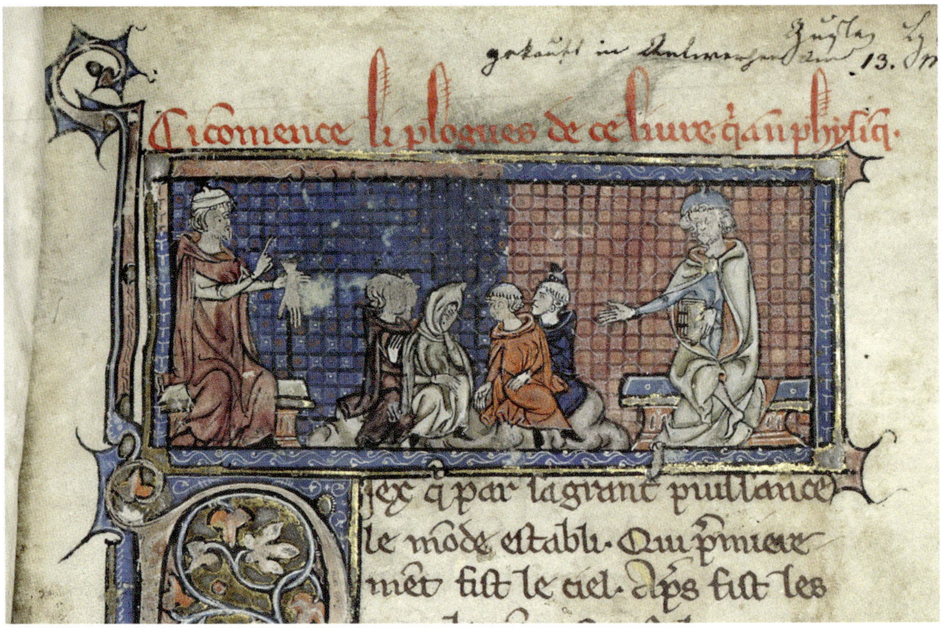

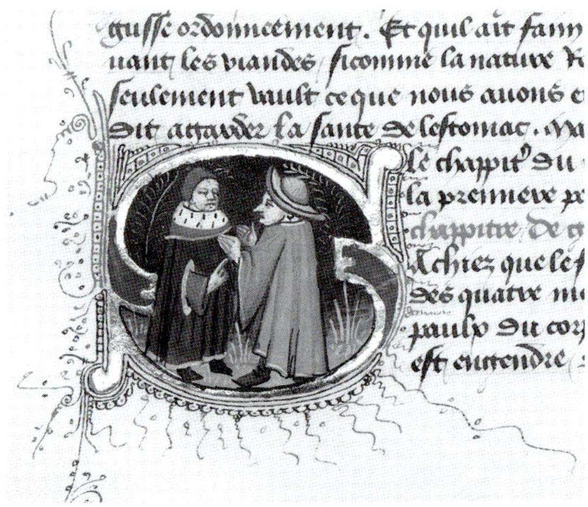

Physicians—that is, men depicted in encounters with patients who wear garments and make gestures that signal elite medical status—appear relatively frequently in the *Régime* images. For instance, in Sloane 2435 the physician wears a long robe with a hood and loose sleeves over a closer-fitting garment with sleeves, and on his head is a minimal, rounded cap (see fig. 54). Comparable distinctions are found in BnF Fr. 12323, in which the physician wears a similar robe and cap, although the "ball" on top of the cap is more pronounced; he often also holds in one of his hands the white gloves he has presumably removed (fig. 55). The physician is similarly dressed, also holding gloves, in the Leipzig manuscript (fig. 56; for other examples, see figs. 38, 47, and 76). In the different period and style of the Morgan manuscript, the physician's garment includes a large ermine collar (fig. 57). As explored more fully in my discussion about

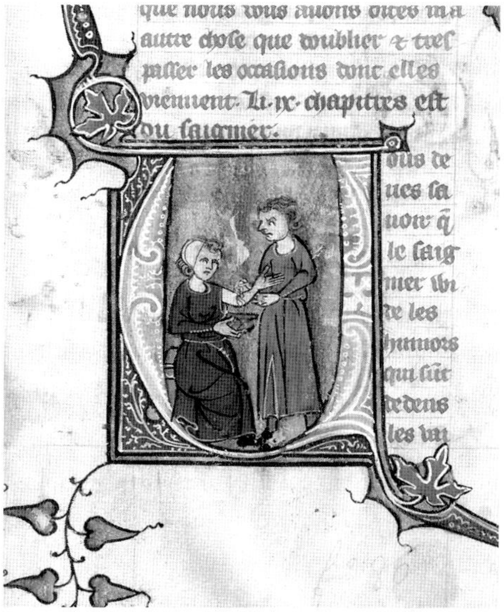

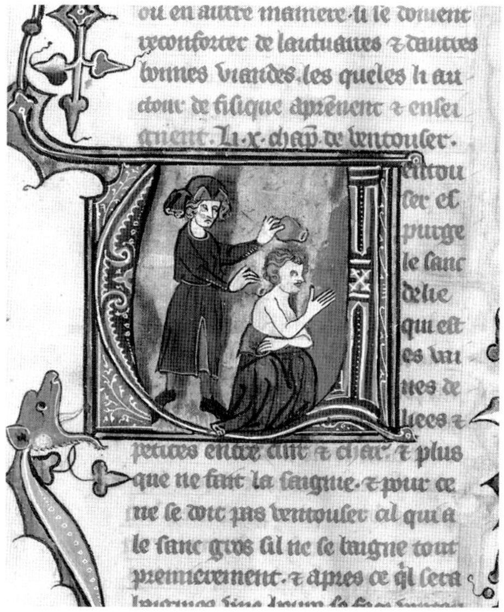

Fig. 58
Bloodletting. *Le Régime du corps*, fourteenth century. Bibliothèque nationale de France, Fr. 12323, fol. 80r, detail. © Bibliothèque nationale de France.

Fig. 59
Cupping. *Le Régime du corps*, fourteenth century. Bibliothèque nationale de France, Fr. 12323, fol. 83r, detail. © Bibliothèque nationale de France.

touch in chapter 1, these men are usually depicted in scenes of consultation, gesturing with authority and generally involved in talking rather than physical contact, although they occasionally administer treatment.

However, such medical figures are not the only caregivers depicted in these manuscripts. Those who are shown administering care such as bloodletting include men in shorter tunics and tights, who often wear coifs—close-fitting white caps that come down over the ears and tie under the chin (recall fig. 1). In BnF Fr. 12323, the practitioner in the bloodletting scene wears what appears to be only an under-robe, and his head is bare (fig. 58), while the figure overseeing this manuscript's scene of cupping wears a shorter tunic, tights, and a chaperon-type head covering (fig. 59).

In the scene that accompanies the chapter on ears from the Leipzig manuscript, several tools of the trade hang in the background, confirming this practitioner's identity as a barber-surgeon, reinforced by his shorter tunic and uncovered head (see fig. 2). In the later Morgan manuscript, the individual engaged in bleeding and cupping patients wears a short, knee-length, belted tunic with full sleeves; he also wears a chaperon, reflecting the changing styles of the fifteenth century (fig. 60). Presumably many of these figures represent barbers or assistants, their more modest clothing distinguishing them from the elite physician figure. In Sloane 2435, this humbler clothing is also identical to that worn by some laborers, such as the fellow stirring mulberries, reflecting the craftsperson or laborer status often granted to barbers and surgeons (see fig. 11).

The existence of different caregivers depicted in the *Régime* manuscripts alludes to the significant diversity within medieval health care itself and reminds us that expertise could be expressed in a variety of ways, including visual, and not exclusively textual, forms. The fancy clothing worn by the most elite practitioners in the *Régime* manuscripts signals a higher status than the other types of providers represented, but even

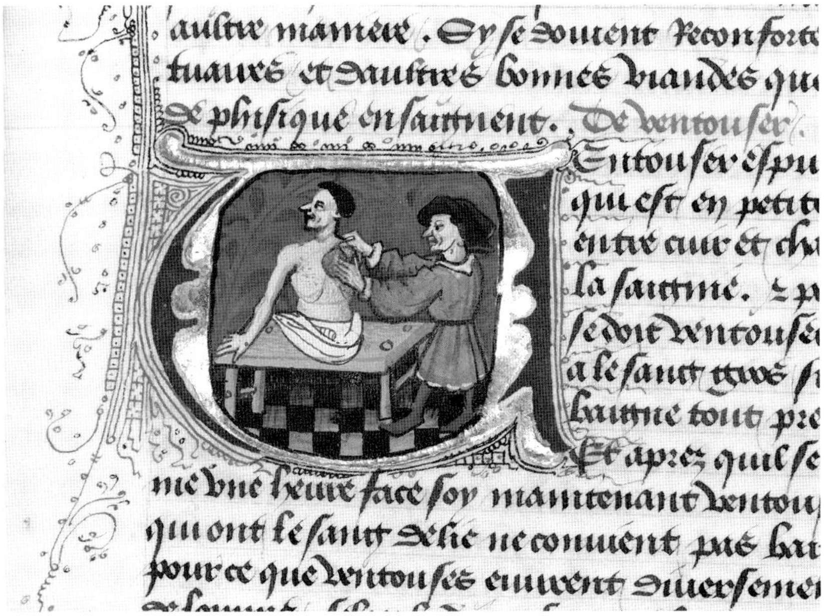

Fig. 60
Cupping. *Le Régime du corps*, ca. 1440–50. The Morgan Library & Museum, MS M.165, fol. 24r, detail. The Morgan Library & Museum, New York. Purchased by J. Pierpont Morgan (1837–1913) in 1902.

the wealthiest practitioners depicted in these manuscripts may not necessarily be officially trained doctors with university degrees. The pictorial expertise of the illustrated physicians in the *Régime* manuscripts, expressed primarily through dress and gesture, is mostly absent from the *Régime* text. Aldobrandino attributes the knowledge he conveys to the authors of the well-established sources he cites and almost never mentions contemporary doctors or physicians as likely readers of his work (a point discussed further below). As such, the *Régime* text demonstrates Aldobrandino's expertise to an elite audience such as Beatrice and her family, while also reflecting the ongoing articulations and rearticulations of medical expertise in this period.

The different types of practitioners we see in the *Régime* images correlate with understandings of professionalization in this period. Across Europe, the thirteenth and fourteenth centuries are often characterized by a noted increase in the number of practitioners as well as greater diversification among them. This shift was driven in part by an increasing demand for university-trained physicians by various communities, especially in upper-class society. Doctors remained rare before 1200, and only a few urban centers could support them; as this highest trained category became larger and more defined, a wider range of alternatives developed as well.[1] In addition to university-trained physicians and surgeons, other health-care providers practicing during this period would have included doctors with partial or no university training (who might also have been surgeons), barbers, apothecaries or pharmacists, midwives, and other types of empirically trained practitioners. Rural areas or smaller towns were less likely to have trained physicians; they would have been served instead by a wide range of practitioners who trained for their craft through apprenticeship, oral transmission, and hands-on learning.[2] While the increased urbanization of the thirteenth century, and with it more robust commercial economies and greater numbers of wealthy citizens, has been linked to the rising demand for trained practitioners, in many regions physicians remained almost completely absent.[3] Barbers' guilds often remained the dominant medical organization, despite the increasing visibility of physicians. For example, in most parts of England outside of London, the barbers' guild oversaw all medical activity without much rivalry from physicians.[4]

Burgeoning universities created the intellectual environment out of which Aldobrandino's text developed; the increased role of university training in medicine can also be tied to the rise of these institutions in the thirteenth century.[5] However, there is evidence that many practitioners did some training at universities without necessarily ever receiving a degree. Take, for instance, the provincial English practitioner John Crophill; he was primarily employed as a bailiff of Wix Priory and was also a part-time ale taster.[6] Even relatively minimal university training could benefit a doctor, who could point to that university training as setting him apart from his untrained competitors. The introduction of university training into the field inevitably affected the public's view of physicians, increasing the ways they could be credentialed. This demand for credentials came not necessarily from university officials, guilds, or licensing bodies but from patients themselves.[7] Especially for the populations with access to physicians—elites with access to personal physicians as well as the urban wealthy—the increased visibility and recognition of a university-trained category of doctor, and thus a wider range of levels of training possible among such practitioners, led to a need to be able to distinguish among those different levels of education. The establishment of this kind of hierarchy based on training and learned knowledge for physicians eventually impacted the stratification of surgical practitioners as well; in Paris, a complex system developed that included learned physician-surgeons, master surgeons who oversaw training through apprenticeships, barber-surgeons, and illicit practitioners.[8] No doubt practitioners at all these levels would have been available to elite patients who were the likely owners and users of many of the *Régime* manuscripts, both illustrated and unillustrated.

The Textual Foundations of the *Régime du corps*

Regimen texts like Aldobrandino's *Régime du corps* did not just appear in the thirteenth century but grew out of a centuries-long tradition that crossed many geographic and linguistic regions. Much of medieval medicine, including that represented by the *Régime du corps* text, was based on the theory of complexion, or the balance of humors, which was essentially derived from the classical traditions of Hippocratic medicine and the later ideas of Galen.[9] The theory of *complexio*, complexion or temperament, proposed that health was related to the balance of the qualities of hot, wet, cold, and dry within a human body. Each person's healthy balance was different, and much of the medical writing from antiquity to the sixteenth century was focused on understanding the connections between complexion and health. It was thought that this balance was impacted by the four humors—blood, phlegm, yellow bile, and black bile—real bodily fluids that had acquired various associations in terms of origin and function. The balance of these humors was tied to characteristics both physical and psychological; *sanguine, phlegmatic, choleric,* and *melancholy* were used to describe an individual's character.

Maintaining that balance was the essence of medieval medical care. An inherent balance was attributed to each person, which varied over the course of one's life depending on factors including age, surroundings, activities, and illnesses or disorders; each part of the body was connected to a specific complexion as well. Phenomena that impacted the body's health were categorized as naturals, non-naturals, and contra-naturals: naturals were elements, humors, and functions seen as intrinsic to the body, and contra-naturals were pathological conditions or diseases. The non-naturals, however, were especially pertinent to the understanding of causes of disease and treatment. These usually included the six factors of air and the environment, food and drink, sleep and wakefulness, rest and movement, evacuation and repletion, and the emotions; sometimes topics such as bathing and sexual activity were added. As the theory developed over the course of several centuries, the six non-naturals became the foundation for medical interventions and the increasing interest in the preservation of health in the later Middle Ages.[10]

The popularity of regimen literature is seen as part of the medicalization observed in this period, and indeed the non-naturals are fundamental to the preventive care promoted in regimens, including the *Régime du corps*. These factors are evident throughout the topics covered in the *Régime*, including chapters on air, sleep, reproduction, bathing, relaxation, evacuation (which includes bloodletting, leeching, cupping, purging, and vomiting), food, and drink. Diet was, of course, the cornerstone of preventive health care; it was also the place to start with a patient's prognosis. It was the least invasive method of treatment, theoretically allowing therapy to take place at home and with relatively little expense. Dietary regulation was a key aspect of medicine, going far back to Hippocrates and other ancient authors. Food and medicine were often one and the same, suggesting the pronounced relationship between health texts like the *Régime* and broader household management guides and recipe books like *Le ménagier de Paris* (a text discussed in more detail in chapter 4). We need only to recall the topic of cheese as discussed in chapter 2; many other consumables are also presented in the text with a similar range of concerns and associations.

The prologue of the *Régime du corps*, which accompanies several copies of the text, is where we are told about the circumstances of the text's creation as a result of the request by Beatrice. This section also describes the organization of the rest of Aldobrandino's text by listing the topics covered in the order they will appear. He claims to have relied on authorities in the three fields of "astronomy, nature, and medicine" and then explains how the text deals with each of these areas; its reliability is based on the fact that his sources are "the best authorities" in these three sciences: "Hippocrates, Galen, Constantine, Johannitius, Isaac, Aristotle, Diogenes, Serapion, Rhazes, Avicenna."[11] Many of these authors were among the most-read authors on medicine in Aldobrandino's time and later.

Aldobrandino does not reproduce complete texts but summarizes and condenses excerpts from these authors into the framework of his composition. Most chapters are relatively short; each one is rarely more than a few folios long. Among the longer chapters is the one on bloodletting (*sainier*), which, for example, runs from 11v to 14r (about six folios of text) in Sloane 2435. Many chapters are shorter than that, and, in many of the illustrated copies, initials that introduce a new chapter appear on nearly every folio. Despite the excerpted nature of the *Régime*, Landouzy and Pépin point out that Aldobrandino transcribes some passages from his sources quite accurately.[12] When he cites a specific author, he often signals this with the phrasing "as Hippocrates says," clarifying the main authority for a particular section. While mentions of contemporary physicians or other types of practitioners are not necessarily uncommon in medical writings, Aldobrandino's text itself makes virtually no such references. The text is written in the imperative mood, and the recommendations in the text are frequently directed in the second-person "vous." For example, the chapter on pregnancy begins, "In order to understand what we are saying to you" [*Pour bien entendre ce ke nous vous dirons . . .*].[13] It is followed by very introductory information, such as reminding the reader that a woman can lose the child at any time during the pregnancy if she does not care for herself. In this chapter he also briefly mentions the role of a midwife, suggesting that in the case of a difficult birth, a midwife (*sage baile*) should turn the infant so that it can be delivered.[14] Whether intentional or not, this form of address does not presume the reader to be a physician and allows for a wide range of audiences. A similar observation has been made by Monica Green about another thirteenth-century French health-care text, a French prose translation of the *Trotula*, *Quant Dex nostre Seignor*. Simple second-person-singular imperatives or third-person generics are used such that the text could be seen as speaking to audiences that did not exclude women caregivers.[15] The language of the *Régime* likewise could have included practitioners without being exclusively for such audiences; for example, Sloane 3525, Bibliothèque nationale de France Fr. 1288, and Wellcome Library MS.546 are all unillustrated copies in manuscripts that appear to have been oriented toward medically focused audiences. The phrase above also demonstrates Aldobrandino's use of "nous" to refer to himself, following a formal singular address that nevertheless has a potential plurality, implying that his expertise comes from being a physician in collaboration with the established authors he cites.

Several centuries of translation were the foundation for regimen literature, which appears in the thirteenth and fourteenth centuries, and of which the *Régime du corps* is a key example. The textual genre of regimens, like most medieval medical writing, developed from ancient Greek texts disseminated through later Arabic translations and compilations that were then translated into Latin. The Hellenistic author Dioscorides (first century AD) is known for his large work on *materia medica*, a key development of herbal pharmacology, that would also have an important legacy in the Middle Ages. Galen, however, is the author with the most substantive and long-term impact on later medieval medical thought. Galen of Pergamum (129–ca. 216) was a physician and doctor to Roman emperors who is viewed as among the important scientists of the ancient world. One reason for Galen's preeminence was his synthesis of many facets of medical thought, including anatomy, physiology, pathology, hygiene, and therapy, in a corpus of more than 350 known titles. His contributions to anatomical knowledge were not surpassed for more than a millennium and remained foundational well into the sixteenth century.[16] Galen's theories were grounded in his own work on anatomy, including his own observations as a medical practitioner; in this work, personal experience was considered valuable evidence as he dealt with a wide range of assumptions and preconceptions of the field. Moreover, Galen's works were based on and forwarded the doctrine of the four humors, or the idea that health was related to the balance or imbalance of these humors in the body.[17]

The next phase of scholarly development in medicine parallels the broader swell of intellectual activity in Muslim regions across the Mediterranean; these advances occurred in the intellectually lively cities of the Middle East and Iberian Peninsula, rather than in the comparatively underdeveloped cities of the Christian West. In these contexts, ancient Greek medicine was translated into Arabic; once this material was absorbed by practitioners, they began to interpret and expand on it. Among the most influential texts translated were Dioscorides and the many writings of Galen.[18] After this initial phase of translation, the concern became how to make this information usable and accessible; thus, in the tenth and eleventh centuries, several important Arabic encyclopedias were written.[19] The Arabic writers most influential in later centuries composed some of these encyclopedias; among them, known by their Latinized names, are Rhazes, Haly Abbas, Albucasis, Averroes, and Avicenna. Several of these key authors and their texts form the foundation of the *Régime du corps*.[20] For example, Abū Bakr Muḥammad ibn Zakarīyā al-Rāzi (Rhazes or Rasis; d. 925) is well known for a text called *The Comprehensive Book on Medicine* (*al-Kitāb al-Ḥāwī fī al-ṭibb*), later translated as *Continens*, which was an assemblage of his vast working files as a practicing physician and a key text for Aldobrandino. ʿAlī ibn al-ʿAbbās al-Majūsī, or Haly Abbas (fl. ca. 983), is known for his *Complete Book of the Medical Art* (or *Kitāb Kāmil al-ṣināʿah al-ṭibbīyah*). Haly Abbas's *Pantegni*, or *Regalis dispositio* in Latin, was a particularly comprehensive encyclopedia that would remain a key text for medical students in the later Middle Ages.[21] Abū al-Qāsim al-Zahrāwī, or Albucasis, composed *The Arrangement of Medical Knowledge for One Who Is Not Able to Compile a Book for Himself* around the year 1000 in Cordoba. The final book of this thirty-volume encyclopedia was devoted to surgery and was especially influential for later medieval surgeons like William of Saliceto (d. 1277) and Guy de Chauliac (ca. 1368).[22] But undoubtedly the most important author for Aldobrandino's text was Ibn Sīnā (Abū ʿAlī al-Ḥusayn ibn ʿAbd Allāh ibn Sīnā), known in the West as Avicenna (d. 1037). Ibn Sīnā wrote what is considered the most influential of these encyclopedias, known as *The Canon of Medicine* (*Kitāb al-Qānūn fī al-ṭibb*).[23] The *Canon* consisted of five books on general medical principles, *materia medica*, diseases in particular parts of the body, broader diseases (e.g., fevers), and recipes for compound drugs. His influence is especially pronounced in the sections of the *Régime* on caring for pregnant women and infants, which reflect the notion that treatments should be tailored to fit the phase of life.[24]

In the twelfth and thirteenth centuries, prominent Arabic medical texts (and through them, therefore, the Greek ones as well) were (re)introduced to Europe primarily through translations by scholars and physicians. Many of these authorities were associated with new medical schools and universities in the cities of Salerno, Montpellier, Paris, and Bologna, and the monastery of Monte Cassino. The founding of universities in Montpellier, Paris, Bologna, Oxford, and Cambridge in the thirteenth century is directly linked to the development of medicine, but less so with this phase of translation.[25] Most of the Arabic tradition that was translated into Latin was Galenic, and "Arabic Galenism" was the foundation of medieval Latin medicine. Among the most common textbooks in use were the *Isagoge* by Johannitius, or Ḥunayn ibn Isḥāq (809–873), a ninth-century translator, as well as the *Canon* of Avicenna.[26]

Through authors such as Constantine the African and Gerard of Cremona, and with the support of various patrons, this new knowledge was presented to the medieval West through two geographic areas: southern Italy and Iberia, especially Castile.[27] Constantine the African (d. before 1098/99) brought the Arabic medical corpus to the Italian cities of Salerno and Monte Cassino, where he developed translations of the works, including the *Pantegni* by Haly Abbas.[28] Toledo, another center of translation by the middle of the twelfth century, was where Dominicus Gundissalinus (fl. 1161–81) and Gerard of Cremona (1114–1187) embarked upon a thorough translation of various Arabic works, including Avicenna.[29] Several secular patrons facilitated translations in the thirteenth century by bringing scholars together in these areas, such as Emperor Frederick II Hohenstaufen (d. 1250) and Alfonso X, king of Castile and León (r. 1252–84).[30] An interest in translation directly from Greek, rather than Arabic, was notable in the thirteenth-century work of English philosophers Roger Bacon (ca. 1220–ca. 1292) and Robert Grosseteste (ca. 1175–1253), as well as that of Nicholas of Reggio (ca. 1280–ca. 1350), the personal physician of Robert I of Naples.[31] Most major works had been translated by the fourteenth century and were still deeply rooted in Galenic theory; Galen's works were being studied in Latin translation across Europe in intellectual centers such as Montpellier, Paris, and Bologna. By this time, a growing body of material had been developed to facilitate the practice of medicine and guide the practitioner. In this intellectual environment regimen literature exploded.

The Genre of Regimen Literature

Primarily written over the course of the thirteenth and fourteenth centuries, regimen texts are broadly characterized by their accessibility, their lay and often elite audiences, and their vernacular languages, including French and Catalan. A more intimate genre frequently tailored for specific patrons, these texts eventually developed into something resembling a "mass-market literature."[32] Changes in this period, including a more commercial economy, increased literacy, and the diversification of society, all contributed to the increasing demand for these kinds of treatises, which, through their prescriptive tone, put the means of preventive health care directly into the hands of lay readers rather than physicians—but only for those who could afford such books. Far from being an obscure or isolated text, the *Régime du corps* was but one instance of this burgeoning genre; as such, it was part of a well-documented movement of learned medicine being shifted into a more accessible, even mainstream, form.

Hygienic or dietetic texts, which focused on the preservation of health as well as treatment in sickness, formed the foundation of the regimen genre. As mentioned already, Avicenna's *Canon of Medicine*, highly influential in terms of regimen texts like Aldobrandino's *Régime du corps*, was founded on Galenic principles, including the six non-naturals and emphasizing the balance or equilibrium of the complexion. Another text significant to the regimen tradition was the *Tacuinum sanitatis*, which was unusual in dealing solely with hygiene and unique for compiling knowledge into forty tables, which provided for easy consultation by a broader public. Written by the Christian physician Ibn Buṭlān in Damascus in the eleventh century, the *Tacuinum* was translated between 1257 and 1266 at the court of Manfred, king of Sicily.[33] The *Tacuinum sanitatis* displays a distinct simplification of the sources on which it is based; it was clearly intended to be appropriate for the knowledge and literacy levels of its probable readers. The *Tacuinum sanitatis* also has a pronounced illustrated tradition that centers on the depiction of domestic spaces, which makes it an interesting foil for the illustrated copies of the *Régime*, as I explore further in chapter 4.[34]

Thus, by the mid-thirteenth century, when Aldobrandino wrote the *Régime du corps*, the prevalent practices of translation and copying had established the Galenic-Arabic medical tradition as the primary model. In fact, regimen literature became the key conduit for the popularization of Galenic theories, including the role of non-naturals not just in illness and disease but also in health.[35] In Aldobrandino's text, for instance, Avicenna (and through him, Galen) was the most significant source. Regimen texts built upon the theory of the six non-naturals, and the extreme popularity of these texts has been linked to the overall medicalization of the later Middle Ages characterized by a focus on a preventive approach to the maintenance of health and the body.

The genre of regimens or rules of health incorporated the Greek and Arabic traditions and was focused on individual health maintenance or hygiene. Popular across Europe by the later Middle Ages, these texts were often written to or for specific, high-ranking individuals interested in preserving their health and avoiding disease.[36] An early iteration of the regimen genre is the *Regimen sanitatis salernitanum*, or *Salerno Regimen of Health*, a highly popular text that first appeared in the late thirteenth century and contained a variety of suggestions for maintaining one's health.[37] An early phase of the genre, which includes Aldobrandino's French text, begins in the mid-thirteenth century and also includes works such as Juan of Toledo's (Johannes de Toleto) *Liber de conservanda sanitate*, which was written in Toledo in the mid-thirteenth century in Latin, but later translated into Catalan.[38]

In the first half of the fourteenth century, we see the creation of texts by Arnau de Vilanova, Bernard de Gordon, and Maynus de Mayneriis. Several of these authors were working for specific patrons, but their works were also translated and disseminated more widely. Arnau de Vilanova, a physician trained in Montpellier and author of several medical texts, became physician to Pere II, king of Aragon, until Pere's death in 1285, and worked intermittently for Jaume II (James) in the late 1290s and early 1300s. Texts he authored include the *Regimen for the King of Aragon* (*Regimen sanitatis ad inclitum regem Aragonum*) drawn up for Jaume II between 1305 and 1308, and *Regimen for Almeria*, the latter a text with health advice for military campaigns (*Regimen Almerie*).[39] These texts, much like the slightly earlier text by Aldobrandino, demonstrate a tone specific to the anticipated lay audience. Arnau's text for the Aragonese king was popular; it was quickly disseminated beyond the king and was translated from Latin into vernacular Catalan.[40] Arnau taught at Montpellier from 1291 to 1303, after having been a student there in the 1260s; Bernard de Gordon, a French physician, also taught at the University of Montpellier, starting in 1285. His best-known works include the *Lilium medicine*, an encyclopedic text completed in 1305, and the *Liber de conservacione vite humane* (1308), which comprised four books often treated as separate treatises (*De flebotomia, De urinis, De pulsibus*, and *Regimen sanitatis*).[41]

The mid-fourteenth century through the fifteenth century saw an increasing number of writings, many of which were aimed at a wider audience, including a wealthier urban clientele. Several characteristics of these texts seem related to their increasing popularity: they were more frequently in the vernacular (though some earlier regimen texts were as well, including the *Régime*), some were also anonymous, and they were increasingly in verse form.[42] Reframing these texts into verse seems likely to have broadened their appeal and thus their dissemination, creating affinities between these texts and other literary genres. Avicenna continued to be a prominent source for these later texts. As this summary of the textual foundations for Aldobrandino's *Régime* demonstrates, the *Régime* tapped into a broad and deep body of medical knowledge. At the same time, it represents a move away from such esoteric traditions, reflecting a period of experimentation and reorganization that allowed a variety of authors, Aldobrandino included, to reconsider the ways in which medical knowledge might be disseminated.

The vernacularization of a variety of textual traditions is often linked to an expanded audience, reaching lay readers who may not have had access to Latin texts. Although vernacular versions were certainly still accessible to university scholars or learned clerical readers, the combination of anthologizing and vernacular translation together in this period seem obviously linked to a wider readership for such texts.[43] In her discussion of the vernacularization and dissemination of *L'image du monde*, the encyclopedic text that accompanies several copies of the *Régime*, Katherine A. Brown demonstrates how that text paralleled vernacularization in romances in the same period, arguing that vernacularization expanded the audience beyond a Latin-reading clerical audience, in part through using literary techniques borrowed from contemporary genres, especially romance narratives.[44] The popularization of vernacular texts—didactic texts and guides as well as broad compendia and encyclopedias—made such knowledge increasingly available to a wider range of readers. This characterization of audience diversification is supported especially by the research of scholars working on manuscripts that include the *Régime* alongside other didactic and encyclopedic works, such as Nathalie Lacarrière's study of University of Pennsylvania LJS 55, a thirteenth-century manuscript that includes a range of encyclopedic works, including *L'image du monde* and an excerpt from the *Régime*, and Theresa Tyers's work on British Library Lansdowne MS 380 and Kassel Landesbibliothek 4° Med. 1.[45] While clearly individual anthologies could reflect quite different levels of complexity or sophistication, it seems likely that these newly developing genres were accessed by mixed audiences and lay readership as well as more scholarly or learned readers.

The Broader Context of Medieval Medical Illustration

A key argument throughout this book is that the illustrated copies of the *Régime du corps* straddle a surprising number of textual, cultural, and artistic traditions. In chapter 1, I explored the dialogue between the visual strategies evident in the historiated initials of the *Régime* and other medieval illustrative traditions, but it is also worth considering the *Régime* initials specifically in relation to medical imagery. The pictorial traditions of medieval medicine include representations of anatomy and other diagrams, scenes of procedures, surgical guides, and herbals; the content and form of the *Régime* illuminations cross over with several of these traditions.[46] Indeed, taken out of context, many of the historiated initials from the *Régime* manuscripts may not appear to be medical in nature. Scenes of food production, sleeping, or bathing, or those that simply depict two people in conversation, do not automatically evoke medicine. While many *Régime* images show medical treatments and other scenes related to healthy living and prevention of illness, these may not necessarily be read as medical illustration.

For many of us, the phrase "medical illustration" first brings to mind anatomical diagrams. But such diagrams are only a small percentage of the illustrations in medieval manuscripts. One explanation for this relative rarity may be the late acceptance of dissection as a medical practice; anatomical knowledge did not have a central place in university medical training.[47] Diagrams of the body certainly do appear at times, communicating information about how different bodily systems worked instead of how the body was literally put together. For example, a series of nine images sometimes circulated together, each one a diagram of a different bodily system, including the veins, arteries, bones, muscles, and nerves (fig. 61). More focused diagrams of the reproductive system, or specific organs, are often also included in the series (fig. 62).[48] The images in the *Régime* manuscripts are narrative rather than diagrammatic, and of course their small scale within the frame of initials limited how much visual information could be conveyed.

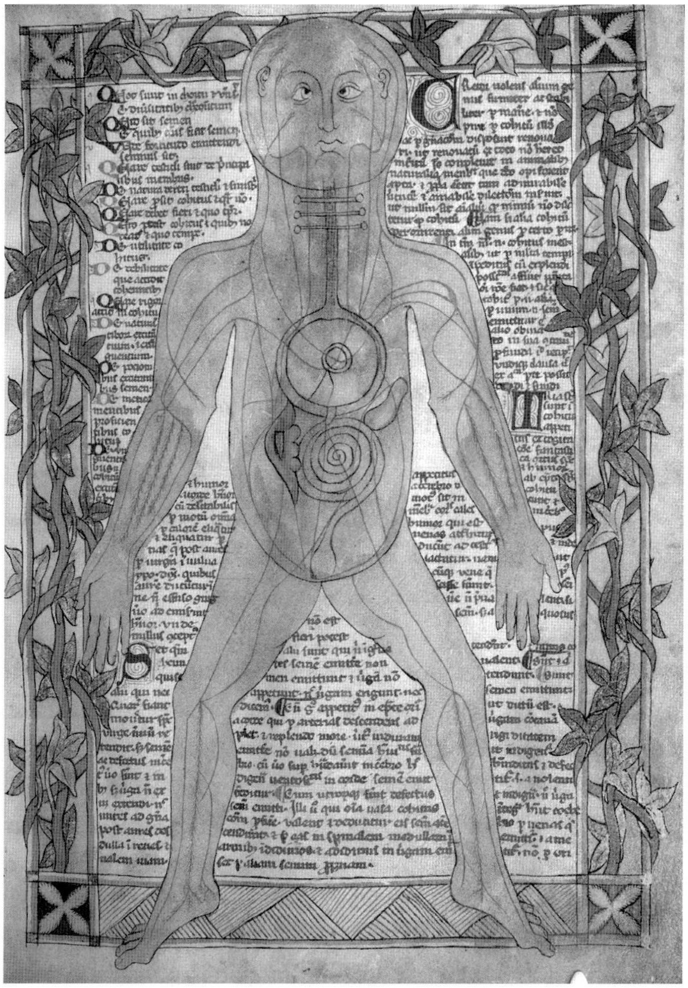

Fig. 61
Diagram of veins. Medical and arithmetical treatises and recipes, ca. 1292. Bodleian Library, Oxford, MS Ashmole 399, fol. 19r. Photo: Bodleian Libraries.

Physicians and other practitioners are depicted in a wide range of genres, from surgical manuscripts like Sloane 1977 (discussed in chapter 1), to the women administering cupping treatment in medical compendia such as British Library Sloane MS 6 or Bodleian Laud Misc. 724, to the "author portraits" that appear in copies of more technical medical treatises. In an early fourteenth-century Latin medical manuscript of a collection known as the *Articella* (British Library Harley MS 3140), historiated initials of doctors and students echo many of the scenes in the *Régime*'s oeuvre and reinforce the identification of a physician-type figure within them. In one initial, a doctor holds up a urine flask, while two students holding flasks look on (fig. 63). The *Articella* includes more complete versions of several texts by the same authors cited by Aldobrandino, including Johannitius, Isaac Judaeus, and Hippocrates.[49] In another example, British Library Harley MS 3745, a medical miscellany of a similar date contains several historiated initials that include a doctor and a patient. Both of these manuscripts are in

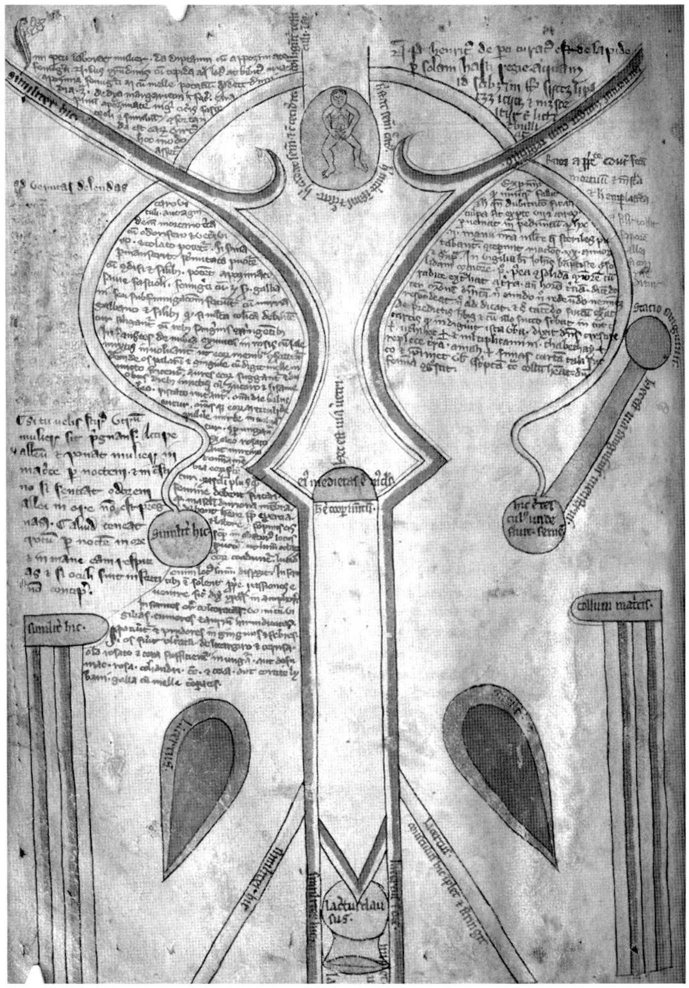

Fig. 62
Anatomy, female reproductive system. Medical and arithmetical treatises and recipes, ca. 1292. Bodleian Library, Oxford, MS Ashmole 399, fol. 15v. Photo: Bodleian Libraries.

Latin, suggesting a more educated, perhaps university-affiliated, clientele. The textual focus in Harley 3140 on prognostic texts such as *Urines and Pulses* indicates this manuscript was intended for a teaching or practicing medical audience, as does the content of Harley 3745. Likely created in Paris in the early fourteenth century, Harley 3140 and Harley 3745 reflect a context of production similar to the illustrated *Régime* tradition, especially BnF Fr. 12323. The connection of these manuscripts to Paris can be linked as well to the development of a key center of medical education at the University of Paris in the thirteenth and fourteenth centuries.[50]

Diagnosis was made in part through the evaluation of various bodily excretions, urine being the most common. In his discussion of a community-contracted physician, Michael McVaugh describes a situation in which urines would have been brought to the physician by town inhabitants; the physician would have looked at a specimen and considered how it informed the advice he would provide on things like bloodletting or diet.[51] Indeed, the preeminence of urine as a tool for diagnosis is evident in the prevalent visual tradition of urine wheels and charts, especially likely to be seen in physicians' almanacs of the later Middle Ages. In an image from a fifteenth-century folding almanac, a rainbow of pigmented containers indicates the range of possible characteristics that would have informed the physician about the patient's health (fig. 64). The accompanying texts attached to each flask provide additional information regarding aspects such as color, translucence, cloudiness, viscosity, and particles.[52] Known substances, such as saffron, gold, and vegetables, are used to describe different colors, and the descriptions are linked to health issues like quality of digestion, fever, infection, and even death, as well as recommendations about treatments such as bloodletting.[53] Citing contracts made between communities and physicians, McVaugh highlights the role of uroscopy in monitoring and maintaining health through diet and phlebotomy.[54] The ubiquity of this diagnostic method is also demonstrated by the fact that the urine flask became the main attribute used by artists to identify a figure as a physician even in a nonmedical context, as shown in a marginal scene in the *Hours of Jeanne d'Evreux* (fig. 65). Although physicians holding urine flasks are not especially prevalent in the *Régime* illustrations, urine texts were often copied with the *Lettre d'Hippocrate* and are included in a number of manuscripts alongside the *Régime*.

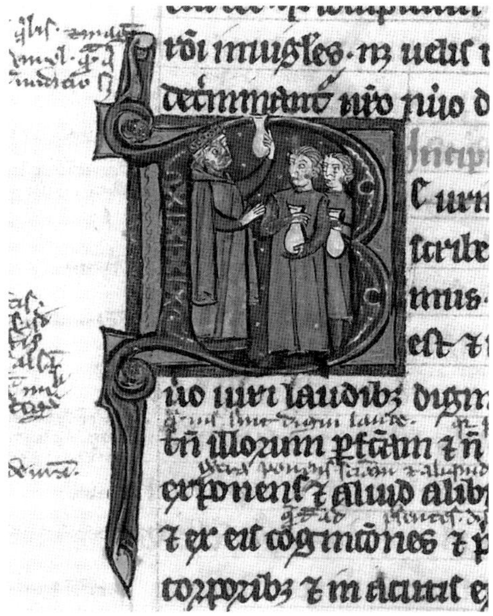

Fig. 63
Doctor and students. *Articella* (medical texts), early fourteenth century. British Library, Harley MS 3140, fol. 32v, detail. © The British Library Board.

Cupping as well as bloodletting, either by piercing a vein or by leeching, are among the procedures that are commonly illustrated in the *Régime du corps* manuscripts as well as in other medical books. Such scenes speak to the range of different types of practitioners seen in the images of the illustrated *Régime* manuscripts, reflecting the diversification of roles that developed over the course of this period and across Europe. The distinctions between physicians and surgeons often correlate with the specific treatments administered by each group: physicians generally dealt with illnesses tied to the inside of the body, while surgeons were responsible for wounds and other traumas visible on the outside of the body. Despite what comes to mind when we think of surgery today, surgeons (and in some cases, barbers) were responsible not only for more complicated procedures such as cataract surgery or limb amputation, but also cauterization, cupping, and phlebotomy.[55] Common procedures like "extraction of teeth; manipulation of dislocated limbs; lancing of boils; treatment of scalds, burns, and skin diseases; setting bones; and suturing wounds" were all usually under the purview of the surgeon.[56] But these separations between the fields were probably less significant on the ground. The existence of learned surgeons highlights that, in some cases, a more important distinction than physician-versus-surgeon was the literate practitioner versus

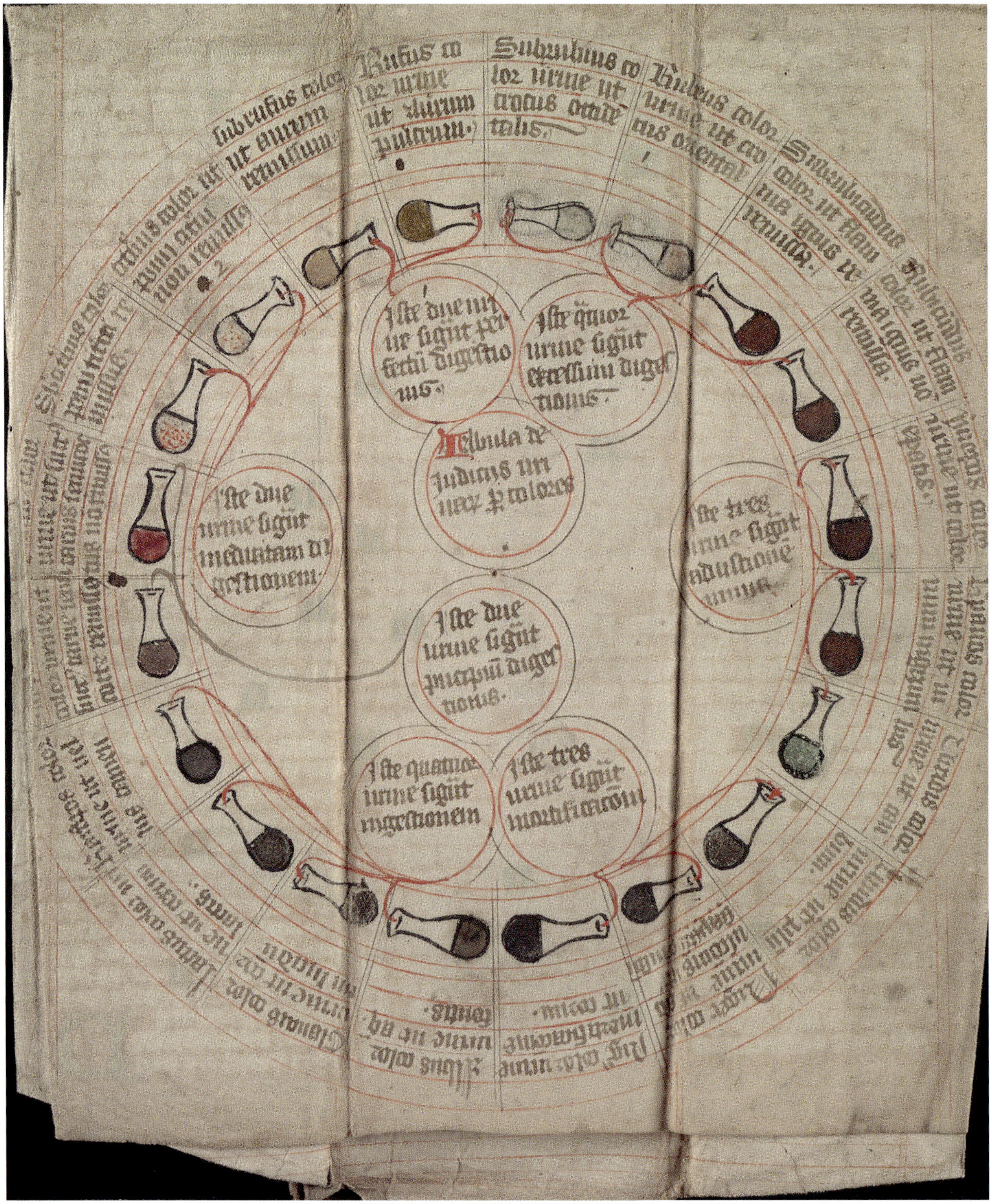

an illiterate empiric; other learned authors argued that surgeons had first to be physicians.[57] The lack of trained physicians in some places would have meant that barbers and surgeons took on more extensive roles as community practitioners. Indeed, even when a community included both physicians and surgeons, they were often expected to work together to facilitate diagnosis and treatment. "Barber" usually refers to practitioners who did some of the same procedures as surgeons, such as phlebotomy, but they were usually less educated; surgeons and barbers often considered themselves independent professional groups and sometimes maintained an antagonistic relationship.[58]

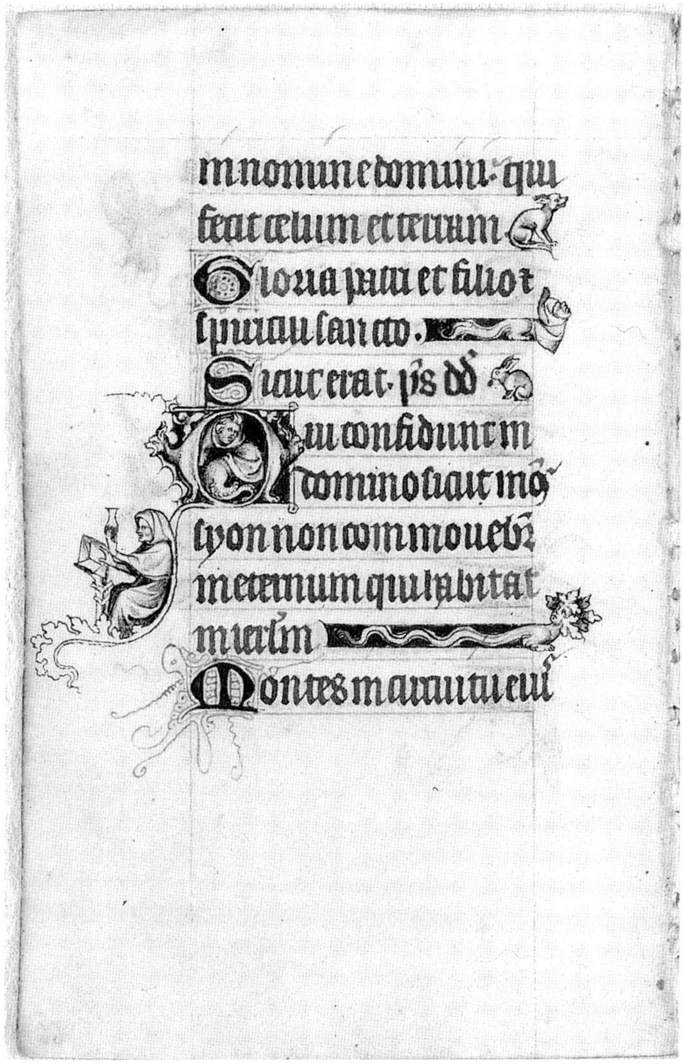

Cautery images, which often depict a complete figure with red dots indicating important points on the body to be cauterized for specific illnesses, are another robust illustrative tradition. Cauterization, cupping, and phlebotomy were manual operations performed by surgeons to rid the body of excess humors, often in combination with other recommended medications. Despite the fact that these treatments were carried out by professionals whose skills were seen as craft and who were usually not university-trained, several tracts eventually circulated that provided guides to these processes, including surgical texts by Roger Frugardi, Henri de Mondeville, and Guy de Chauliac. The physicians who wrote these texts were advocating for seeing surgery as a learned field, leading to the professionalization of surgery as well as the stratification of different types of surgical practitioners.[59]

Fig. 64
Urine wheel in almanac. Almanach, tabula festorum, mobilium ab anno 1364 usque annum domini 1462, 1406–24. Rosenbach Library, Philadelphia, MS 1004/29, fol. 9v. The Rosenbach, Philadelphia.

Fig. 65
Marginal figure of physician with urine-flask attribute. Jean Pucelle, *The Hours of Jeanne d'Evreux*, ca. 1324–28. The Cloisters Collection, fol. 65v. © The Metropolitan Museum of Art. Image source: Art Resource, New York.

For example, the illustrated medical manuscript Sloane 1977 contains relatively technical, sophisticated textual content, including Roger Frugardi's *Chirurgia* (Surgery), Matthaeus Platearius's French translation of the *Circa instans*, and a surgical text attributed to Galen and Hippocrates.[60] It includes scenes of practitioners listening to and advising patients and also depicts rather complex medical and surgical procedures, including cranial surgery, closing arrow wounds, treating genital ailments, and setting broken bones, as well as a scene of an apothecary's shop (fig. 66; see also figs. 22–23). Although this manuscript's text is written in French rather than Latin,

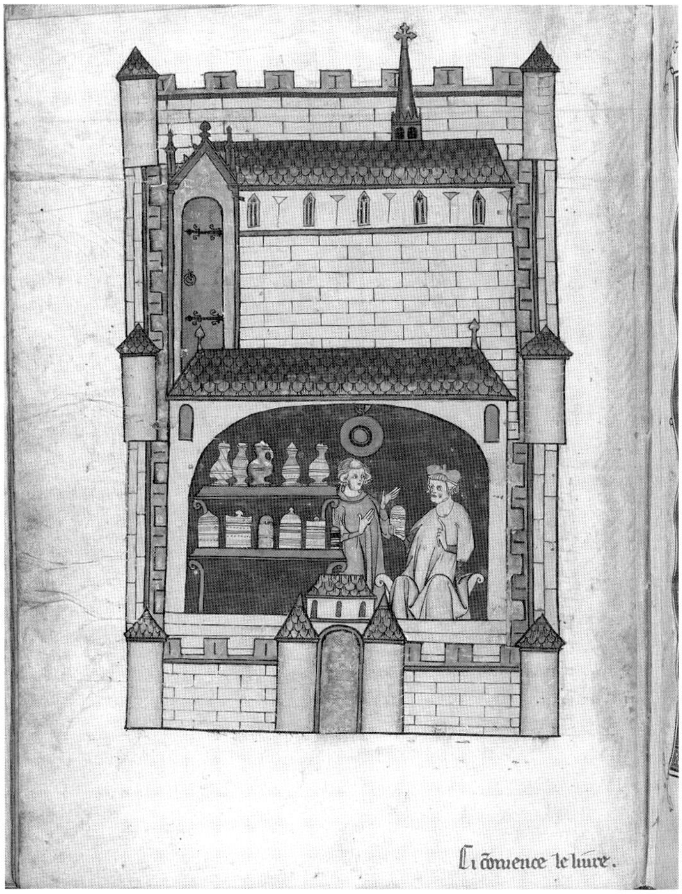

Fig. 66
Apothecary shop. Surgical texts, early fourteenth century. British Library, Sloane MS 1977, fol. 49v. © The British Library Board.

questions remain about its intended audience. Clearly a wealthy patron commissioned such an extravagant work, but the manuscript appears too luxurious to be used by a physician during actual practice; it is also possible that it may have even been intended for a religious, rather than a lay audience like that of the *Régime*.[61]

There are numerous instances of surgical texts being accompanied by illustrations, though they rarely contain the level of specificity one might expect as necessary for a surgical manual, suggesting other purposes for the images. For example, illustrated copies of Roger Frugardi's *Chirurgia*, a surgical text, exist despite the fact that readers of the manual were already knowledgeable about the procedures discussed, so that pedagogical images were not really necessary. Such illustrations are commonly brief snippets of scenes without great detail, suggesting other purposes for their inclusion. Helen Valls argues that such images functioned as visual markers; surgical scenes that are integrated throughout the text act as "cueing images" that "provide sufficient information for the contents to be speedily recognized."[62] But in the case of Sloane 1977, where the pictures are separated from the text, the images function differently. Whittington suggests that the full-page grid of images in this manuscript could have served as a general reminder for the surgeon of "the best approaches and sequence to various operations" (see figs. 22–23 and 66).[63] Other surgical manuscripts include illustrations of instruments; the precise illustrations of British Library Additional MS 29301, a copy of John Arderne's treatise on *fistula-in-ano*, demonstrate how to treat fistula with specific surgical tools (fig. 67).[64] This image is just one example of the diagram that commonly accompanies Arderne's text and is remarkable in showing several stages to the procedure. Each step is marked by a symbol, such as a star or asterisk, that also appears in the text describing the actions in the image. This unusual visual system is understood to be remarkably innovative compared to most other surgical images from the period.[65] In another example, Sloane 6, an illustration of multiple surgical tools is included alongside scenes of phlebotomy and cupping (this manuscript is discussed in more detail in chapter 4). Although no complex surgeries are depicted in the *Régime* initials, the inclusion of simpler treatments, such as bloodletting and cupping enacted by barbers or surgeons, suggests the prevalence of such practices, often conducted by figures who appear to have less status than a physician and sometimes even practiced by women.

In contrast to the interventions made by surgeons, the medicinal treatment of illnesses—the cornerstone of medieval health care—was a complicated and challenging method for healing patients in the Middle Ages. This primary method of intervention was also indelibly linked to the medieval European pharmacy. The medieval textual tradition of herbal medicine, or botanical pharmacology, was built on the inheritance of Greek medicine and throughout the Middle Ages remained one of the pillars of medical writing, to the point that medical recipes are among the most common types of medical text.[66] The text of the *Régime* itself contains no recipes, but recipe texts are often among those that are bound into the same manuscript with the *Régime*. Among just the illustrated copies, BnF Fr. 12323, Arsenal 2510, Sloane 2401, Cambridge, and Ajuda all include recipe collections alongside the *Régime*; in at least BnF Fr. 12323, Arsenal 2510, and Sloane 2401 they appear to be original. On-the-ground practice of "kitchen-garden" medicine was probably a combination of simpler remedies based on tradition and experience, with some knowledge that originates in the written tradition.[67] Tyers, in her discussion of the recipe collections included in the unillustrated Kassel manuscript, points out that such compilations brought together diverse materials that were nevertheless "practical and useful to families with ambition"; the inclusion of recipes does not rule out such nonacademic readers.[68]

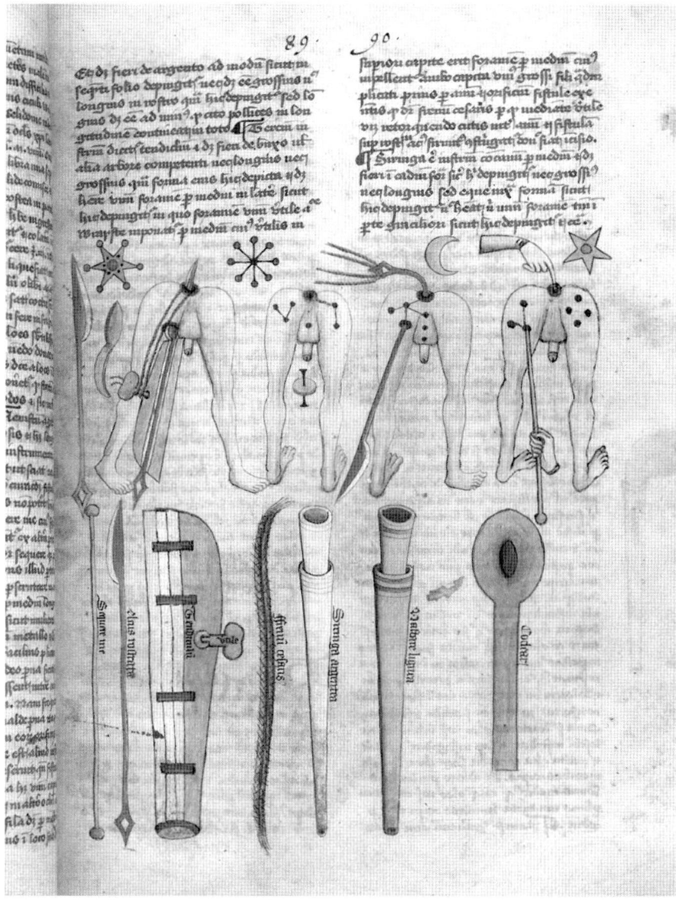

Fig. 67
Diagram of *fistula-in-ano* and tools. John Arderne's *Practica*, fifteenth century. British Library, Add. MS 29301, fol. 25r. © The British Library Board.

There were also problems of defining, measuring, and describing medicinals, further complicated by the fact that, by the latter part of the thirteenth century, practitioners were not involved in gathering most of their own *materia medica* but relied instead on tradespeople and pharmacists.[69] On the one hand, such trade meant that physicians were not limited to locally available substances; on the other hand, they were subject to other facets of the commercialization of medicine and beholden to those who provided the substances. The establishment and expansion of pharmacies over the course of this period is another phenomenon related to the professionalization and diversification of practitioners and is also occasionally reflected in the extant visual culture. Like barbers and surgeons, pharmacists often worked in collaboration with physicians and sometimes even established contractual agreements with them.[70]

The primary types of botanical texts circulating in this period were herbals or medicinal recipes. Herbals were encyclopedic texts listing a vast array of substances, generally based on Dioscorides's *De materia medica* and various translations and reinterpretations of that text. Herbals with illustrations circulated from an early period, the earliest surviving example being the Vienna Dioscorides from the sixth century, which was probably made for Anicia Juliana, daughter of a Byzantine emperor, and continued over the course of the Middle Ages, extending well into the fourteenth and fifteenth centuries with examples like the Carrara Herbal (ca. 1390–1400) and the Roccabonella Herbal (ca. 1445).[71] Although the *Régime* should not be considered an explicit part of the herbal tradition, it does contain sections on foods, including plants, which are illustrated in some of the illuminated copies. These herbal texts focused on individual substances and their general attributes, rather than specific recipes for combining substances. Compound recipes for medicines are essentially a different genre that is not part of the *Régime* textual tradition.[72] In line with the theories behind Galenic medicine, which espoused evacuation as a means to achieve humoral balance, laxatives and emetics were among the recipes included in these compilations. Indeed, this facet of humoral medicine was well illustrated in the illuminated copies of the *Régime*. Regardless of the popularity of such texts, the technical literature does not adequately reflect the use of simpler remedies on the ground. Prescriptions of local herbs were probably common, though likely tailored to the patient depending on their economic status: rarer and imported substances would be used for the rich, but more easily found treatments recommended for more everyday citizens.

The pictures in the *Régime du corps* may not conform to what broadly comes to mind with medical illustrations, but then very few medieval medical images do. These images are not present simply to facilitate understanding of an accompanying text—to illustrate textual concepts visually. As Peter Murray Jones has pointed out, the relationships between medieval medical imagery and texts are significantly more complicated; in many cases, a given medical image has an "ambiguous or even non-existent relationship to the words of the text."[73] In some cases, medical or scientific images circulated in manuscripts without any text at all; in others, the images clearly take significant precedence over the text, which is present to help understand the image, rather than the other way around. The acknowledgment that most medieval medical images do not adhere to a single style or way of functioning releases the *Régime du corps* images from similar expectations. With the understanding that they are as much part of other genres as they are part of the medical tradition, we can begin to see their implications for health care and household management on a much broader level.

The Texts That Accompany the *Régime* and Their Audiences

As my discussion in this chapter has sought to demonstrate, the *Régime du corps* is fundamentally connected to both the textual and pictorial traditions of medieval medicine. It was the product of centuries of textual tradition as well as the contemporary trend of summarizing, condensing, and repackaging elements of that tradition into more accessible, often vernacular, formats. These connections are also demonstrated when we consider the kinds of texts that appear alongside the *Régime*. A range of complementary texts suggest how the *Régime* was perceived in each particular manuscript: as a medical or scientific text, as a novelty text for an elite collector, or as a tool for domestic management that brought together devotion and health care. In these various contexts, the *Régime du corps* displays a pronounced flexibility and malleability, creating associations between genres that are rarely discussed together.

The diverse readers of the *Régime* were interested in material that was general as well as specialized, secular as well as religious. These textual companions indicate audiences ranging from physicians or those interested in specialized medical and surgical content to more general audiences who read the *Régime* alongside prayers and charms intended to aid in the maintenance of good health. Its repeated appearance with particular texts indicates that the *Régime du corps* was consistently understood as a text that fit within these different genres. Many of the texts that accompany the *Régime du corps* were among the most popular of the Middle Ages. The *Secret of Secrets*, which purported to be a letter from Aristotle to Alexander the Great but was probably written in Arabic in the tenth century and translated into Latin the twelfth, is included in several manuscripts with the *Régime*, and a letter from Pseudo-Hippocrates to Caesar (*Lettre d'Hippocrate à César*) is a collection of remedies that appears at least nine times in the corpus of *Régime* manuscripts.[74] Another copy includes the *Bestiare d'amour*, an allegorical love poem written by Richard de Fournival in the mid-thirteenth century that was incredibly popular.[75] While the *Régime du corps* may have resonated differently depending on whether its accompanying texts were formally medical in nature, focused on more practical health uses, or compiled as tools for moral advice or spiritual guidance, it was consistently copied with texts that were notably popular with lay readers.

In fact, even among unillustrated copies, several examples reinforce the likelihood of domestic use by families focused on household health. Some of the texts that accompany the *Régime*, such as the *Image du monde* discussed in chapter 2, have strong connections to users who included women. The audiences that were likely for the illustrated copies—lay households that included women and men—are also evident across the larger corpus of manuscripts that include the *Régime du corps*. The elite households that can be tied to the illustrated copies did not have a monopoly on this information or on the concerns that were managed within their homes; rather, the texts reflect broad interests that concerned many types of readers across society.

The *Régime*, based as it is on the theory of *complexio*, was inevitably informed by the practices around astrological medicine. In the text, Aldobrandino indicates the need to establish the right time for doing specific procedures, but these recommendations are generalized in terms of months, seasons, or ages; they do not provide information for precise calculations. Even though astrological diagrams are not among the *Régime* illustrations, scholars have pointed out how blurry the lines are between the different facets of health care represented by astrology and the medicine of the regimen texts.[76] The theory of "critical days," which asserted that certain days in the progression of an illness signify a crisis or change and that knowing those days is key for planning treatment, was a fundamental consideration for medical treatment largely based on what we would today call astrology; this kind of astrological medicine was a fundamental part of late medieval health care. Based on Galen's treatises *On Crisis* and *On Critical Days*, this approach was handled by a number of Arabic authors and, later, Latin medicine.[77] Such texts offered a variety of guidelines: foods to be eaten by a patient before or after a procedure as well as recommended seasons, moon phases, and times of day for initiating various treatments. The encyclopedic nature of UPenn LJS 55 provides just one example of a context that reinforces the *Régime*'s value as a knowledge source, as does the practice of copying it with the *Image du monde,* another encyclopedic text that includes astrological and related information.

The intersections of the *Régime du corps* with a variety of scientific traditions, such as astrology and astronomy, suggest that they were seen as logical textual companions. Lay audiences were often quite well read on such topics, especially when patrons of regimen texts were also collecting other types of medical and scientific material. Astrological medicine was a major component of medical practice in the Middle Ages and thus culturally prevalent among those making use of the *Régime*. The pictorial traditions associated with astrological medicine include charts depicting the cycles of the sun and moon, urine wheels, and diagrams known as the Zodiac Man and the Bloodletting Man (fig. 68; see also fig. 64). Such images appear together in a variety of manuscript genres that contain calendrical content, from books of hours to physician's almanacs, the latter reflecting information about a specific set of years. The images associated with astrological medicine appear frequently in a type of small, folded almanac; around thirty of these survive, all made in England during the fifteenth century and thus contemporary with the later *Régime* manuscripts.[78] The practicality of astrological texts in the context of domestic health-care manuals is also made clear through compilations such as Kassel, a fifteenth-century manuscript that includes the *Régime*.[79] In another compilation from the fourteenth century, Trinity College Library Cambridge O.2.5 (1109), astrological material is presented alongside medical texts, prayers, recipes, and other content, demonstrating the interconnections between health, astrology, astronomy, and prognostication for household health and well-being.[80] The *Régime du corps* likewise corresponded to astronomical, astrological, and broader scientific manuscript trends.

Among the larger *Régime* corpus that extends to unillustrated copies, several manuscripts suggest audiences with a pronounced interest in health care that likely included

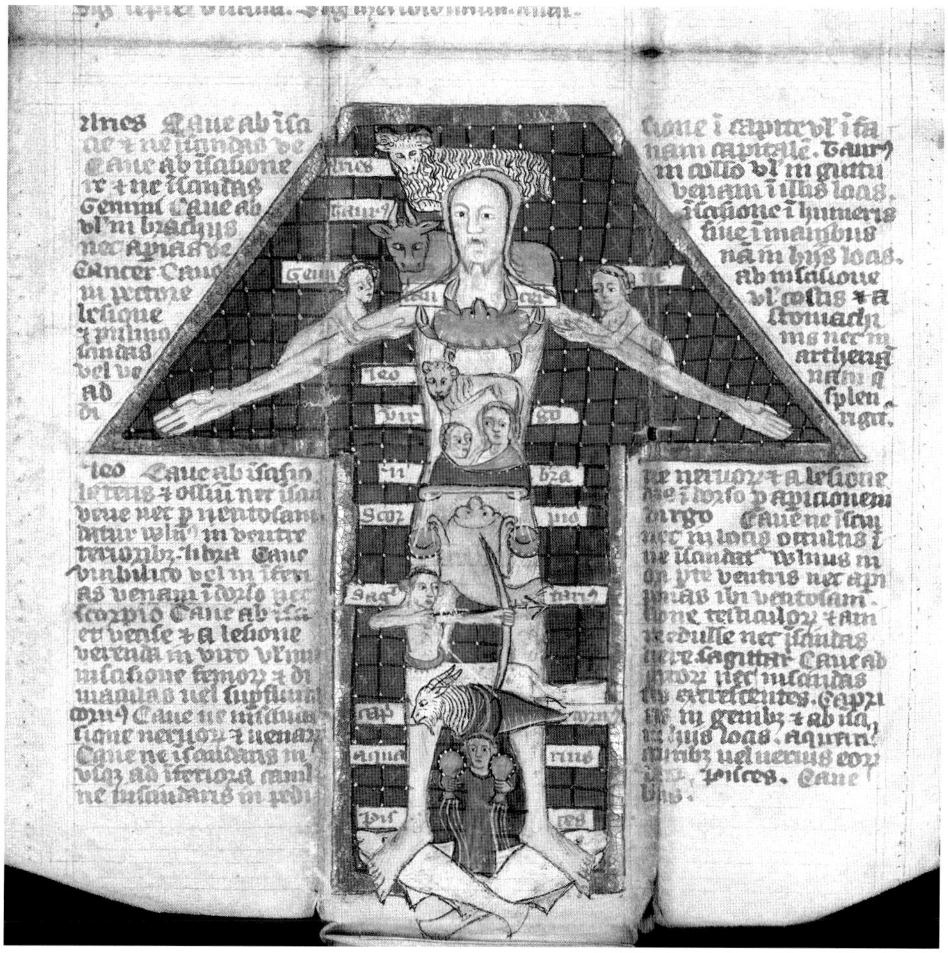

Fig. 68
Zodiac Man. Folding almanac, ca. 1415–20. Wellcome Library, MS.8932, fol. 5r, detail. Photo: Wellcome Collection.

both lay users and more learned or academically inclined readers. Copies such as BnF Fr. 1288, Sloane 3525, and Wellcome MS.546 present the *Régime* alongside notable medical texts. The text has been included with medical or scientific texts such as Roger Frugardi's *Chirurgia* (Surgery); the *Circa instans*, an herbal of simples written by Matthaeus Platearius in Salerno in the twelfth century; a plague tract written by Parisian physicians in 1348; work by the Montpellier doctor Bernard de Gordon; urology texts; medical recipes, including those attributed to Jean Pitart; and excerpts from the *Trotula*.[81] The inclusion of medical texts, however, is not necessarily an indication of exclusively scholarly or medical readers. For example, in Wellcome MS.546, a fourteenth-century example, Gilles de Corbeil's *De urinis, De dietis* by Isaac Judaeus, and an abridged version of Trota's *De passionibus mulierum*, all in French, are included alongside the *Régime* and other health-oriented texts that focused on infertility.[82] Noteworthy as a medical compilation, this manuscript nevertheless shows signs of an elite, and possibly female audience. In addition to the focus of the content on fertility issues, of significant concern to lay readers, Tyers has connected the small size and deluxe nature of the book to a readership that was more plausibly domestic than academic.[83] Even when the *Régime* is couched among traditional medical texts, its audience remains linked to a wider range of readers that likely included women and others outside the medical profession.

In two other unillustrated manuscripts, Kassel and Lansdowne 380, the *Régime* is featured alongside health texts, including portions of the *Trotula*, that seem focused on fertility and procreation. Lansdowne 380 is a late-fifteenth-century manuscript containing an extensive collection of moralistic, liturgical, and didactic texts, many associated with health-related advice, a condensed version of the *Trotula*, and the copulation chapter of the *Régime*.[84] Contrary to the assumption that such texts were intended for male medical professionals only, scholars have argued that that this manuscript's focus on fertility and related topics suggests instead a domestic, household use of practical medical knowledge. Tyers asserts that educated women did have access to textual medical knowledge, and that they provided information that facilitated joint involvement by women and men in fertility and related family concerns.[85] In her thorough description of this manuscript, Kathleen Sewright asserts the affinities between the manuscript's texts and the didactic conduct literature often collected for young women, including those of the merchant-gentry class.[86] There is a reference to "E. de Kyngstone" in the manuscript, presumably Elizabeth de Kyngstone, a wife of Sir William Kyngstone (1476–1540), who was a courtier of Henry VIII. Later female owners of this manuscript also seem to be genealogically related, suggesting a continued use in domestic female contexts.[87] Tyers argues for a similar non-scholarly and female audience for the Kassel manuscript, another extensive fifteenth-century compilation that includes many of the same texts, including the *Régime* and the *Trotula*.[88] Close analysis of the text and consideration of regional genealogy demonstrates the relevance of such texts for families and communities. These examples further support my assertions in chapter 2 about the likely domestic audiences for the illustrated copies, not only for Sloane 2401, which shares much with Kassel and Lansdowne 380, but also for most of the manuscripts discussed.

Religious texts also occasionally accompany the *Régime*, including the Psalms and a variety of other prayers, sometimes alongside charms and recipes. Copies such as BnF Fr. 1109, Biblioteca Apostolica Vaticana Pal.lat.1990, and British Library Sloane MS 1611 are all noteworthy unillustrated examples. Sloane 1611, a thirteenth-century copy, includes a variety of religious texts alongside the *Régime* and other medical texts. Among its contents are liturgical texts containing hymns and psalms, a moral verse, a sermon, and a verse version of the Life of St. Margaret, as well as the popular letter from Pseudo-Hippocrates to Caesar.[89] Paul Meyer suggests the book was written in thirteenth-century France, with fourteenth-century annotations written in England. The wide-ranging nature of these texts, potentially relevant to pastoral care in a variety of ways, indicates that the manuscript may have been collected by a cleric or other person in religious service, possibly a woman. The manuscript's folios are quite dirty and contain many marginal annotations throughout, suggesting it was engaged in significant use by its owner(s).[90] The inclusion of the Life of St. Margaret is a compelling feature, as the story of her bursting forth from the belly of a dragon evolved into her role as an important saint associated with successful childbirth.[91] Furthermore, preceding Margaret's life are recipes and charms that include several for female ailments, beginning with one focused on difficult childbirth. Sloane 1611 epitomizes interconnections between devotion, religious practice, and reproductive well-being; the *Régime* in this context provides additional guidance for managing household health.

It is necessary to accept that not everything is known about the medieval readers of the *Régime du corps*, but, as this chapter has demonstrated, the reach of its knowledge was vast and its position as a valued text seems clear. Taking into consideration not only the illustrated copies but also the larger group of manuscripts connected to the dissemination of the *Régime*, this medical text was *not* exclusively intended for the medical establishment. Much of the content in the *Régime*, based as it was on various canonical texts, would have been available to scholarly audiences in other forms; medical content, especially focused on the management of fertility, family planning, and household health care, was pertinent to many types of users. While physicians would have valued the text of the *Régime* for a number of reasons, some might have seen it specifically as a tool for communicating with patients, as a resource for translating advice into terms laypeople would understand; the abundance of copies associated with lay readers reinforces our understanding that it had a wide readership. Among the unillustrated versions, there are good reasons to assume domestic, household use by audiences that included women.

When it comes to the illustrated copies, the audiences seem even less likely to be physicians. These volumes are filled with scenes that depict physicians being consulted by the same populations that would have owned and used these books, instead of presenting scenes intended to convey information for the procedures done by physicians themselves. Furthermore, if an illustrated copy was theoretically intended for a physician as a tool of authority and prestige, why include other types of caregivers? The inclusion of a diversity of practitioners of various status—physicians, surgeons, and barbers, men and women—undermines the idea of complete academic authority. On the contrary, these images present the multiplicity of different health-care practices used within the medieval domestic sphere.

Conclusion: Privileged Patients as Health-Care Consumers

Across Europe during this period, elite and royal patients took advantage of their access to trained physicians. Significant evidence points to wealthy patients seeking out the most qualified and well-known doctors of the elite medical establishment. Whether this was because they resided near large urban centers that provided such access, or because they hired physicians themselves to work for them or be part of their courts, these patient groups were clearly driving the demand for a medical elite mostly trained at universities across Europe.[92] Beatrice of Savoy and her family members were exactly this sort of elite patron, maintaining their health and thus their success through developing relationships with, and procuring the exclusive services of, physicians like Aldobrandino. Although medical substances were also limited in availability for most of the population, pharmacists thrived alongside trained physicians; those with financial resources always fostered demand for rare drugs. It is exceedingly plausible that similar resources were available to Beatrice, her daughters, and their courts.[93]

However, the greater diversity of practitioners, the vernacularization of health texts, and the rising literacy and upward mobility of the urban wealthy and gentry all complicate the prominence of the physician and his authority while demonstrating the increasing independence or commercial power of families and patients. In her exploration of several gentry families, Hannah Ingram has demonstrated that, while members of the gentry or merchant classes sometimes consulted physicians, they also often managed their own health care without a physician's involvement. Furthermore, she documents evidence of an occasional mistrust of doctors by such families, who opted to take more control over their household health management.[94] Indeed, the greater personal involvement of a patient or their family with the decision-making around health care has altered how scholars understand the patient-practitioner relationship. Instead of seeing the relationship as one predicated on the doctor's authority and the patient's passiveness, such an interaction is better described as a "negotiation" or "exchange," indicating the more pronounced role of the patient.[95] Many of the images in the *Régime du corps* corroborate this assessment, in which the depicted action is often a verbal conversation. The notion of the patient-practitioner relationship as a negotiation, sometimes even involving a contract, also highlights the economic power of the patient; the patients, especially wealthy ones, had at least some choice about their health care. The onus was on the physician to establish not just authority but also trust, since the very nature of humoral medicine, which concerned all aspects of a patient's life, was often rather intimate.[96] The practitioner could become a kind of personal advisor as much as a physician, giving recommendations on aspects of life that might not seem immediately to be medical in nature. The consultation images in the *Régime* manuscripts also potentially provided guidance for when to consult a practitioner and what type of practitioner was appropriate for a medical issue—an example of how such books supported the user's personal involvement in their own health care.

Precisely the same types of households that commissioned or owned illustrated copies of the *Régime*—the nobility and the wealthy elite—were most likely to have access to the expertise of trained physicians. Both McVaugh, writing about Iberia, and Carole Rawcliffe, focusing on England, explore the high status that court physicians could attain, wealthy to the point that they were paid more than knights.[97] Indeed, Aldobrandino himself, as the personal physician of a countess, Beatrice, may have experienced some of that status. A similar status was likely granted to physicians in a number of the royal households for which illustrated copies of the *Régime* were made. For instance, Queen Eleanor of Provence, Beatrice's daughter, had several doctors available for her family who were consulted during the illnesses of her children.[98] According to Green, "it would probably be difficult to find a high-ranking woman who was *not* attended by a male practitioner at some point in her life" in the fourteenth century and later.[99] But these numerous examples of wealthy and high-status physicians working for specific courts still represent unusual circumstances compared to the average range of providers in urban centers or more common rural and small town contexts.

Indeed, upper-class women often had access to the most highly regarded, university-trained physicians, who often served as their personal doctors; as Green points out, such women were also the ones who were likely to own books.[100] In fact, several women known to have owned medical books also employed professional practitioners. Far from upsetting professional authority, such manuscript ownership potentially reaffirmed the status of those women. The *Régime du corps*, ostensibly composed by a personal court doctor for a countess, is an obvious example of such a circumstance; derived in part from the canonical medicine of physicians, it was found to be highly relevant to domestic audiences. Access to physicians and ownership of medical books were not mutually exclusive. In the cases of several *Régime* manuscripts, written medical knowledge was embraced by household members involved in caring for the health of their families.

The lavishly illustrated copies of the *Régime* may also have served to facilitate the decision about when to take another route.[101] Neither the status of physicians nor the status of their patients would have precluded other forms of health care, including a variety of home remedies, folk traditions, magic, and religion. Indeed, the landscape of medical care in this period, both for the wealthy and for a wider body of patients, was a complicated and diverse terrain. Most medieval health care would have involved a multi-pronged approach that included amuletic charms read aloud or written on small parchment scraps and placed on the body; the wearing of jewelry, gems, girdles or belts, pilgrim badges, and other talismans for protection or cure; visits to saint's shrines or other holy places; and self-medication.[102] Many of these alternative forms of care were used across social strata and often took place in the home; unfortunately, such practices are also largely undocumented. Ingram's work on documenting the responses to illness and treatment in the private letters of three gentry families represents a productive approach to accessing attitudes and practices regarding household health management. She determines that, in some cases, a "medical matriarch" was primarily responsible, and that women were often involved in decisions even when physicians were consulted.[103] Despite fewer options, patients in rural and poor areas probably sought skilled empirics when possible, while also looking to their own communities for treatment, frequently relying on various forms of folk medicine that were often administered by women.[104] No doubt many people among the peasantry and urban poor were treated by their family members or neighbors, since only a small percentage of people lived in cities with access to other kinds of practitioners, whether empirical or professional.

Many forms of health care were already employed when university-trained physicians became an additional choice for the wealthy, and those physicians inevitably had to contend with such practices. These activities were not necessarily seen as contrary to or in conflict with more official medicine, and medical texts often recommend charms or the creation of amulets as part of treatment. The appearance of new kinds of trained medical practitioners did not guarantee their immediate success or that they would necessarily overtake existing modes of healing and treatment. Surviving physicians' contracts make clear that "the novel authority claimed by medical practitioners was fragile and required continual reinforcement."[105] Such practitioners likely made use of a variety of techniques to communicate their expertise to potential patients.

The wealthy no doubt valued expertise and may have chosen to seek a doctor first when illness occurred; such patients would not have sought only a single remedy. As Rawcliffe puts it, "during a period when master surgeons commonly had recourse to charms and prayers when attempting difficult operations, and herbalists were well versed in humoral theory . . . the patient was rarely disposed to maintain rigid distinctions: for him or her the rich diversity of physical or spiritual treatment offered a continued hope, desperately sought, of relief from suffering."[106] Not wishing to delegitimize the other treatments valued by their patients, doctors referenced and even prescribed other forms of medical treatment. Such practices included many forms of self-treatment that would have been based within the domestic sphere and are reflected in the diversity of health-care approaches used by many in the late Middle Ages.[107] The wide range of texts accompanying the *Régime du corps* in surviving manuscripts further demonstrates how household health would have been supported not only by traditional medicine but also with other forms of encyclopedic knowledge, devotional practice and prayer, informal charms and recipes, and more. From noble audiences such as Beatrice and her family, to the gentry and wealthy merchant classes, elite readers would have taken advantage of their access to professionals while also making use of a wide range of other health-care methods, many of which were based in the home and are found depicted in these books.

The maintenance of the household, including the health care of those living within it, is at the center of both the *Régime* text and its accompanying images. Household management is not simply something that fell under the purview of regimen literature like the *Régime*. A variety of textual traditions, including household guides, conduct literature, and dietary texts dealt with many of the same concerns while being more overtly geared toward the domestic sphere. Indeed, both pictorially and textually, the *Régime* manuscripts are in dialogue with a much wider range of genres, and a consideration of them solely as medical texts fails to reflect their complexities. The diversity of genres with which the *Régime* images and text engage helps us understand how they fit into the culture of care, which is distinguished by a wide range of tactics for maintaining health and well-being, including, but not limited to, professional medicine. As these wider contexts are explored in chapter 4, the roles of women in domestically oriented health care, especially within the *Régime* copies and their images, becomes increasingly visible.

4

HOUSEHOLD MANAGEMENT, STATUS, AND THE CARE OF THE BODY

One of the most memorable images from any of the illustrated *Régime* manuscripts depicts a poor soul in the throes of vomiting (fig. 69). A very large and multicolored stream rushes from the man's mouth, immediately communicating the content of the chapter. Despite the Arsenal manuscript's limited color palette, the artist was clearly unencumbered, scaling the vomit to be nearly the same size as the patient's body and removing any background objects that might be distractions. As viewers today, we are inclined to respond to this image with entertained surprise or even mild disgust at the volume of material spewed forth, both responses that suggest that we were not expecting to see this image in such a fancy book.

This scene of vomiting is not limited to the Arsenal copy, although different moments are depicted across the *Régime* manuscripts. In BnF Fr. 12323, this chapter is introduced with an image that shows a practitioner aiding a person who has presumably been given an emetic for this purpose, while the patient kneels in front of a bowl and prepares himself (fig. 70). In Sloane 2435, the patient leans forward, assisted, while several white dashes modestly indicate his sickness (see fig. 24). In the later, fifteenth-century manuscript of the *Régime* at the Morgan Library, two figures are depicted, and this time they are both women (fig. 71). Clearly, vomiting was a legitimate subject for illumination.

The juxtaposition of mundane topics and ostentatious manuscript design is a key contradiction inherent in the illustrated *Régime* manuscripts, and one I explore further in this chapter. How should we square the luxurious nature of many of these books and the status they afforded owners with the everyday nature of many of their scenes? In the Middle Ages, of course, we know that the demarcations between private and public spheres were far less established than they are for us today, and that the daily activities of bodies were much more prevalent and visible. Even so, that does not mean such activities necessarily had to be illustrated. The inclusion of scenes like those of

ou en la fin. Si doit on
le fourciele froter. et
escaufer par mouvoir
le cors et par toulles cha
udes. Et si se haste on
dou conforter. de dou
ner brouet de geline.
et doindre lestomac de
bure et doille violat. p(or)
cou quil ia peril de mo
rt. Et sil avient quil
ait trop g(ra)nt soif. Si
fera cuire en aige go
me arrabie. gôme adra
gant et siliû. Et de ceste
aige buvera tiede. Se
constractions li avi(en)t
par tout le cors. par tr(es)
fort medecine. si ni a
nul conseil. Si come
dist ypocras. Car ces
te est mortaus. Se li cô
stractions est par par
ties. Si estuet oindre
lesl[…]e deriere par
tout le dos. de dialte de bu

re doile violat. Et puis
baignier en aigue ou se
ront cuites mauves ibi
mauves voletes brens
perresins. Et a lisir dou
baing. oindre de lait de
feme. En tel maniere
pora le peril de medeci
nes trespaser. Li tresime
chapitres qui nos apr(ent)
a coi li vomirs est bon(s)
et a coi il puet grever.

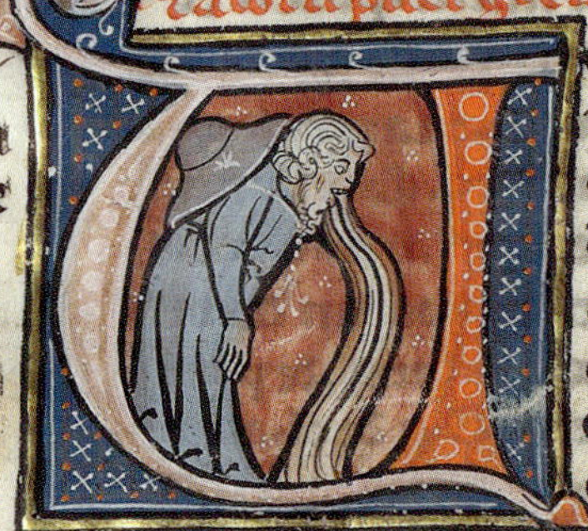

Omi
rs. si
come
dist
avi
cene.
Cest
espe
ciaus medecine. pour
purgier lestomac. et le
chief et le cors. Et qui le
fait si com il doit. Si ga
de le sante et aide lesto
mac a cuire le viande

vomiting and defecation, in addition to other routine household activities such as preparing food, offers insights different from those gained by the consideration of audience or patronage. I also explore how the images reflect economic or other social stratification. In the end, of course, these books depict household activities in the same domestic environments in which the manuscripts themselves resided. The presence of the household, as a place in which users engaged with these books, and in terms of the pictured world constructed by the manuscripts' images, is central to understanding how health care was practiced in the elite domestic sphere.

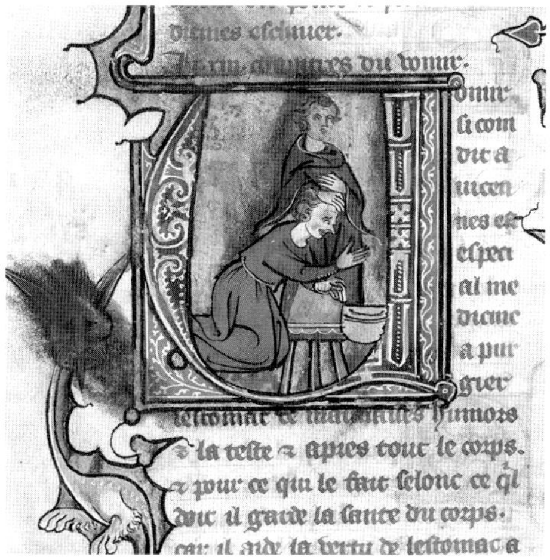

Fig. 69 (opposite)
Vomiting. The Bute Painter, *Le Régime du corps*, ca. 1285. Bibliothèque nationale de France, Arsenal MS 2510, fol. 17v. © Bibliothèque nationale de France.

Fig. 70
Vomiting. *Le Régime du corps*, fourteenth century. Bibliothèque nationale de France, Fr. 12323, fol. 89v, detail. © Bibliothèque nationale de France.

While the *Régime* manuscripts are undoubtedly informed by the established medical traditions discussed in the previous chapter, those contexts clearly provide an incomplete picture of the *Régime*'s reach and its relevance to a wide range of audiences. By considering the *Régime* not just as a medical text but also as an encyclopedic text like the *Tacuinum sanitatis*, or as a household guide in the tradition of *Le ménagier de Paris* or Christine de Pizan's *Le livre des trois vertus*, we can see its complexities more clearly and have a more complete view of the context in which the manuscripts existed and were used. The images and text of the illustrated copies reflect the place of the *Régime* at the junction between a wide range of illustrative and literary genres, demonstrating a kind of genre hybridity. The *Régime* images and text maintain the centrality of health care within household activities, bringing professional medicine into dialogue with the practices of the domestic realm. While household health care is more difficult to document, a variety of sources, not the least of which are the *Régime* images themselves, can be brought together to generate a view of the household world in which these manuscripts circulated.

Many of the images of the *Régime du corps* seem to reinforce the authority of the physician, but the inclusion of female practitioners and caregivers complicates that authority and offers a glimpse into a more diverse picture of medieval health care. Such household-based health care is depicted in both the images and the text of the *Régime*. The language used in the *Régime* text leaves open which individuals would be following the directives, an ambiguity reflected by the pictorial inclusion of female providers and treatments in domestic spaces. Women's household authority is prevalent in these manuscripts not only through images of women administering treatments and other kinds of care but also through other scenes depicting a variety of conversations, food or drink production, or consultations, such as the wet nurse scenes. Across the *Régime* illuminations, signifiers of status and authority denote the complexities of power relations in these households, which reflect back onto the possible owners and

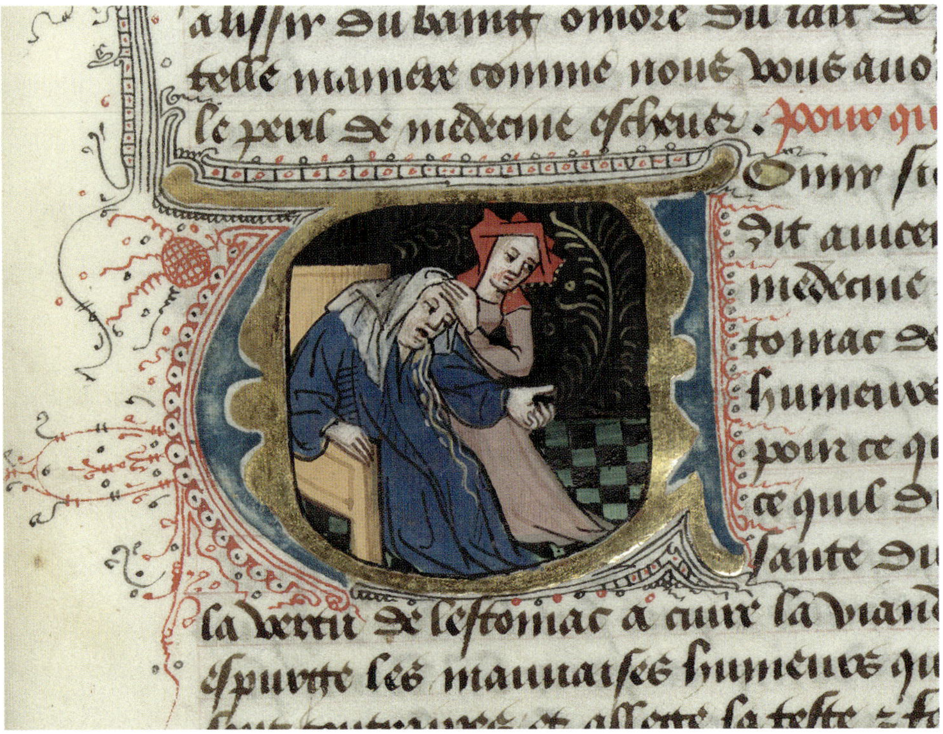

Fig. 71
Vomiting, with woman aiding. *Le Régime du corps*, ca. 1440–50. The Morgan Library & Museum, MS M.165, fol. 33r, detail. The Morgan Library & Museum, New York. Purchased by J. Pierpont Morgan (1837–1913) in 1902.

users of the books. The six non-naturals—that is, those various environmental factors that impacted health such as cleanliness, sleep and wakefulness, evacuation, and food and drink—were a foundational aspect of medical knowledge in the Middle Ages, central to how physicians and academics theorized the treatment of illness. But obviously, knowledge of these factors was neither exclusively available to educated readers, nor set only in the purview of physicians. The non-naturals also happened to be among the quite ordinary actions maintained within a household.[1] The forms of health care in which women were involved were often the kind left unrecorded, made up of everyday activities within the house.[2]

There is little question that the *Régime du corps* reflects engagement with academic medicine, especially as part of the trend of regimen literature that, although oriented toward more general audiences, was developed on a solid foundation of established medical tradition. But the *Régime* also engages with a number of other late medieval literary traditions, including household guides, conduct literature, and recipe collections, that would have catered to similar audiences but that dealt specifically with the domestic rather than the academic sphere. The popularity among women of collecting all of these genres, health care included, is linked to status, in which the aspiration for or maintenance of a certain social or cultural standing was tied to conditions of ownership and access to knowledge.

The *Régime du corps* speaks to a variety of potential audiences and experiences; especially in the case of the illustrated copies, the diversity of household members is reflected in the images themselves. Closer consideration of late medieval households in general, including who was in them and what went on within them, provides context for the *Régime*'s scenes of domesticity. Elite illustrated books like the *Régime* manuscripts were in and of themselves markers of status, but they were part of an array of other types of conspicuous consumption and wealth, such as food, clothing, and access to physicians—all expressions of status that are connected to the care of the body and literally on display in the *Régime* illustrations. The overt display of household wealth was often made through bodies, the same bodies whose mundane but essential activities were being managed and cared for within the home.

Household Guides, Conduct Literature, and Recipes

The *Régime du corps* clearly appealed to multiple audiences, including lay readers, in part because of the aura of knowledge and authority it gave owners. Much of it seems addressed to the upper classes, not just through the circumstances of its creation but also through its content. Discussions of wet nurses, imported spices, or wild game would all have signified a sophisticated and wealthy reader. The illustrated copies, which further embellished subject matter already associated with an elite lifestyle through abundant illuminations and gold leaf, clearly distinguished the *Régime* as a status text. Indeed, the illustrated copies of the *Régime* provide the reader with much more than information and imagery about medical treatment and advice.

When they are considered in the context of the broader textual traditions of household management, which include conduct literature and other courtesy texts, it becomes clear that the *Régime* manuscripts also communicated ideals of household management and social status. Texts such as *The Good Wife's Guide* (*Le ménagier de Paris*; ca. 1394), Christine de Pizan's *The Treasury of the City of Ladies* (*Le livre des trois vertus*; ca. 1405), *Le livre du Chevalier de la Tour Landry pour l'enseignement de les filles* (1371–72), or John Lydgate's poem "Dietary" (1400–1450) provided guidance for managing the complexities of upper-class, late medieval households like those in which the illustrated *Régime* manuscripts would have appeared.[3] Such literature often contains the implications of upward mobility, as they were especially popular with bourgeois collectors at a time when social movement was most possible. These genres and the *Régime* flourished during a period in which book collecting and literacy across numerous social classes was increasing, extending the messages of these texts to a wider range of audiences. Access to books and access to health professionals and medical substances went hand in hand, and the dialogue among different late medieval genres reiterates the interconnectedness of health care, household management, and conspicuous consumption.

Le ménagier de Paris is a household guide, written anonymously in French near the end of the fourteenth century.[4] Addressed to a fifteen-year-old bride, it is written from the point of view of her new husband, an older man who was a wealthy bourgeois in Paris. Its content guides the new wife in both moral conduct and the household duties that she would need to know; it is remarkably comprehensive and practical, covering topics such as gardening, care for horses, recipes and feast menus, advice for getting rid of fleas, and suggestions for hiring servants.[5] The text provides a window into an affluent urban Parisian household, and such a household's material culture and intellectual interests. It offers a compelling view of what a wife could anticipate in such a home, in which she is expected to be competent but also obedient, and it reflects a certain tension around her independence or authority in the course of her management of the household and ultimately of her husband's needs. The male-centric focus of *Le ménagier* highlights the relatively neutral language and information of the *Régime*. In fact, the Kassel manuscript, a compendium that includes the *Régime,* has been indirectly connected to one of the four surviving copies of *Le ménagier*, further supporting the notion that these texts circulated in similar contexts among shared audiences. Bibliothèque nationale de France Nouv. acq. Fr. 6739, a fifteenth-century copy of *Le ménagier*, was owned by Pierre of Roubaix and Herzelles and his wife, Marguerite of Ghistelles (d. 1495), family members with ties to the composition of other advice literature connected to *Le ménagier* and the Kassel *Régime* manuscript.[6] As Theresa Tyers points out, there is compelling support for thinking about the *Régime*, *Le ménagier*, and other accompanying texts as complementary, aimed as they were at those managing households and caring for the health of a family.

Christine de Pizan's works are among some of the best known and most popular of the later Middle Ages, including her allegorical response to Jean de Meun's *Roman de la Rose*, *Cité des dames*, in which she made the case for the significance of women throughout history. A companion to that text completed the same year, *Le livre des trois vertus,* was written for Princess Margaret of Burgundy (1393–1442), the young wife of the dauphin Louis de Guyenne (1397–1415).[7] Indeed, Christine had an extensive elite audience, which contributed to her pronounced success as a writer; this success, especially remarkable for a woman, occurred even during her lifetime. *Le livre des trois vertus* is divided into three parts and addresses three different audiences about appropriate behavior, dress, and household adornment: Part I is for the princess; Part II for ladies-in-waiting and ladies of the manor; and Part III for bourgeois women, prostitutes, and the poor.[8] Rosalind Brown-Grant describes the *Trois vertus* as a text that employs the form of the courtesy genre to provide women with lessons in how to use their actions to "prove misogynists wrong" within the constraints of contemporary society.[9] The text was one of Christine's most popular works and was copied prolifically in manuscripts and early print. Both apparently commissioned for noblewomen, the *Régime* and the *Trois vertus* are steeped with insights about class stratification in the domestic sphere of the household.

Other examples of such texts include "Dietary" by John Lydgate and *Le livre du Chevalier de la Tour Landry pour l'enseignement de les filles*, both of which emphasized moderation. *Le livre du Chevalier de la Tour Landry* was written by a provincial aristocrat for his daughters; it generally advocated restrained and subdued behavior and included warnings about the dangers of vanity.[10] Lydgate's "Dietary," first written in

Middle English, focused on food and thus health as it related to food. The text argues for moderation and the control of consumption and was probably geared to an audience of wealthy urban or rural householders.[11] The morality of restraint espoused by these texts does not really appear in the *Régime*, which maintains the comparatively neutral, informational tone of an encyclopedia or other fact-based guide.

These examples speak to conduct literature's broad popularity, crossing class lines as the most powerful members of the urban elite aspired to behave like the nobility and display their wealth in similar ways. The proliferation of these kinds of texts in this period "directly connected to the social mobility of the emergent bourgeoisie for whom possessing conduct books became a marker of its ascendency."[12] Indeed, books in general became markers of that ascendency, as did fashion, interior decoration, and food—all themselves topics that would appear in the content of conduct or courtesy texts, as well as in the *Régime*. Although many of these conduct texts espoused restraint and moderation, as do the rather ineffectual sumptuary laws of the period, the prolific copying and dissemination of these texts demonstrates a pronounced preoccupation with material consumption, display, and self-presentation: "Both communally and individually, the newly empowered urban elite were seeking a recognition hitherto reserved for the noble class, and in pursuit of this honor were acquiring and displaying objects and behaviors of authority that were traditionally noble."[13] In her discussion of fashion in the *Ménagier*, *Le livre du Chevalier de la Tour Landry*, and *Le livre des trois vertus*, Roberta L. Krueger demonstrates that both conduct books and fashion moved from the courtly environment to the households of the lower aristocracy and urban bourgeoisie and, through that travel, became possessions associated with status.[14] Indeed, several scholars have pointed out that some of these texts were also at times richly illustrated, unequivocally marking them as objects of distinction.[15] In such cases, the content of a book might have been less important for evoking status than the book considered as an object itself. Inventories such as that of Clémence of Hungary, in which books are identified by their material characteristics such as coverings, decorations and clasps, as well as their value in monetary terms, rather than their content, speak to the inherent value of book collections.[16]

In the context of household guides and other conduct literature, the *Régime du corps* becomes a text that is as much about the management of a household as it is about medicine. The management of health within a household relied not only on medicine per se, but also on a wide range of activities that do not initially appear to be related to health care at all. In her assessment of women as patrons, owners, or readers of medical material, Green asserts that very little academic medicine, that is, the traditional texts composed by and used by university-trained physicians, made its way into the collections of lay women. She finds that relatively few medical books appear in the collections of women, and that they are a small percentage of all books associated with women.[17] But regimen texts seem to be an exception; they are often considered as examples of medicine made more accessible for lay audiences through abbreviation and vernacularization, and often such readership may have included women.

Especially when couched with other types of texts, including medical works such as versions of the *Trotula* that highlight fertility and family health care, the *Régime* was one of a range of texts that reflected the interests of female readers.[18]

Broadening the textual category of health care to include recipes and charms as well as household guides provides a more complete picture of health knowledge. The kind of health care that women were most involved in was often less likely to be written down, being preserved instead through oral transmission; however, textual evidence of this tradition does exist. Recipes in the Middle Ages were not significantly different from what comes to mind when we think of recipes today: short, anonymous, repetitive, nonnarrative, and adaptable texts usually related to the making of things we consume.[19] And they were ubiquitous. Michael McVaugh points to exactly this type of ephemeral text, a scrap of paper used by a notary inscribed with a recipe from the recipe book attributed to Arnau de Vilanova, arguing for its importance because it gives us a rare glimpse into how learned medicine expanded beyond books and reached patients.[20] Some recipes deal with preserving or cooking food, but others involve techniques for scenting the air, purgatives, painkillers, plasters, eye drops, and procedures for improving skin and hair. Recipes appear across manuscript culture, though paradoxically, as Cabré explains, "their omnipresence makes recipes historically hard to handle, for they are copied here, there, and everywhere."[21] They were flexible, constantly modified, and have a high degree of adaptability that complicates how we think about originality and the production of knowledge.[22]

Indeed, numerous scholars have suggested that recipes, especially those which marginally appear in other kinds of books or in letters, provide a much better representation of women's learning and expertise: "Rather than dismissing the occasional medical recipe scrawled into the back of a book owned by a woman as irrelevant, therefore, perhaps it is time we started paying attention to these snippets of medical lore as evidence for a much broader and wider medical discourse shared orally among medieval women."[23] Recipes can and should be seen as women's texts; "by doing so we bring into historical existence a world of knowledges and practices that we often assume to exist but can rarely trace."[24] While the *Régime* itself was not a text of recipes, recipes and related types of texts often appear alongside it. This occurs in the illustrated copies Arsenal 2510, BnF Fr. 12323, Sloane 2401, Cambridge, and Ajuda; numerous unillustrated copies also contain some kind of additional recipe text.[25] The *Régime*, at a fundamental level, is focused on household care of the body; women as the key to the dissemination of the text as patrons makes sense, because they also oversaw so many of these facets of the household care of the body covered on its pages.

By shifting our perspective to expand what we think of as medical, a more nuanced version of household medicine comes into view. Women may not have been prevalent consumers of traditional medical texts for reasons that include literacy and access, yet it is certainly likely that elite, book-owning women often had access to that expertise through the practitioners themselves, alleviating a strong demand for books on such topics. A consideration of the domestic sphere is essential to understanding the agency of women in health care as well as medicine more broadly, despite the fact that it is more often than not left out of discussions about the history of health maintenance or the treatment of illness. Demonstrating the inadequacy of using readership or ownership alone as a marker of access to knowledge, Cabré points out that "[w]omen's authority does not come from a written text, but surfaces in descriptions of what they do."[26] While such activities are somewhat removed from historical documentation, scholars have been able to construct household health practices from sources such as letters. As Hannah Ingram points out in her discussion of the letters of three fifteenth-century gentry families, household care in middling and higher-status contexts "increasingly fell under [the] purview of experienced female members" in this period.[27] The practice of sharing recipes was "firmly inscribed within women's roles as managers of households," unquestionably seen as part of domestic medicine even as the phenomenon is difficult to access.[28] Those actions are often literally depicted in the *Régime* images, showing book users how they might take a role in their own households and providing us with a particular window into that world.

The Medieval Household and Its Depiction in the *Régime*

The growth and diversification of book audiences on both sides of the Channel in this period points to just one of the many ways that the cultural habits of the court impacted a much wider range of society. Indeed, the scholarly work on medieval royal and elite households provides a strong reminder of the large network of people affiliated with courts.[29] These courts would have included people whose names have survived, such as the children, siblings, in-laws, knights, squires, and *damoiselles*; those who held major offices in the household (and were often nobles), including chamberlains, chaplains, ushers, grooms, keepers of the Wardrobe, the Armoury, the Mint; as well as those whose names rarely survive, such as the workers in the kitchen, cellar, bake house, buttery, and chandlery.[30] A late medieval household might encompass hundreds of people and was made up of individuals from numerous social classes.

What was a household in the later Middle Ages, and why is it relevant to the illustrated copies of the *Régime du corps*? The term "household" can mean a variety of things, including the physical space in which people live, or the group of people who converge and reside in that space. As Sarah Rees Jones points out, "'household' might seem self-evident but [is] actually quite hard to define."[31] The illustrated *Régime* manuscripts may have circulated in households of both the aristocracy and the increasingly wealthy bourgeoisie, two groups that would have had the means to own such rich books. Those households would have in themselves encompassed a spectrum of social classes—from the householders themselves, to family members, officers, and servants, both men and women. In fact, the fourteenth and fifteenth centuries saw a rise in the economic power and social status of the bourgeois, made up of successful merchants and other professions. Such upward mobility was accompanied by a demonstrable drive to attain the same trappings of wealth as the nobility, and these markers of status included consumables like food, clothing, and, most notably, books.

The household is literally on display in the illustrated *Régime* manuscripts, as the activities and scenes that we see in these books—sleeping, bathing, laundering, food preparation and consumption, the disposal of refuse, the delivery of and care of children, and medical care—all took place primarily within the household sphere. Most of these activities contributed to the care of the body, which Felicity Riddy has argued was the primary purpose of the household. Looking after "the concerns of the household" meant servicing the demands of the body; it was precisely that "everyday body" that was the focus of the home.[32] In an effort to think about how medical care took place in the household, and how that is reflected in the *Régime*, it is productive to note that these activities essentially addressed the six non-naturals of humoral medicine. Health care was not exclusively made up of medical treatments or remedies once a person was sick; the maintenance of health considered more broadly includes ongoing care within the home and the preventive care that happened every day.

Those household activities that focused on cleaning, food production, and childcare in one way or another were the responsibilities of women. Depending on the size of a household, these activities were done by servants, who were often managed by women, or more directly handled by the wife and mother of the house.[33] Royal women would have overseen servants who managed many of these activities, and Beatrice's daughters would have been knowledgeable about these concerns. By 1256, all four daughters had been married for some time; they would have been quite familiar with these duties by the time they might have received a copy of Beatrice's text. At the same time, this broad interpretation of health care can be difficult to document, in part because it folds in so seamlessly with the regular activities of home management. Cabré argues that "neither medieval medical resources or women's health agency can be accurately mapped without thorough consideration of the domestic sphere, normally left outside the histories of the art of maintaining health and alleviating illness."[34] Book ownership is undoubtedly an important way to assess an interest in medical information, especially as book collecting expanded with the increased literacy and new purchasing power of the aspiring bourgeoisie. Examining the range of literary genres that overlap with the concerns of household management, including conduct literature, household guides, and recipe compilations, makes women's engagement with health care more pronounced and visible.[35]

The historiated initials of the illustrated *Régime* manuscripts present us with numerous opportunities to think about human interactions in the context of household health care. Conversations or other kinds of exchanges between two people appear primarily in part 1, which focuses on the six non-naturals as well as treatments, and part 2, which deals with body parts and their ailments. In these two sections, we see patients, usually elite, consulting with physicians, as well as with more humbly dressed practitioners, barbers, and physician's assistants administering treatments. The physicians are always men, but the other practitioners appear as both men and women, and the

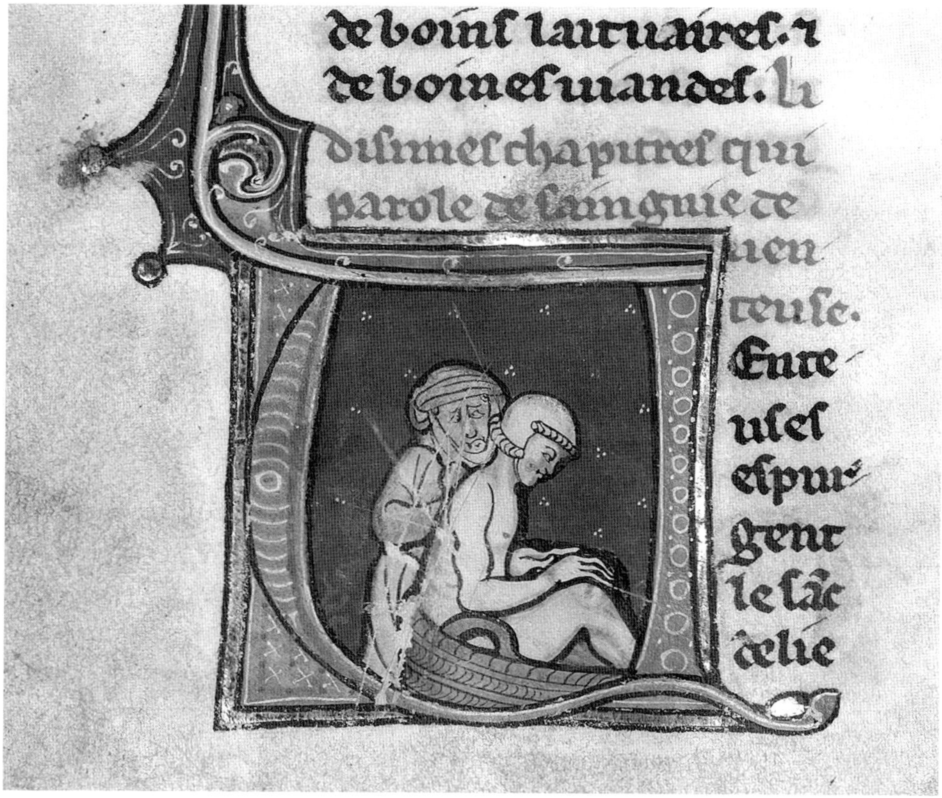

Fig. 72
Cupping, administered by a woman The Bute Painter, *Le Régime du corps*, ca. 1285. Bibliothèque nationale de France, Arsenal MS 2510, fol. 13v, detail. © Bibliothèque nationale de France.

patients are depicted as both men and women as well. In a scene from Arsenal 2510, a woman administers a cup to the back of a man wearing only a coif on his head; her substantial headdress covers her forehead and includes a thick strap that runs under her chin, resembling the fillet-and-barbette style seen in the other earlier *Régime* manuscripts (fig. 72). A handful of other types of encounters are also seen in these manuscripts; the scenes of wet nurse selection would be such an example (see figs. 8, 26, 27). In these first two sections of the *Régime*, most actions are focused on bodies: bodies being treated, or bodies being maintained through clean water, rest, and other environmental factors.

The established medical tradition laid out in my previous chapter, and the university-trained physicians associated with the promotion of that tradition, were clearly just one of the spheres of knowledge that informed the *Régime du corps*. Physicians are depicted in the imagery from the *Régime* manuscripts, but so are other types of practitioners, reflecting how households, including elite ones, engaged with a diversity of treatments. The *Régime* brings together a broader range of knowledges and engages with household guides and other domestically oriented texts as well as the medical tradition. These multivalent sources parallel the wide range of health-care practices in use during the later Middle Ages. A richer understanding of the activities taking place within the household that contributed to health and well-being facilitates

Fig. 73
Cupping, administered by a woman. Medical treatise, ca. 1425–50. British Library, Sloane MS 6, fol. 177v, detail. © The British Library Board.

a fuller appreciation for how the household care is depicted in the illustrated manuscripts' images themselves. All patients, from poor to wealthy, made use of a plethora of practices to maintain health, many of which have a less concrete documentary record because of their ephemerality. Of course, it comes as no surprise that these are often forms of care associated with women's work and women's concerns.

The depiction of female health providers in *Régime* images points to precisely this diversity of medical experience. Some of these women administer treatments that are done by men in other manuscripts, suggesting that women may have been professional health-care providers in some sense; in other cases, they are probably meant to depict members of a household rather than medical practitioners. In Sloane 2435, for instance, we see a female practitioner as she applies heated glass bells to the bare back of a male patient seated in front of her, drawing out the toxins through suction with a method called cupping (see fig. 40). A similar scene shows a woman conducting the cupping procedure in Arsenal 2510 (fig. 72). This depiction of a woman conducting the treatment is unusual, but not unprecedented, and is not limited to the illustrated *Régime*.

Numerous scenes of women conducting cupping treatments exist in other medically related manuscripts, including Sloane 6 and Laud Misc. 724 (figs. 73–74). Sloane 6 is a fifteenth-century English compendium of texts including works by William of Saliceto and John Arderne. It includes a wide range of illustrations, including four of a female practitioner doing a cupping procedure on both male and female patients. A similar series of four scenes appears in Laud Misc. 724, a medical miscellany made in England around 1400. Women help with other treatments, too, as in the scene in the Morgan manuscript in which the vomiting patient is offered aid (see fig. 71). In other cases, the activity is something always administered by women, including the scenes that accompany the chapters on birth and childcare.[36] The inclusion of women alongside men as practitioners in the *Régime* manuscripts encourages consideration of many different types of health care practiced in this period, especially in households in which these books likely circulated and in which women were key participants.

In part 3, which focuses on food and drink, we see household activity from another perspective. While many of the chapters in this section of the *Régime* are represented with still images of foodstuffs—renderings of static plants or individual animals—some of the subjects are illuminated with more active scenes. For example, we see servants actively making cider and beer or sifting grain; another scene shows a cow being milked rather than simply showing a container of milk. Although these are relatively straightforward depictions of food production, such images remind us of the extensive range of activities that would have been taking place in and around medieval aristocratic households. Although these manuscripts' images allude only minimally to the various kinds of mundane labor necessary to run medieval households, that work is not completely absent from the illustrations. Indeed, the unassuming manner in which human waste is evoked in the scenes of vomiting and purging indicates the intimacy inherent in the medieval home.

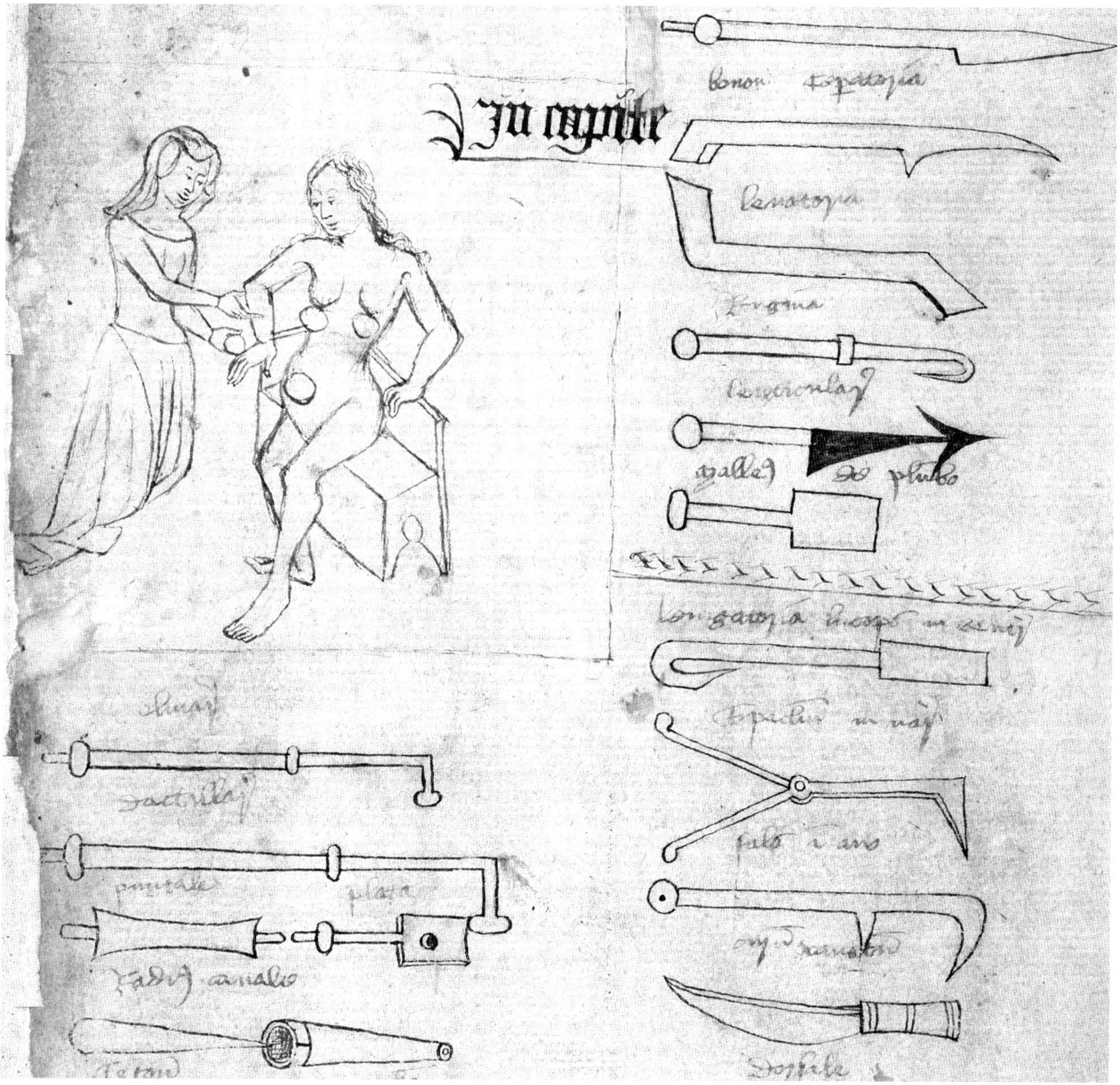
de plumbo

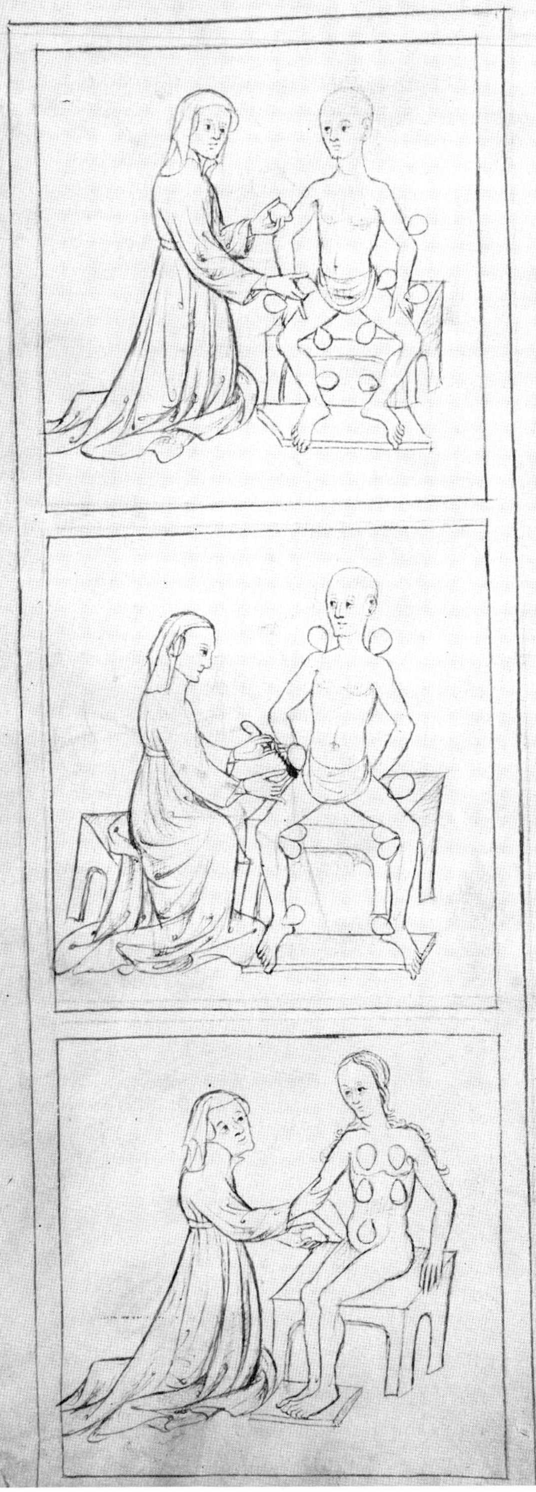

Even with the brief glimpses of the labor that would have permeated the household, the illustrative programs of the *Régime* are unquestionably preoccupied with the people in the household with the most status. Although these historiated initials are consistently small and leave little space for depicting a background or other details, the artists consistently manage to provide remarkable specificity in clothing to establish the status of the people depicted; occasionally even the surroundings indicate status (such as the canopy beds in some of the fifteenth-century childcare scenes). These small details indicate how status was visually constructed within the actual household while also speaking to what the original commissioners of these illustrated copies demanded.

Fig. 74
Cupping, administered by a woman. Surgical treatises, ca. 1400. Bodleian Library, Oxford, MS Laud Misc. 724, fol. 96v. Photo: Bodleian Libraries.

Late Medieval Households and Status

As numerous scholars have pointed out, it can be challenging to pin down just what we mean when we use the term "household." The Middle English word "household" came into use in the late fourteenth century; according to Riddy, it partially replaced the French word "meinie," which referred to a group of people rather than a place.[37] "Household," in contrast, was tied to place, and thus "to the idea of co-location, if not co-residence."[38] The term "referred mainly to a group of people," but people "who lived and worked under the same roof."[39] Maryanne Kowaleski and P. J. P. Goldberg concisely articulate the word's focus on both space and relationships, stating that it "alluded to a particular space (the house where they all lived) as well as to the relationship between the co-residents (relationships often overlaid with the ties of kinship), particularly such everyday routine activities as eating and sleeping."[40] That proximity of people within a shared space is key to our understanding of household health care as well.

Malcolm Vale, in his study of princely courts in the late thirteenth and early fourteenth centuries, contrasts "the household" with "the court," asserting that they should not be seen as synonymous and pointing out that the organization of the household was a necessary part of the court. The household moved around with the itinerant and peripatetic courts of the later Middle Ages, so that, wherever royalty set up their residences, the household was also present.[41] The court was "a protean place, as well as a gathering of people, often fluid in composition and constantly changing," but one that required the ruler to reside in this space; in contrast, the household was a more clearly defined formal body made up of components including the chamber, the wardrobe, and the hall, as well as other types of departments.[42] The household, or at least the royal household, refers primarily to those various offices, staffed by nobility, knights, and family members, that are required to make the court possible (and presumably the servants who did the work of these offices). The court's locational instability distinguishes it from the households of the gentry or urban bourgeois elites, which do seem to be defined more precisely by the established space of the home.

These various definitions point out the different ways we might conceive of households when considering a wider range of social classes. A more stable and spatially defined notion of the household can be tied to the groups slightly lower on the social scale, including the urban wealthy and their peers in the country; these homeowners were far less likely to live an itinerant lifestyle, in contrast with the nobility. The larger houses of the gentry, in contrast to more compact urban homes, would have allowed dwellers more space between people and their bodies. Therefore, the role of the physical home in the creation of the household changed depending on these factors. That the moving household of the court promoted a particularly pronounced change is no surprise, because visitors and temporary residents came and went as the court moved. However, even the stationary household was characterized by permeability, involved as it was in the negotiation of private and public space: "The household functions as a liminal space between the intimate bodily needs of the individual on the one hand and the wider needs and demands of society on the other."[43] In her discussion of the urban households of the burgesses in late medieval English towns, Riddy describes such spaces as a "domestic geography," implying movement between private and public.[44] Within the controlled environment of such spaces, households managed hospitality and private activity along with the various routines necessary for daily life.[45] Living and working happened together in these spaces, and as such, the private and the public merge in a particular kind of domestic living.

What did households look like in this period? How big were they; who was in them; what did those people do; and how were they organized? How many people would have been present at any given time? Obviously the numbers would vary, but here are some basic descriptions to set the stage for my discussion. Bourgeoisie, well-off artisans, and merchants lived in multi-room houses, on several floors and with rooms that had separated, designated purposes. One estimate suggests these homes would have had roughly four to eight rooms, on two or three floors; while not large, they were certainly more spacious than the very small homes (one to two rooms) of the poor.[46] These homes also included an open hall, similar to the aristocratic hall but on a smaller scale. Increasingly these were built of the timber-frame construction that developed in the thirteenth century.[47] These homes were family homes and included parents, children, servants, apprentices, and possibly other temporary workers, such as journeymen. In great houses, many of the concerns of the household were managed by servants; in smaller homes, they were more likely the responsibility of the household's wife and mother.[48] But just because servants facilitated that oversight does not mean that such women were not involved. For instance, Eleanor of Provence, Beatrice's daughter and Queen of England, maintained her own household, the operations of which were dedicated specifically to sustaining the queen and her entourage.[49] There is no question that in this case, she was directly involved in overseeing her household. She was particularly engaged with the lives of her children, including the oversight of their health; she was close with many of her ladies in waiting and consulted frequently with advisors of various kinds.[50] A key difference between bourgeois homes and a great estate seems to have been that, in the former, the woman of the house likely had an even more direct hand in household management; indeed, the immediacy of all aspects of living were probably more pronounced in such homes.[51]

For princes, kings, and other royals, household expenditures were vast, household members numbered in the hundreds, and many visitors made visits to the courts as they traveled. Vale points to instances in which wages were paid over a year to more than one hundred household members in one court, and itineraries that suggest tens if not hundreds of travel days in the course of a year.[52] Estimates for the royal household's size in late fourteenth-century England are around four hundred people.[53] The great houses of rural lords, dukes, and earls would have been smaller, perhaps between forty and 150 or so; wealthy bishops and abbots forty to eighty; with households of barons or rich knights estimated at between twelve and thirty.[54] Eleanor of Provence moved between numerous royal residences in England (Windsor, Winchester, Clarendon, Woodstock, Havering, Guildford, Marlborough, Westminster, and occasionally other manors or hunting lodges) that were very richly furnished and decorated.[55] Anne Rudloff Stanton has mapped a similar "personal geography" across England for Isabella of France, Eleanor's daughter-in-law.[56] Margaret Howell creates a remarkable picture of the extravagant spaces of Eleanor's residences, and mentions many of the individuals who would have been involved in managing their different facets.[57] Eleanor's personal household was physically based in the queen's apartments at Windsor and had its own accounts and people, possibly around one hundred people at its largest: "ladies, knights, *valetti*, senior domestic functionaries such as marshal and steward, cooks and tailors . . . nurses and laundresses, messengers, grooms and carders, together with many serving in much more humble capacities," as well as clerks, doctors, and chaplains.[58]

Although it is difficult to fully represent the income or expenditures of aristocratic households, Christopher Dyer provides a few examples that suggest that incomes could be several thousand pounds.[59] Expenses would also have been extremely wide-ranging at these upper echelons of society. As a way to create a picture of a household like those of Beatrice and her daughters, we might consider the examples of Eleanor of Provence or other members of England's royalty. In late medieval England, the single highest cost for aristocratic households was food, which occasionally approached as much as 50 percent of disbursements, but was usually closer to 25 percent.[60] From November 1304 to November 1305, Edward I's expenditures were around 12,860 pounds, of which around half was related to the kitchen.[61] In another example, Eleanor of Provence's personal household accounts show that she spent one thousand pounds a year on food-related departments, which was more than 50 percent of her receipts in those years.[62] Food preparation was a huge focus for many of the servants in any given household. Certainly, part of this large expense had to do with the many household members and servants who required sustenance themselves, but the cost also reflects the importance of food as a display of wealth. Extravagant feasts featuring foods associated with luxury—fine, white bread, meat (especially game), wine, and spices—were markers of wealth, and the visible exhibition of such foods was seen as the epitome of the aristocratic way of life. As we have seen, food plays a key role in the health care of the *Régime*, and the foodstuffs mentioned are often the kind that should be almost exclusively tied to royal or aristocratic households.

While food and related expenses were a significant expenditure through which one's wealth could be expressed, a number of other kinds of household objects functioned in similar ways, including textiles, clothing, jewelry, silver, and even books. Textiles still made up a significant expenditure, in part because they included everything from bedding and hanging fabrics to sheets and towels, clothing for servants, and clothing for the aristocrats themselves and their families. Items like jewelry and silver, while serving as important display items expressing wealth, were less frequently bought because they were inherited or received as gifts, and they were durable.[63] Books were relatively rare belongings, even among aristocratic owners; Eleanor of Provence stands out as a particularly avid collector of books.[64] While the earlier group of illustrated *Régime* manuscripts probably came out of the royal households of women like Eleanor of Provence or her sister Margaret, the fifteenth-century copies have associations with a wider range of upper-class and wealthy households that were not necessarily of the nobility: rural lords, the gentry, or urban bourgeois patrons.

The Body, Status, and Sartorial Display

As established in chapter 2, the later, fifteenth-century group of illustrated *Régime* copies can be tied to royal owners as well as members of the non-noble upper classes. This trend, which suggests that the popularity of the *Régime du corps* shows an interest in the text from audiences beyond its aristocratic origins, correlates to well-known shifts taking place in the fourteenth and fifteenth centuries. As the urban bourgeoisie grew in status and power with new economic successes, they also aspired to many of the trappings of the nobility. These newly successful members of society naturally employed their newfound wealth for social gain, and we can see numerous ways in which conspicuous consumption increased in this period. The audiences using the illustrated copies of the *Régime du corps* definitely understood them as objects of display and signifiers of wealth. The manuscripts depict the households in which the books themselves were stored, used, and shared. Book collecting and fashion were both ways for participants to indicate their wealth in the domestic sphere or household. The books also display status in their images, on the bodies of those represented through their clothing. Household finery, the popularity of household guides, and a growing participation in book culture and fashion all indicate the ambitious nature of consumption and display among members of this class.

In many ways, the increased buying power and aspirational display of the newly wealthy classes was a threat to the nobility, who had much at stake in maintaining the existing hierarchical class structures. Indeed, in this period upward mobility, especially from the wealthy bourgeoisie to the nobility, was increasingly possible as the line between these classes became blurred. Such mobility was tied to the display of wealth and the consumption of rare products and items made with lavish materials. The increased display of wealth by such consumers, which represented the instability of the distinction between the nobility and the urban wealthy, led to the creation of sumptuary laws. In both France and England in this period, laws were enacted to reinforce existing hierarchical structures and to prevent various groups from encroaching upon the position of the elite.[65] Although these laws varied in content, they generally articulated regulations about who was able to wear certain kinds of clothing, textiles, materials, or jewelry. It is commonly thought that these laws were largely ineffectual, and their rearticulation for more than two centuries indicates as much. It is not a coincidence that an increased interest in fashions and the proliferation of conduct books happened simultaneously; as Krueger points out, these were "contingent phenomena" that speak to "the ambivalence and volatility of social identity in a period of intense historical change."[66]

Clothing and jewelry were clearly important markers of status, and, as newly wealthy groups attempted to express their burgeoning power, they inevitably mimicked the popular fashions of the social elite. Before the mid-fourteenth century the clothing of virtually everyone was similar and relatively modest. Such clothing most commonly started with a long, plain undergarment, called the chemise or chainse, often made of linen. Over this, a finer bliaut was worn, essentially a long, flowing robe. The bliaut was often worn by women with a loose belt, with slits or loose sleeves, and a simple, unrevealing neckline.[67] One of the most popular styles of headwear for women was the fillet and barbette; the fillet was a stiff band of linen or silk worn around the head, and the barbette was a band of linen that went under the chin. These were sometimes combined with a hairnet around braided or bundled hair, sometimes called the crespine (or crespinette).[68] This description of thirteenth-century dress generally aligns with the clothing of most of the figures in the earlier group of illustrated *Régime* manuscripts and, for the most part, seems to have been the fashion in both regions; Margaret Scott, for instance, describes the headdress with the chin strap as typical of Franco-English fashions during this period.[69] Supporting this assessment, the women in Sloane 2435 generally wear long robes with long sleeves, punctuated only by a thin girdle or belt that sits loosely over the hips (fig. 75; see also fig. 16). The collar of this garment is at the neck and unadorned, and the sleeves are long and fit close to the arm. The distinctions between lower- and upper-class women are relatively minimal and are most pronounced in the images in which the women appear together, such as the wet nurse scene (see figs. 8, 27). In this case, the primary difference is the headwear; both women seem to wear a hairnet, but the more elite figure also wears a fillet and barbette. We see similar styles in BnF Fr. 12323, which is expected, since the illustrative programs of these two manuscripts have so much in common (see fig. 26). In the pregnancy scene from BnF Fr. 12323 (see fig. 38), the woman consulting the physician actually resembles the wet nurse in the following chapter's scene with two women, reinforcing the class differences that are often articulated by clothing throughout the manuscripts.

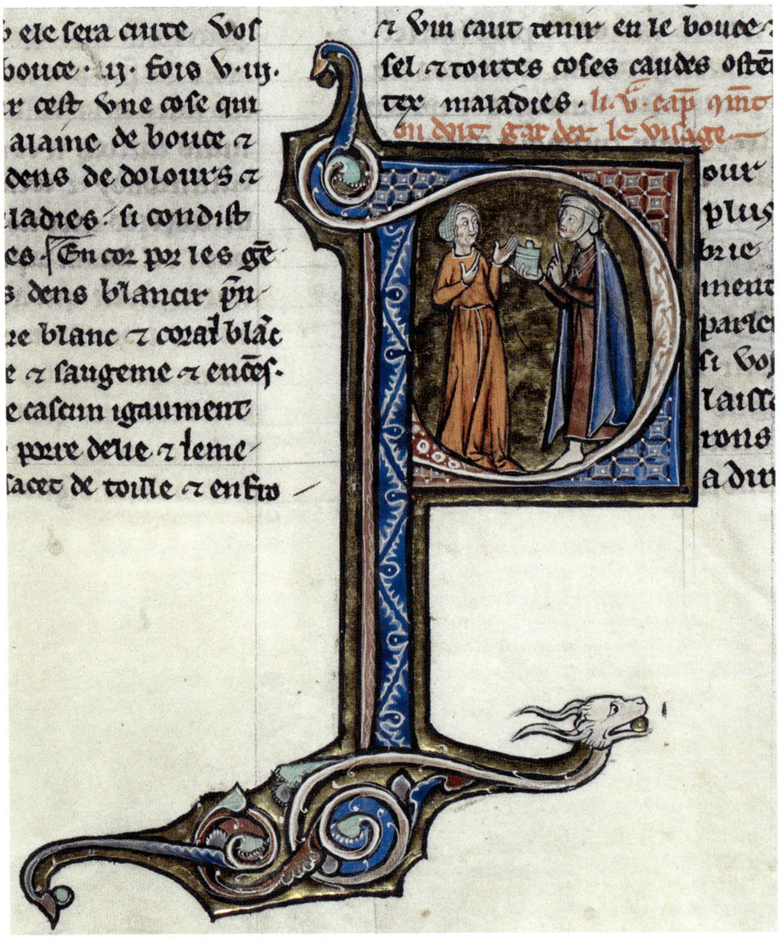

In Sloane 2435 and BnF Fr. 12323, the physician is usually shown wearing a brightly colored robe over another long garment, with slit armholes that expose the arm underneath; occasionally he also wears a hood over the shoulders of this garment. The headwear of the physician is also distinct from other figures; in both of these manuscripts the doctors wear a puffy, round, beret-like hat, often with a ball at the top (fig. 76).[70] Furthermore, in BnF Fr. 12323, various figures hold a pair of white gloves, presumably removed to facilitate the procedure. At times these gloves are held by the physicians, and in some cases they are held by patients.[71] Some male figures hold removed gloves in the Leipzig manuscript as well (see fig. 56). Throughout these manuscripts, male workers often display shorter tunics, with simple white coifs covering their heads. The close-fitting coif was an extremely common headdress, appearing abundantly in medieval art across media; usually covering the ears and laced under the chin, it could be worn alone but was also worn underneath another type of headdress (for example, see figs. 1, 11, 14, 22–23, 40, 58, and 72). In Arsenal 2510, uncovered heads are more common, and generally fewer markers of status are exhibited than in Sloane 2435 and BnF Fr. 12323 (see figs. 7, 34, 69, and 84). A practitioner with an uncovered head and shorter tunic is also seen in some scenes from the Leipzig manuscript, but other markers of identity appear in the images. For example, in the image from the chapter on ears, the knives and other tools seen in the upper left corner indicate that this is a surgeon or barber (see fig. 2).

The later group of illustrated *Régime* manuscripts clearly reflects the social changes taking place in this period. As Krueger and others point out, the fourteenth and fifteenth centuries were a period of great instability and upheaval in which distinctions in status between the nobility and the increasingly wealthy bourgeoisie shifted.[72] (Of course, some of that upheaval was the result of health-related chaos, including pandemics.) As aspiring urban elites sought to replicate aristocratic life, they appropriated many of the newest fashions. In the mid-fourteenth century, the tunic went out of fashion and more fitted garments with round sleeves became popular, while elite men's and women's clothing became more distinct along gender lines. Men's clothing

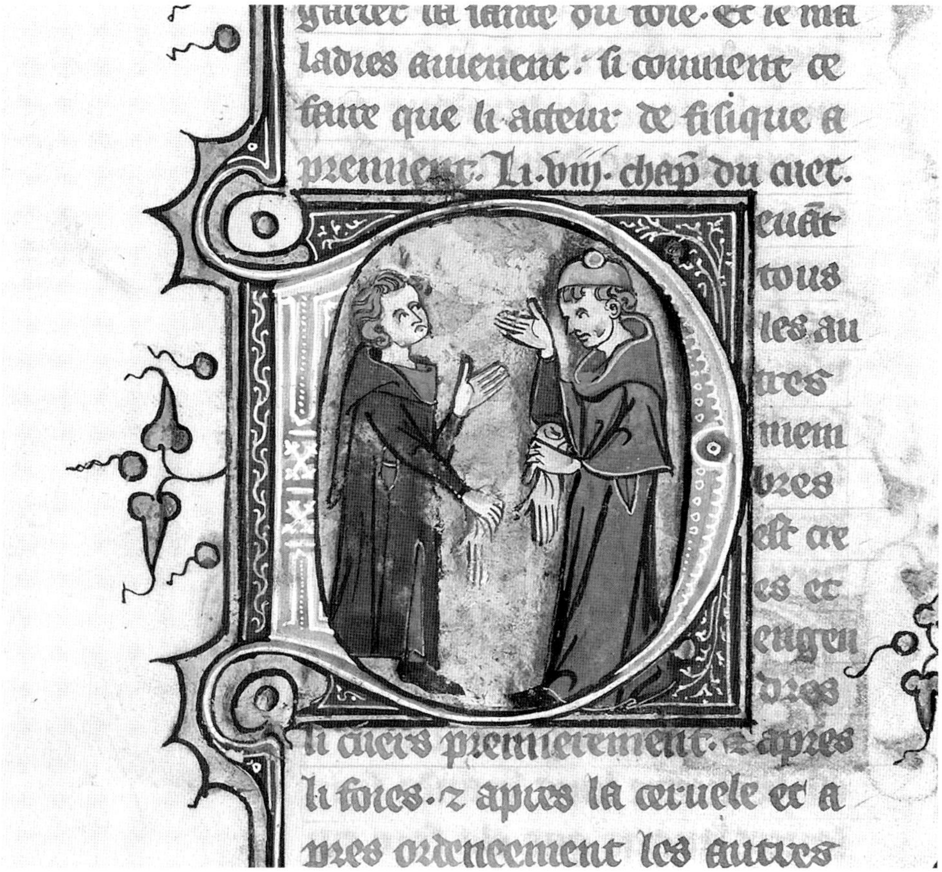

Fig. 75 (opposite)
Complexion. *Le Régime du corps*, ca. 1265–70. British Library, Sloane MS 2435, fol. 37r, detail. © The British Library Board.

Fig. 76
Heart. *Le Régime du corps*, fourteenth century. Bibliothèque nationale de France, Fr. 12323, fol. 105v, detail. © Bibliothèque nationale de France.

moved toward short, formfitting pourpoints or doublets with legs showing.[73] In the popular dress for women, we see a tightening of the bodice and plunging necklines. Both men and women are depicted wearing a showy outer garment called a houppelande. Increasingly elaborate headdresses also appear, like the built-up or padded bourrelet, as well as various spherical, cylindrical, or two-horned shapes; men wore increasingly complex chaperons, while women donned horned or padded headdresses.[74] Most of these styles appear in some form across Europe, demonstrating the "unity of style" in the years between 1380 and 1420, and similar fashions were popular in both England and France.[75]

Indeed, many of these fashion trends can be seen in the fifteenth-century illustrated copies of the *Régime*. For example, many women in these manuscripts wear the somewhat horned headdresses prominent in this period; they also wear robes (or cotehardies) that are more fitted and tightly belted high on the waist, which often have lower and more elaborate necklines. In the image of the book-holding woman from the pregnancy chapter of the Morgan manuscript, the woman's cloak has long sleeves that appear to be lined in ermine (fig. 77). Many of the upper-class men don the latest fashion of shorter robes that display their stockinged legs, although physicians are

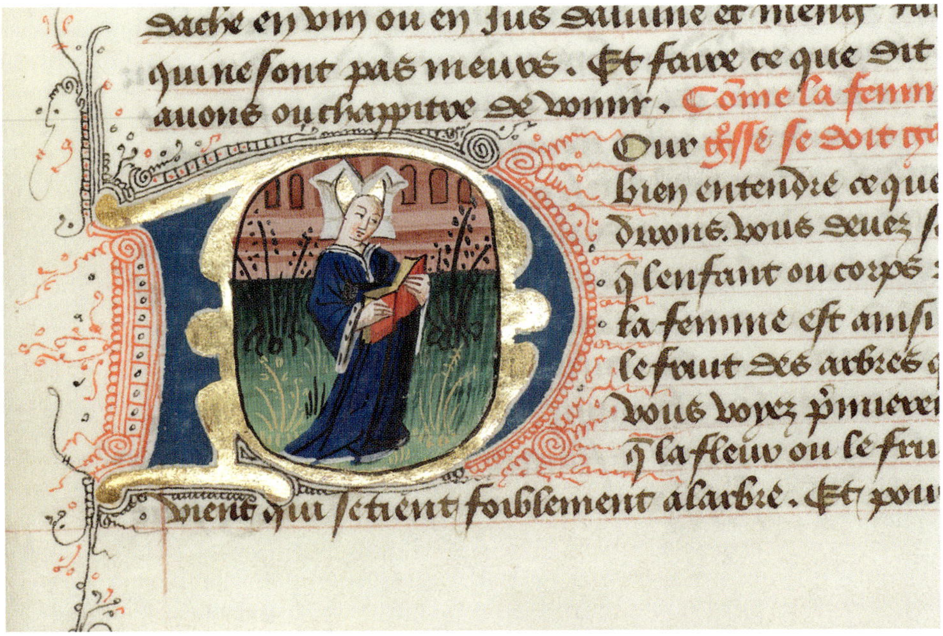

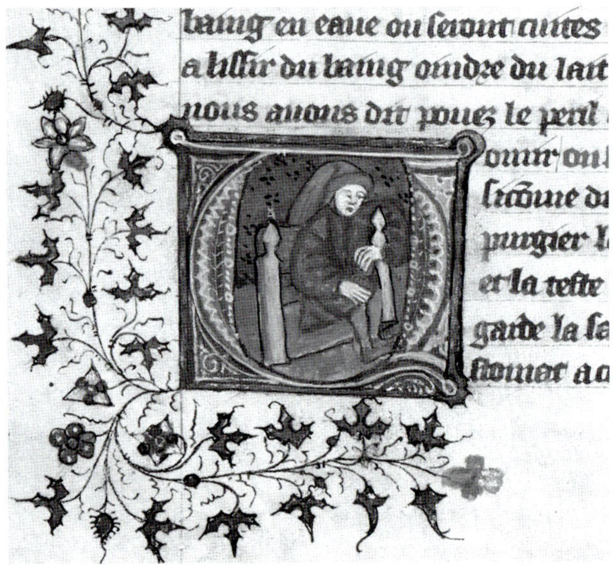

Fig. 77
Pregnancy. *Le Régime du corps*, ca. 1440–50. The Morgan Library & Museum, MS M.165, fol. 42r, detail. The Morgan Library & Museum, New York. Purchased by J. Pierpont Morgan (1837–1913) in 1902.

Fig. 78
Vomiting. *Le Régime du corps*, ca. 1450. Cambridge University Library, MS Ii.V.11, fol. 26v, detail. Reproduced by kind permission of the Syndics of Cambridge University Library.

shown in different instances wearing both the shorter style and longer robes (see figs. 35, 36, 60). In other examples, physicians wear robes with a tall collar, and even some that sport an ermine lining (see fig. 57).[76] Hats for men seem to be primarily floppy chaperons worn in various configurations; female servants also wear wrapped headwear resembling the chaperon (fig. 78).[77]

What should we make of these observations about various styles of dress found in the illustrated copies of the *Régime*? Obviously, representations of people in manuscripts like these do not necessarily depict either specific patrons or even real, lived experience. Nevertheless, the inclusion of these figures, with their fashionable dress and air of elitism, probably does gesture toward the audiences for these books: either the nobility in general, or perhaps the increasingly wealthy bourgeois consumers of books who were becoming more abundant in this period. Nonroyal audiences were potentially involved in collecting these books, and these images demonstrate the popularity of these fashions. The illuminations may not be complicated enough to depict elaborate textiles or jewelry, but they still contain enough markers of status to reflect the importance and social standing that fashion gained in this period. As Kreuger points out, the widespread popularity of conduct books followed the distribution of clothing and textiles, which were all signifiers of status; such books "followed the pan-European journey of stylish textiles, through whose changing designs elite women and men attempted to negotiate the instabilities of late medieval culture."[78] The role of fashion in conveying status is reflected not only in the content of conduct books or household guides but also in the ownership and copying of the books themselves—something we can also point to in the case of the illustrated *Régime* manuscripts as well as other kinds of illustrated books.

Illustrated Encyclopedic Guides

The emphasis on fashion as a marker of status is certainly not limited to the images from the *Régime du corps* manuscripts. Ostentatious sartorial display often accompanies luxurious books, including books that, like the *Régime*, provide insights into household practices or health management. For example, late medieval illustrated copies of the *Tacuinum sanitatis* are a related but independent tradition that makes use of similar devices couched in a different visual format. As two texts with robust pictorial traditions, the illustrated manuscripts of the *Tacuinum sanitatis* and those of the *Régime du corps* both contain a variety of subjects that addressed household practices that range widely beyond medicine. The pictorial traditions each visualize the world in which these books were likely used, although the *Tacuinum sanitatis* prioritizes growing, harvesting, and preparing foods, as well as general practices for maintaining the space of the home, while the *Régime* focuses on how such preparations support wellness and health treatment, often facilitated through human interaction. Each tradition depicts the domestic spaces of the household, conjuring an environment similar to that with which numerous conduct and household guides were concerned. Indeed, both the *Tacuinum sanitatis* and the *Régime* engage with both medical and nonmedical textual and pictorial traditions, bridging similar generic divides but doing so with different results.

The *Tacuinum sanitatis* describes guidelines for healthy living that are similar to the *Régime du corps*; it was also the result of a thirteenth-century translation of an older Arabic text. The eleventh-century Arabic text *Taqwīm al-ṣiḥḥa* was compiled by Ibn Buṭlān, a Christian physician working in eleventh-century Damascus; the text was translated in the mid-thirteenth century at the Sicilian court.[79] The original text presented its information in the form of forty tables (*taqwīm*), which provided for easy consultation by a wide range of readers.

The later illustrated *Tacuinum* manuscripts reduced the text and in its place added large, nearly full-page illustrations, with the *mise-en-page* including an identification word at the top of the page and a few brief sentences below the image. These highly decorated copies were produced in northern Italy around 1380–1400 and were probably commissioned by Giangaleazzo Visconti, count of Milan, or those connected to his court.[80] Cathleen Hoeniger asserts that these illustrated *Tacuinum* manuscripts would not have been used for gaining medical or scientific knowledge, since so many copies of important scientific treatises were already in the Visconti Library through Giangaleazzo's avid collecting.[81] While the *Régime du corps* was clearly seen as a text that contained valuable knowledge, with its initials being useful through their indexical qualities, both extensively illustrated traditions were likely intended as display objects and status symbols for wealthy owners.

The illustrated *Tacuinum sanitatis* tradition covers many of the same topics as the *Régime* manuscripts, including a variety of non-naturals (such as coitus, bathing, vomiting, and climate or the seasons) and substances (plants, herbs, animal meat, cheese, and dairy). Additionally, related topics such as chatting, summer and winter rooms, clothing, dancing, horsemanship, fencing, and hunting are included in the *Tacuinum*; for the most part, the *Tacuinum* leaves out direct references to specific medical treatments or procedures such as bloodletting, leeching, or cupping. Entries on meat show an entire butcher shop, rather than simply the animal isolated in empty space, and even the copulation scene, on some level similar to the tradition informing the *Régime* images, includes not just the bedroom but the entire architectural structure in which the activity takes place. At the same time, many more substances, in particular plants, are covered in the *Régime*, especially in the more abundantly illustrated copies of the fifteenth century.

The *Tacuinum* images are notably different from those in the illustrated *Régime* manuscripts, especially in terms of size and form. Most obviously, the *mise-en-page* of the *Tacuinum* manuscripts provides for a much larger image size and thus space in which to embellish the surroundings of the scene depicted.[82] Some of these expanded backgrounds are landscapes, while others display elaborate architecture, often cutaways that offer the viewer the rich details of a busy interior space. In contrast to the *Régime* images of cheese (see figs. 41–43), the Paris copy of the *Tacuinum sanitatis* displays several separate scenes on the topic—new cheese and old cheese, as well as ricotta—with complete views of interior rooms where cheese is being produced or stored (fig. 79). Although these interior scenes do not provide absolute clarity about all the steps that go into making cheese, they give us a sense of certain aspects of the process, such as how the space was organized and decorated, or how much cheese might be produced at one time. Thus, in these nearly full-page images with extensive backgrounds, which often include multiple figures, the *Tacuinum* manuscripts offer a relationship between text and image that is significantly different from the historiated initials and more extensive text of the *Régime* manuscripts. The *Tacuinum* images seem crafted to foster slow looking and admiration; the *Régime* initials, on the other hand, while they certainly display markers of luxury and some whimsical, entertaining scenes, still function as chapter headings and potential finding aids at which a reader might only glance.

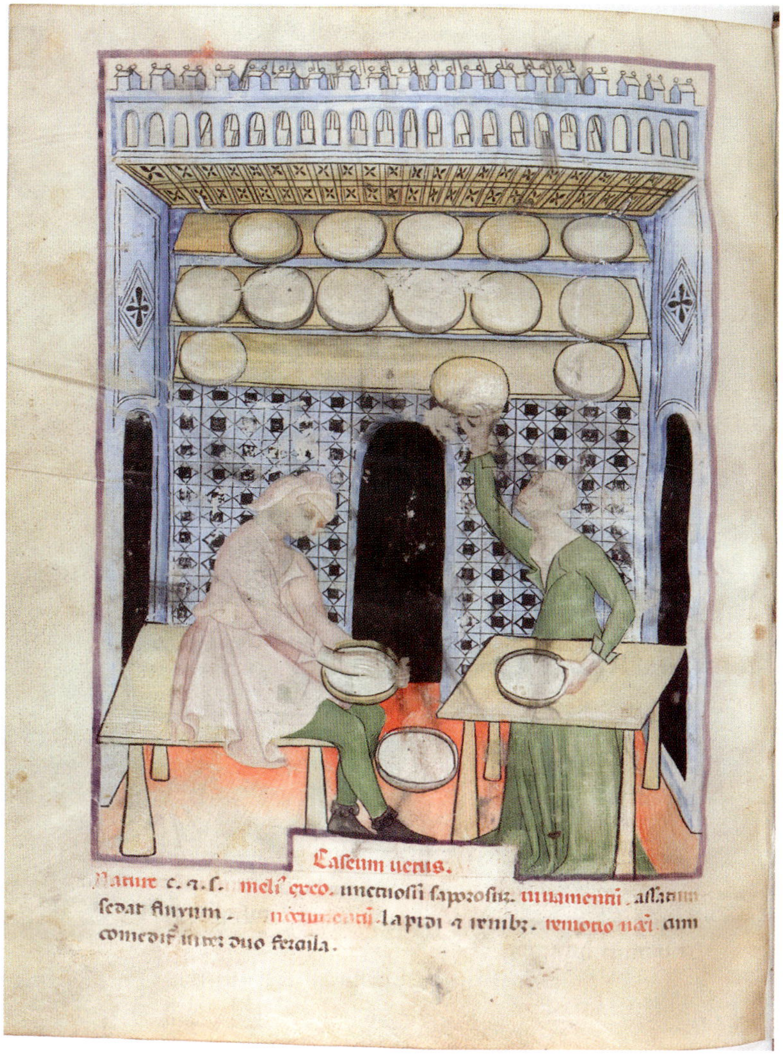

Fig. 79
Old cheese. *Tacuinum sanitatis*, late fourteenth century. Bibliothèque nationale de France, MS Nouv. acq. lat. 1673, fol. 59v. © Bibliothèque nationale de France.

Although plants are the focus of numerous images in illustrated *Tacuinum* manuscripts, and scholars have made connections between them and the images in herbals, they seem far removed from the herbal tradition. As in the *Régime*, a kind of genre hybridity can be seen in the *Tacuinum*. Hoeniger connects it to herbals, courtly love and romance literature, and the iconography of the idealized feudal estate.[83] In some sense, the herbal tradition seems more pronounced in the *Régime du corps* manuscripts, where chapters present a repetitive series of images of plants without people. In the *Tacuinum*, for example, a scene of harvesting depicts two people dressed in extremely fine clothing and jewelry (fig. 80). On the left, a woman in a pink robe with a long skirt, loose, fringed sleeves, and a fitted bodice reaches toward the man. The dress and her pearl necklace emphasize her pale skin and hair. To the right, a man holds a melon; he wears fitted hose and a blue tunic, a fashionable ensemble complemented by the large chain around his neck and a golden crown. This manuscript's focus on "love themes and fashionable dress" implies a strong tie to pictorial models in the chivalric tales of romance narratives, emphasizing an idealized courtly life amid the natural world.[84] Even in the images of crops that include laborers, the workers seem dressed in unexpectedly refined and brightly colored garments. Paralleling a common interpretation for the idealized world portrayed in the *Très riches heures* of Jean, Duke of Berry (produced between 1412 and 1416 in France by the Limbourg Brothers), the portrayal of happy workers contributes to the overall utopian picture of well-managed and successful rural estates. These affinities with such romance traditions further emphasize the wide range of sources, medical and

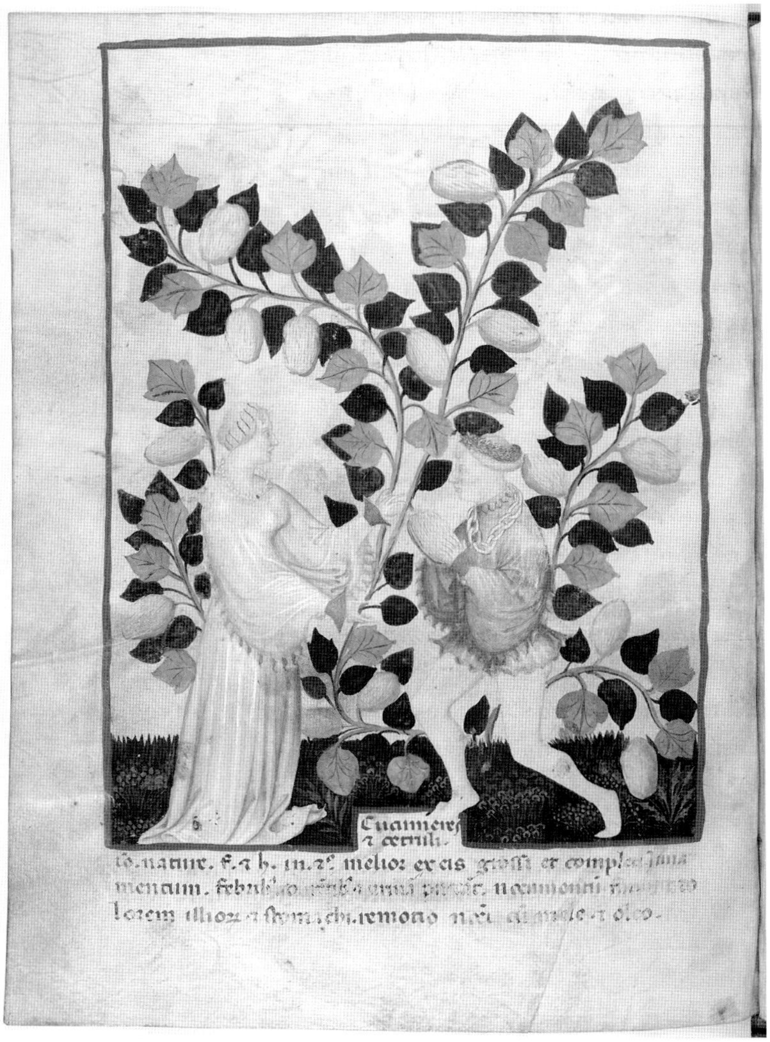

Fig. 80
Watermelon, cucumber. *Tacuinum sanitatis*, late fourteenth century. Bibliothèque nationale de France, MS Nouv. acq. lat. 1673, fol. 38v. © Bibliothèque nationale de France.

Fig. 81
Theriac. *Tacuinum sanitatis*, mid-fifteenth century. Bibliothèque nationale de France, MS Lat. 9333, fol. 51v. © Bibliothèque nationale de France.

nonmedical, that inform the illustrated *Tacuinum*.

One of the *Tacuinum sanitatis* manuscripts includes a particularly evocative scene for "Theriac," which depicts three men in a shop that includes an entrance for customers and an open counter behind which two purveyors stand (fig. 81). Theriac was a compound substance used for any number of different ailments (most notably poisons and the plague). Sometimes involving as many as eighty ingredients, including notable substances such as opium, it was apparently challenging to prepare; it is unsurprising that it was also under tight professional controls.[85] The illustrated scene displays the somewhat expected characteristics of a medieval pharmacy, including rows of bottles and jars lining the shelves in the background. A well-dressed customer stands in the doorway, involved in an exchange with a bearded man we may assume is the pharmacist; another figure, a beardless assistant in more modest attire and his head uncovered, is in the background preparing a medicine. Both the customer and the apothecary wear fashionable chaperons on their heads, a sign of their relative status as part of a wealthy merchant class. This pharmacist is the closest we get to a medical practitioner in the *Tacuinum sanitatis*, and his clothing suggests a somewhat similar social rank to that of the successful physician shown in the illustrated copies of the *Régime*.[86]

This image epitomizes the differences between the illustrated traditions of the *Régime* and the *Tacuinum*. Apothecary scenes are not prevalent in the *Régime du corps*, nor is theriac the topic of a chapter.[87] One of the few instances of such a scene can be found in Besançon Bibliothèque municipale MS 463, a fifteenth-century copy of the *Régime*; the manuscript's only image appears at the beginning and depicts a woman, her hand reaching for her purse, at a shop overseen by a male apothecary holding a jar (fig. 82). The woman shopping for *materia medica* in this scene demonstrates the likelihood that such women facilitated domestic medicine in their homes. In fact, guidance for exactly this action—obtaining ingredients from the apothecary—is provided with instructions for a compound remedy that accompanies Sloane 2401, another illustrated copy of the *Régime*.[88] Despite the full-page expansion of the topics included in the illustrated *Tacuinum* manuscripts, they provide virtually no representations of caregivers, physicians, or treatment scenes in their depictions of a refined lifestyle.[89] This absence is especially pronounced alongside the illustrated copies of the *Régime*, in which we see a noteworthy prevalence of physicians and other practitioners in the comparatively small images.

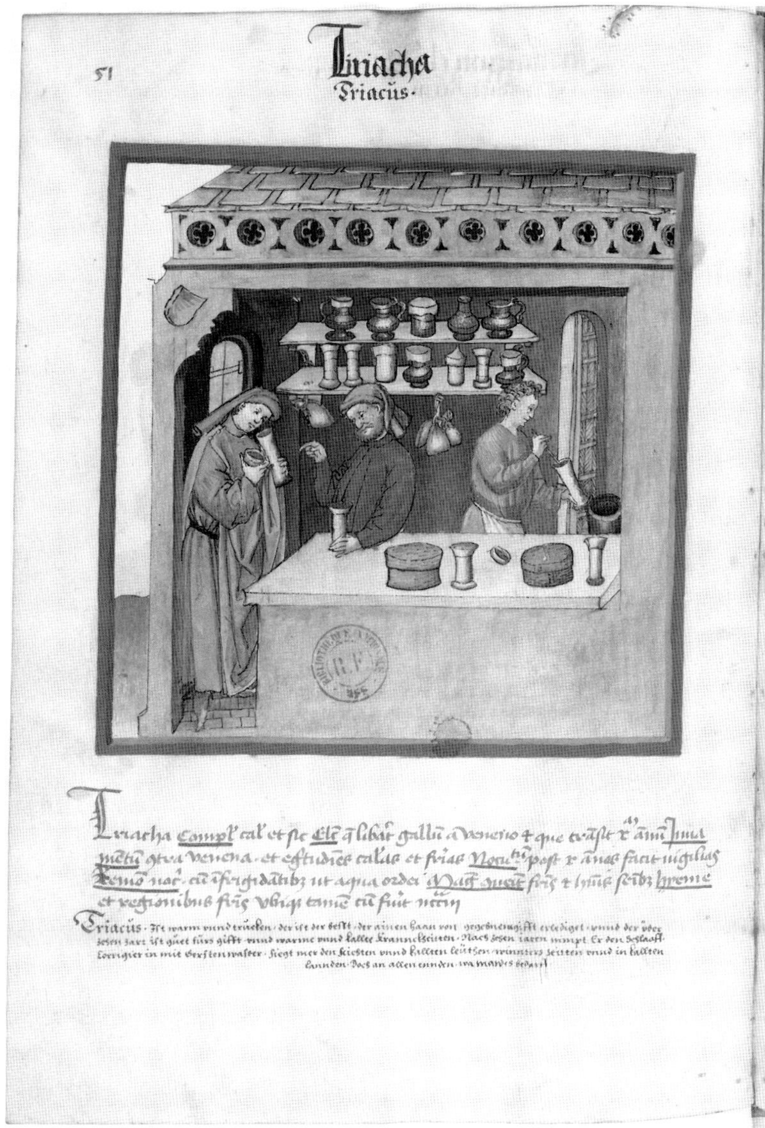

These contrasts reflect, at least in part, the different contexts and purposes of these two illustrative traditions. The Visconti court of Milan, characterized by overt luxury, commissioned these picture books in the tradition of chivalric literature, herbals, and other types of encyclopedias rather than as a medical aid, whereas the *Régime du corps* manuscripts, presumably created to facilitate household health management, required more extensive, useful text along with illustration. Historiated initials, which inherently serve to guide users through a manuscript's content, signal a fundamentally different pictorial role and relationship to the text in the book.[90] The minimal text and picture-book format of the illustrated *Tacuinum* manuscripts emphasize ostentatious display, and the content of those images further reinforces that association with opulence. While this is certainly a factor in how we read the illustrated *Régime* manuscripts, the inclusion of physicians as well as numerous treatment and related scenes makes clear their prioritization of health and wellness.

Household Care of the "Everyday Body"

Everyday activities are *the* central focus of the image programs in the illustrated *Régime* manuscripts, celebrated by way of both the high quality of illuminations and the sheer number of scenes in each book. This bringing together of the luxurious and

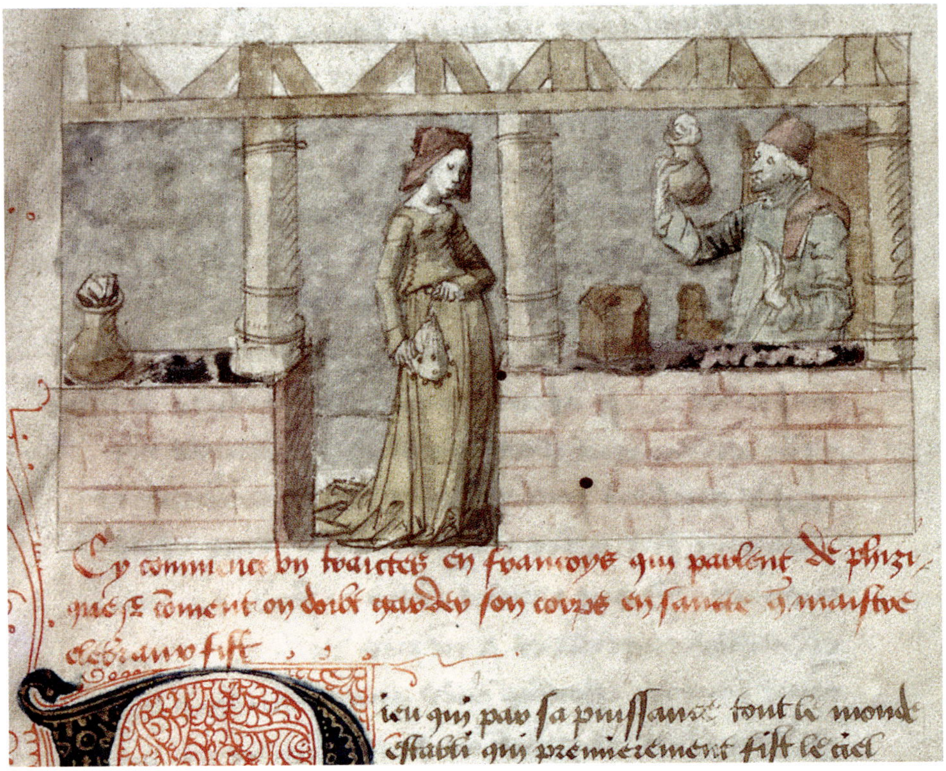

Fig. 82
Frontispiece with pharmacy scene. *Le Régime du corps*, fifteenth century. IRHT-CNRS, Bibliothèque municipale de Besançon, MS 463, fol. 1, detail. Bibliothèque municipale de Besançon.

the mundane is less perplexing, however, if we think about the actual experiences of people within upper-class households; indeed, the mundane (food, for example) could simultaneously be an expression of status. As Riddy has described it, the care of the body, "the everyday body," was the center of the late medieval urban household.[91] By this she means that most of the activities that took place in the household, many of which were routine, were involved somehow in the management of bodies, either directly through actions like feeding or indirectly through supervision of the environment in which those bodies lived. By "servicing the demands of the body," households were spaces in which their members oversaw and facilitated many essential activities: "eating, sleeping, washing, getting dressed and undressed, preparing the food and clearing it away; raising the children; tending the sick and dying."[92] Many of these aspects of bodily care reflect almost verbatim the six non-naturals of humoral medicine, which included air quality, movement and rest, sleeping and waking, food and drink, excretions and waste, and the passions or emotions. The content covered by the text of the *Régime du corps* closely reflects the six non-naturals, as the different sections of the text make clear. Despite the long legacy of the six non-naturals in the history of medical thought, however, the everyday quality of many of these activities have no doubt contributed to the characterizations of regimen texts as unsophisticated or made up of commonsense practices. But within these manuscripts, these less celebrated topics are handled with the same importance as other topics that might seem more appropriate for illustration. They benefit from the level playing field created by the format of the historiated initial; all the scenes appear at the same size and are emphasized to the same degree. The illustrated *Régime* manuscripts provide an unequivocal demonstration of the value of these household activities that support the care of the body. They may not always be especially action-filled scenes, but they remain fraught with potentiality for health or the loss of it.

Food is abundantly represented in the illustrated *Régime* manuscripts; in Sloane 2435, for example, forty-four of the seventy-two initials depict food or its ingestion, and in the later Cambridge manuscript, 115 of 143 do so. These foods include grains, meats, dairy, beverages, and spices—many of which would have been consumed primarily by the wealthy of society. The production and consumption of food was a primary focus in the medieval household; the majority of servants' time was dedicated to food preparation and serving, and food was usually the largest expenditure for aristocratic households.[93] Eating food was not just about sustenance and nutrition, though obviously those essential needs were being met; as the significant focus on it in regimen literature suggests, food was the primary tool moderating the humors and thus preserving health.[94] Related to this, balance or moderation—not overindulging—was a virtue espoused by late medieval conduct literature. For example, in "Dietary," a relatively popular fifteenth-century conduct poem likely oriented toward wealthy householders, Lydgate repeatedly comes back to the notion of being measured in one's consumption, especially in terms of private eating (as opposed to conspicuous public display). Claire Sponsler has argued that this shift in consideration from public to private consumption illuminates the changes in the "self-fashioning bourgeois consumer."[95] In the *Ménagier* too, the author advocates for restraint and responsible behavior, despite the ostentatious lifestyle indicated by the text as a whole.[96] Such recommendations appear in the *Régime* as well; we might recall the reservations about cheese discussed in chapter 2.

Of course, those who had access to many of these foods—meat, fish, game, spices—were already in a privileged position, and food's association with status is abundantly evident in texts such as the *Ménagier* or the *Tacuinum sanitatis* as well as the *Régime*. Aristocratic households had a focus on meat, fish, and game; the latter in particular was associated with an aristocratic lifestyle, since hunting was well established as a solely aristocratic privilege. Some of this focus had to do with the rarity or availability of substances.[97] For instance, venison was deemed especially valuable, as was signaled through its use as a gift as well as its selective consumption at special occasions. Such value was also attributed to a number of spices and other imported substances, while the range of spices used depended on the wealth of a household. Even somewhat modest houses could afford some imported items, such as dried fruits, almonds, or rice; cinnamon, cloves, ginger, mace, pepper, and sugar were more expensive (and saffron especially so) and therefore were seen primarily in magnate households.[98] In one documented instance, expensive spices, wild animal meat, and gold leaf for the

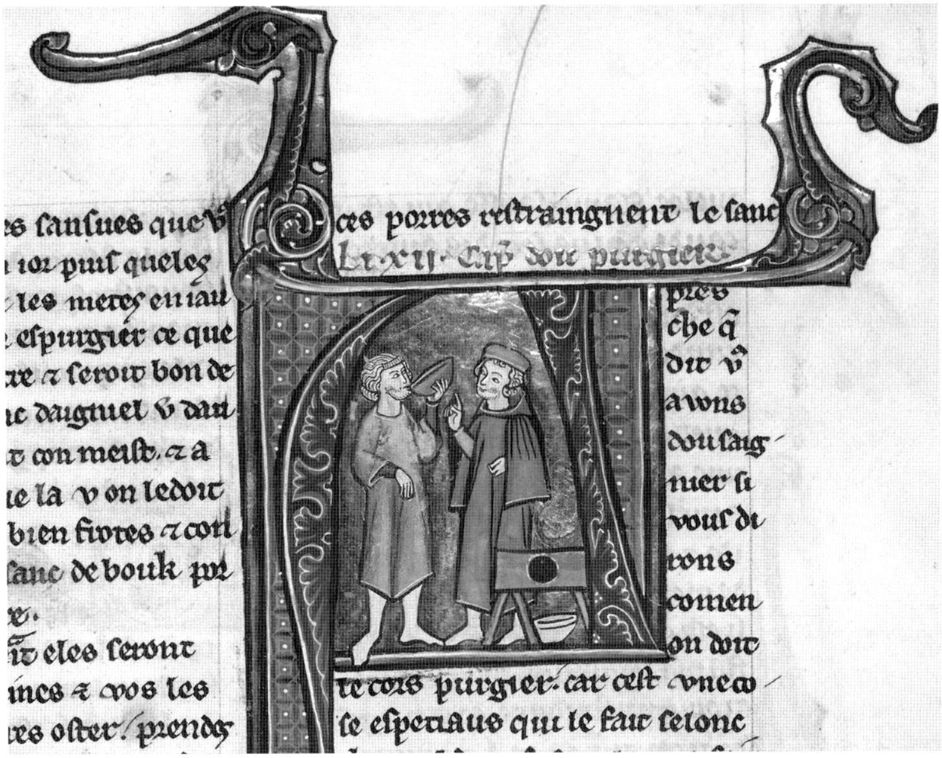

Fig. 83
Purging. *Le Régime du corps*, ca. 1265–70. British Library, Sloane MS 2435, fol. 16r, detail. © The British Library Board.

decoration of food were ordered for a large feast.[99] This example eloquently demonstrates the interrelatedness of different forms of conspicuous consumption, including the shared materiality of books and food. The menus and recipes detailed in *Le ménagier de Paris* also show these practices. Although aimed at a wealthy bourgeois audience, these recipes were clearly modeled on aristocratic traditions; just the cost of the spices required by the recipes would have been substantial.[100] Feasts were an essential part of upper-class culture, and despite the call for moderation in some forms of conduct literature, overabundance and the display of wealth were clearly used as indicators of status.

Food production in an upper-class bourgeois or aristocratic household affected not just the elite members of the household, of course, but also servants and other household workers, many of whom would have also been deeply involved in the preparation of these consumables. For larger households, a significant volume of food needed to be produced, and an equivalent amount of labor went into that production. Many of these activities were no doubt rather mundane and repetitive, in part because they needed to happen every day. The focus on the display of large feasts masks the labor that went into these kinds of special events as well as everyday eating. Such labor does appear occasionally in the images of the illustrated copies of the *Régime*, in scenes of food preparation such as stirring apple mush for cider or sifting rice. Even more invisible than such preparatory labor would have been the accompanying work of cleaning up after food preparation and meals, disposing of waste, and dealing with the human waste of food consumption.

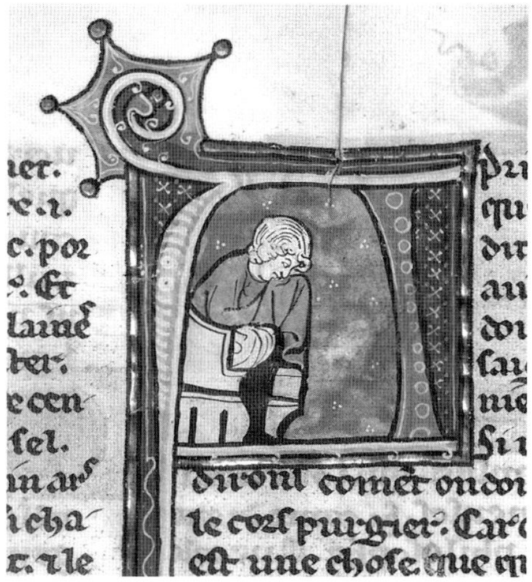

Fig. 84
Purging. The Bute Painter, *Le Régime du corps*, ca. 1285. Bibliothèque nationale de France, Arsenal MS 2510, fol. 15v, detail. © Bibliothèque nationale de France.

Food preparation and consumption obviously led to other activities that were just as prevalent in households. As Riddy points out, "eating and defecating are central activities to be managed by household routines; they are the business of the kitchen and the privy."[101] Especially in more compact urban bourgeois homes, these activities would have been simply a familiar part of living in close quarters, in which people inevitably had close-up and intimate knowledge of their coinhabitants. That embodied intimacy, which we see in a general lack of squeamishness, indicates an awareness of a shared humanness that might be one reason we see a surprising frankness in topics covered in conduct literature and in some of the scenes depicted in the illustrated *Régime* texts. Comfort with this level of intimacy and messiness no doubt facilitated the care of bodies that were understood to be "needy, vulnerable, hungry, cold, growing up and growing old, endlessly leaky"; indeed, everyday bodies.[102] Perhaps if regimen texts like the one ostensibly commissioned by Beatrice were intended to facilitate the care of exactly these kinds of bodies, it should not be a surprise that some of these activities are also depicted.

In the *Régime* initials, defecating and vomiting are treated as significantly as bloodletting or sleep. For instance, in the image of purging from Sloane 2435, one man holds a cup up to the other man, who drinks from it; the figure on the right asserts his authority with a gesture of command (fig. 83). The particular subject of this image might be missed with only a cursory glance, but the diminutive seat and bowl depicted in the lower right of the image clearly indicate the next step in this particular narrative. In contrast, the image of this scene from Arsenal 2510 shows the patient actually sitting on the seat (fig. 84). The frankness of these images, even though they reflect the specific context of health treatment rather than everyday evacuation, asserts a comfort with bodily intimacy when it came to the maintenance of health in the domestic sphere.

The act of defecation also occasionally appears in other kinds of manuscripts, for example in the margins or *bas-de-page* of a book of hours. In a highly decorated Flemish example of this popular genre from around 1300, one man defecates while another collects the results and offers them to a lady (fig. 85). According to Michael Camille, an image like this is meant to present a parodic commentary on courtly culture; rather than being offensive, the success of such images lies in a certain comfort

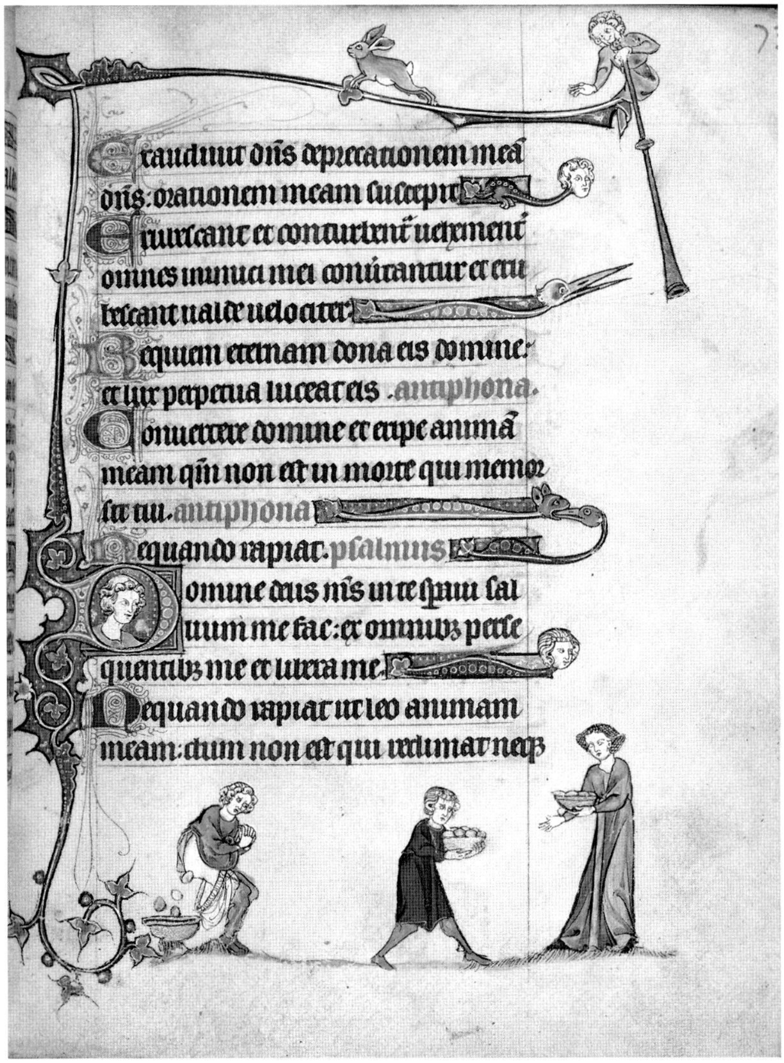

Fig. 85
Bas-de-page defecation scenes. Book of hours, ca. 1300. Trinity College, Cambridge, MS B.11.22, fol. 73r. © Master and Fellows of Trinity College, Cambridge.

with excrement, which did not necessarily have the associations with infection or dirt that it has today.[103] In his eloquent words, "shit had its proper place in the scheme of things," which allows for this image to be a cheeky critique without being totally offensive to the reader.[104] The disruptive tone of the scene from the book of hours, however, is absent from the comparable scenes in the *Régime* manuscripts, which are not intended as humorous commentary but as matter-of-fact experience.

Many of these different facets of household management were primarily the responsibility of women. While women in smaller, bourgeois households probably dealt more directly with many of these duties, elite women clearly also managed these facets by organizing staff who oversaw activities related to the care of the body. Even if some evidence implies that women were not formally entrusted with the care of the whole household's health, it is likely that many levels of medical care were simultaneously in use in a given household.[105] Riddy reminds us that household care is often "disruptive of hierarchies and unimpressed by status," complicating how authority over health care played out in medieval domestic spaces.[106] Knowledge and the authority it generates are central to medieval health care and to the *Régime du corps* more specifically. As the accompanying images suggest, a wider range of household knowledges existed than conventional thinking about medicine suggests.

Conclusion: Expanding Women's Medicine

The generic nature of the *Régime's* advice is clearly one reason the text was copied as much as it was, and for so many different types of readers or users. These audiences likely included upper-class men and women managing their families and their fertility, clerical readers seeking to provide guidance on devotion and health, physicians eager to connect with potential patients, and bibliophiles drawn to the novelty of encyclopedic knowledge. But even as it is clear that some adaptations of the *Régime* had multiple audiences, female ownership and access is probable for several of the copies, and there are good reasons to assume that it continued to be seen as a "woman's text" as it circulated.[107] Among the numerous copies associated with women owners, both illustrated and unillustrated examples are found, including Sloane 2401, Kassel, and Lansdowne 380.[108] The lavish illustrated copies were certainly status items for enthusiasts: abundantly decorated manuscripts of relatively novel and unusual material, and far less common than a bible or prayer book. Owned by the kind of collectors who had other encyclopedias and scientific or medical compendia, they also dealt with concerns that related more to household management. Although royal women would have overseen servants who did the actual work in many of these activities, women like Beatrice's daughters would have been quite familiar with these concerns. The household sphere, a socially complex realm largely overseen by women, is well represented in the initials of the illustrated *Régime* copies.

On the one hand, we clearly cannot assume that these manuscripts were exclusively women's books; many men have been tied to them one way or another. But, as Tyers's work suggests, such manuscripts were valuable to families—with all the diversity of different genders, ages, and perspectives—in which women undoubtedly played a key role. Furthermore, such households had many people with access to the books, including children and other family members who might be the next generation of owners or users. Admittedly, few medical texts can be tied to female owners, creating challenges to linking such manuscripts to the domestic sphere of women. However, as numerous scholars have pointed out, a limited conception of what we consider medical may be causing a false distinction. As this chapter has suggested, household care of the body was broader and more encompassing than medicine in the traditional sense, and at the same time central to everyday activities in the home.

Despite the minimal evidence of women owners of manuscripts of learned medicine, elite women were clearly clients for both the rising medical profession and books in general. This increased collecting speaks to a growing interest in books and inevitably ties in with maintaining one's current prestige as well as the aspirations of upward status. The *Régime du corps* shares much with the conduct books and household manuals that became especially popular in the fourteenth and fifteenth centuries. All of these genres are evidence of conspicuous consumption, especially among aspirational bourgeois book collectors. They gave advice for the maintenance of a good household while also reflecting the ideals of aristocratic life, and they were of particular interest to, if not exclusively geared toward, female audiences. Considered in this context, the illustrated copies of the *Régime du corps* should be seen as books that informed household health management by elite women while also participating in the expression of status. The luxurious nature of these manuscripts does not negate their connection to the mundane, everyday activities depicted in their images that occurred within the domestic sphere. The households represented in the *Régime* manuscripts, after all, are also the households in which the books themselves resided. Such households may have had access to physicians, but the books also reflect a wide range of other practices that focused on the care of the body within the home. Those practices, which took place in domestic sphere, were activated by the agency of women.

CONCLUSION

The late medieval illustrated copies of the *Régime du corps* are compelling objects, delivering insights on the domestic environments in which they were created, used, and shared. By shining a light on these fascinating but understudied manuscripts, my goal has been to demonstrate the potential inherent in studying manuscripts that exist outside the canon and about which much remains unknown. This book shows that all images, even small historiated initials like those of the *Régime* manuscripts, have surprisingly abundant content worth unpacking. This illustrative tradition informs how we might think about a number of aspects of medieval life, including class and gender dynamics, household management, domestic health care, and perceptions of knowledge and authority—encouraging us to make use of and also to go beyond a focus on patronage or iconography. This study also challenges how we frame the visual culture of medieval medicine, and it does so by acknowledging the interconnectedness of the diverse health-care practices represented in these books. Indeed, these manuscripts reflect the nature of power in the late medieval world, in which privileged access to and control over knowledge were essential; such claims to authority were often gendered, as is provocatively pronounced within the *Régime* tradition.

This book also offers readers an example of methodological promiscuity, experimenting with approaches that come out of areas as diverse as narrative theory, cinema studies, anthropology, and geography in addition to the methods of art history and other historical fields, in an effort to broaden our insights into these manuscripts as well as the medieval cultural spheres they inhabited. Indeed, throughout this book I have embraced speculative approaches that make the most out of the evidence that survives. Particularly useful for projects like mine—that is, on manuscripts with significant lacunae—have been the concepts of "domestic geography" and "object itineraries," both of which encourage thinking about images and objects in relation to their movement in time and space, on both small and large scales.[1] From their localized environments in the home to their travels across bodies of water and over centuries, these objects created effects both intimate and vast. They impacted household habits of care and acted as drivers that spread the text and images across Europe for hundreds of years.

In thinking about how Beatrice and her daughters might have engaged with the *Régime* manuscripts and the information they contained, we should consider how women were involved in the passing down of not only objects or things of monetary value but also of household practices—the methods or routines that kept a household running smoothly. These might include the knowledge of when to seek out the expertise of a physician and when one could rely on other types of practitioners or household staff instead. Such handed-down knowledge might advise on the types of treatments to arrange for one's household members, what considerations or decisions might impact a couple's reproductive capacities, and how to find and work with a wet nurse. It might include the foods and beverages that are best to have on hand to maintain a healthy household, and how to acquire and prepare those provisions. And of utmost importance would have been the actions necessary to maintain a clean and orderly household, including the management of waste, washing of clothes and other linens, bathing, and other activities. Of course, many of these practices are essentially ephemeral, transitory, and only minimally discussed in medieval texts or documents. They were the repetitive and ongoing, persistent aspects of living in a household that traditionally get short shrift in surviving sources and are thus underemphasized in scholarship as well. In contrast, these mundane, everyday practices are pronounced, and even emphasized, in the images of the illustrated *Régime* manuscripts, which boldly insist on their importance through the visual emphasis of vivid colors and gold leaf.

Previously unknown copies of the *Régime* occasionally surface, adding to the body of research on the text, and can lead to new information about known copies. More information on the patrons of the illustrated manuscripts would indeed be exciting, but new revelations seem relatively unlikely. A more promising route involves continuing studies that explore women as consumers of books, and specifically of health-related materials. Future research may very well alter how we discuss women readers and their roles in the dissemination of medical ideas. Such ongoing work encourages us to continually reassess what constitutes a "medical" text or book. Is "medicine" too limiting a term? Is the term "health care" any better? What other terms, if any, might apply? We as scholars can further open up our understanding of what constitutes medicine in the Middle Ages to be more inclusive; we can also move toward terminologies that account for the diversity of health care. What are the ramifications of describing the *Régime du corps* as a household health guide rather than a medical text? Such a characterization might seem an apology for the *Régime*'s lack of scholarliness, an acknowledgment of the text's social and cultural milieu. Rethinking our terminology in relation to these manuscripts offers a more accurate and encompassing way to understand not just the *Régime*, but all the multivalent components of health management in this period.

To facilitate a deeper understanding of how academic, religious, and lay audiences consumed and manipulated the same texts, and how they related them to other types of treatises or literature, a broader study of all the surviving manuscripts that include the *Régime* is needed. My study is admittedly limited by focusing on a group of illustrated copies, and a new assessment of the full archive of *Régime* manuscripts would be welcome, as would a new transcription or even English translation of the text. Admittedly, many of the illustrated copies share a similar type of audience: elite lay readers with a particular perspective on the content of the books, often paired with a pronounced interest in collecting deluxe books as status objects. A broader study of all the copies of the *Régime*, with special attention to the other texts that accompany Aldobrandino's work, would give us a more thorough understanding of how the *Régime* was perceived and used by practitioners, academicians, the clergy, and other types of readers, as well as by the nobility. Case studies like those by Theresa Tyers on Lansdowne 380 and Kassel—two late, unillustrated copies that are robust compilations including some of the *Régime* text—are excellent models for the potential of this type of scholarship. The insights from such projects would further illuminate the cultural and intellectual associations that audiences of the deluxe versions might have had with their copies.

Medical imagery continues to be underexplored in art history, in part because it is often characterized as being a separate tradition independent from more common visual narratives. The illustrated *Régime* manuscripts, however, display clear evidence that the designers of their images were fully engaged in contemporary artistic practices. The pictorial programs offer numerous instances in which images have been modeled on existing types. But the abundant images and complexities of the illustrated *Régime* manuscripts also required innovation and creative solutions that went beyond existing models. As this study and many others have argued, the visual traditions we see in medieval medical manuscripts fully participate in artistic norms of the period while they also demonstrate that different expectations of their imagery necessitated additional pictorial strategies.

That those creative pictorial strategies happened within the frameworks of historiated initials is probably another reason for the somewhat limited art-historical engagement with manuscripts like the illustrated *Régime*. Seemingly straightforward historiated initials were used often, in a wide range of manuscripts, but the most robust studies still focus on deluxe volumes with full-page illuminations. As I have argued here, the simplicity of the historiated initials in the *Régime du corps* disguises their sophistication. They are often stunning examples of artistic efficiency, in which scenes have been whittled down to their most basic elements for the sake of clarity. Another aspect of their efficiency is how they necessarily capture a particular moment in time, often a moment that is especially fraught or charged. Their capacity to render visible the uncertainty of health care is one of the more poignant aspects of these books, even while they are admittedly extravagant objects that might also be characterized as frivolous and superficial.

While their owners and users may have been a relatively limited group, those owners also probably used the *Régime*'s information to help with the well-being of other people: their children, various members of their households, the caregivers of their children, servants, and even neighbors. These images also depict a range of individuals of different socioeconomic groups, and participants interact with one another, alluding to the actual networks of people engaged in the household's care of the body. The everyday maintenance of health in medieval households did not apply only to the head of the household and his family; rather, everyone's bodies were cared for in that shared space. Everyone within the household hierarchy was impacted by the treatments and advice included in the *Régime* and depicted in its accompanying images. The historiated initials make profound connections between the content of the books, the bodies and spaces in the images, and the lived space in which the books themselves circulated and real bodies moved. They may show an idealized view of elite households, but they nevertheless prioritize the work that bodies were doing in such a context.

Beatrice, her daughters, their descendants, and other owners of the illustrated manuscripts of the *Régime du corps* were not just chance patrons or recipients. These books were collected and copied because they contained or expressed something valuable, whether that was useful information, knowledgeable authority, relatable domesticity, privileged refinement, or elite status. More likely, however, these manuscripts embodied multiple values at once, serving as tools of knowledge as well as objects associated with wealth. Despite the challenges of assessing their reception and use, the illustrated *Régime* manuscripts clearly encapsulate the variety of concerns and priorities central to household management in the later Middle Ages. They offer us a window into domestic spaces where health maintenance was of paramount importance, and where the care of the body was recognized to have serious consequences as well as often unknowable futures.

Appendix 1: Summary of Illustrated Copies

Manuscript	Estimated date	Location of production	No. of illustrations	Additional texts in MS (additional images in parentheses)	Associated names or owners / provenance	Measurements
Sloane 2435	1265–70	Northern France (Cambrai?)	72 initials	*Image du monde* (27 diagrams; 13 historiated initials)	Benoit de Florenche (unknown); Artist: Aldebrandin Master	295 × 190 mm
BnF Arsenal 2510	1285	Northern France (Cambrai, or possibly Tournai or Saint-Omer)	37 initials	A few folios of recipes	Artist: Bute Painter; Jehan Neriot, 16th-century possessor (loaned by House of Madame of Vendôme)	232 × 165 mm
BnF Fr. 12323	1350	France (Paris?)	52 initials	Several medical recipes (by Jean Pitart, Jean de Chalon, Jean d'Aunoy, and others); *Image du monde* (7 diagrams, 12 historiated initials); tract by Parisian "masters of medicine and astronomers" on the pestilence of 1348	Charles of Valois (1270–1325)—in reference to Charles's patronage of physician Pitart, not as patron of BnF Fr. 12323	290 × 195 mm
Cambridge Ii.V.11	ca. 1450	Northern France (Rouen?)	143 initials, plus 1 frontispiece and 1 folio with heraldry	2 folios of French and Middle English recipes (85–86)	Later owners: King Henry VII (1457–1509) and Queen Elizabeth of York (1465–1503)—arms on fol. 6v	277 × 207 mm
Morgan M.165	ca. 1440–50	France (Rouen)	147 initials, plus 1 frontispiece	Letter to Caesar by Pseudo-Hippocrates (1 initial); the book of Galen (1 initial); zodiac and planetary tables (1 chart); excerpts from the *Flos medicinae Scholae Salerni*	P.P. (Rouen binder for English, early 16th century); Thwayte (probable 16th-century owner)	260 × 180 mm
Sloane 2401	ca. 1450–1500	France	137 initials	Letter to Caesar by Pseudo-Hippocrates; the book of Galen; miscellaneous medical recipes	Conjoined coat of arms of Margaret, wife of Richard Brydges, of Ley, Weobley, Herefordshire (16th century)	245 × 170 mm
Ajuda Cod. 52-XIII-26	ca. 1470s	Flanders (Bruges)	147 initials, plus 1 frontispiece	Letter to Caesar by Pseudo-Hippocrates (1 initial); the book of Galen (1 initial); *De mundo* in Latin (1 initial)	Inscription "No. 1291", a number from library of Henry VIII; arms of Thomas Boleyn (ca. 1477–1539); possible artists: Master of the Harley Froissart (Philippe de Mazerolles), Master of the London Wavrin	280 × 200 mm

Manuscript	Estimated date	Location of production	No. of illustrations	Additional texts in MS (additional images in parentheses)	Associated names or owners / provenance	Measurements
Universitäts-bibliothek Leipzig Cod. Haen. 3478	ca. 1270–1300	France	No initials, 35 miniatures			175 × 120 mm
Vatican Reg. lat.1256	15th century		No initials, 21 miniatures, plus 1 frontispiece		Ex libris de Bourdelot (17th century?)	230 × 165 mm
BnF Arsenal 2894	15th century		No initials, 81 miniatures	Medical compilation; amalgamation of numer-ous treatises		286 × 210 mm

Appendix 2: Scenes Depicted in Each Illustrated Copy

Chapter	Sloane 2435	BnF Arsenal 2510	BnF Fr. 12323	Cam-bridge Ii.V.11	Morgan M.165	Sloane 2401	Ajuda Cod. 52-XIII-26	Leipzig Cod. Haen. 3478	Vatican Reg.lat. 1256	BnF Arsenal 2894[*]
Heraldry				6v						
Prologue/ Introduction	1r Plus 1 framed scene	1r (Physi-cian with urine flask in margin)		7r Plus half-page illumina-tion	5r Plus half-page illumina-tion		1r Illumina-tion and heraldry	2r	1r	
Part 1									2v	
Chap. 1: Air	2v	3r	71v	8v	7v	9r	4r		3r	
Chap. 2: Eating	3r	3v	72r	9v	8r	9v	5v	6r	4r	
Chap. 3: Drinking	5r	5r	74r	11r	11r	12r	8v	9v	6v	
Wine				12r	12r	12v	10r			
Chap. 4: Sleeping and waking	7r	6v	75v	13r	13r	13v	11v	12v	9r	
Chap. 5: Working and resting	7v	7v	76v						10r	
Chap. 6: Bathing	8v	8r	77r	14v	15v	15v	14v	15r	11v	
Chap. 7: Living with a woman (copulation)	9v	9r	78r	15v	17r	16v	16v	17v	13r	
Chap. 8: Avoiding anger	10v	10r	79v					19r	14v	
Chap. 9: Bloodletting	11v	10v	80r	17v	19v	18v	19v	20v	15v	
Chap. 10: Cupping	14r	13v	83r	20v	24r	22r	24v	26r	20r	
Chap. 11: Leeching	15v	15r	84r	21v	26r	23v	27r	28v	21v	
Chap. 12: Purging	16r	15v	84v					30r	22v	
Chap. 13: Vomiting	21r	17v	89v	26v	33r	29r	36r	39v	29r	
Chap. 14: Avoiding pestilence	22r	19r	90v	27v	34v	30v	37v	41v	30v	
Chap. 15: Four seasons of care	23r	20r	91v	29r	36v	31v	40r		32r	
Chap. 16: Living safely in cities	25r	21v	93r	30v	38v	33v	43r	47r	34r	
Chap. 17: Care on the road	26r	22v	94r	31v	40r	35r	44v	49v	35v	
Chap. 18: Pregnancy and childbirth	27v	24r	95v	33r	42r	36v	47r	52r	37v	
Chap. 19: Caring for a newborn	28v	25v	97r	34v	44r	37v	49r	54v	39v	

Chapter	Sloane 2435	BnF Arsenal 2510	BnF Fr. 12323	Cam-bridge Ii.V.11	Morgan M.165	Sloane 2401	Ajuda Cod. 52-XIII-26	Leipzig Cod. Haen. 3478	Vatican Reg.lat. 1256	BnF Arsenal 2894*
Chap. 20: Caring for oneself in four ages	31r	27v	99r	36v	47r	40r	53r	59r	42v	
Part 2										
Chap. 1: Hair	32v	29v	101r	38v	49v	42r	56r	62r		
Chap. 2: Eyes	34v	32r	103r	40v	52r	44v	59v	66r		
Chap. 3: Ears	35v		104r	41v	53v	45v	61v	67v		
Chap. 4: Teeth	36r		104v	42v	54v	46r	62v	69r		
Chap. 5: Face/complexion	37r			43v	56r	47r		71r		
Chap. 6: Stomach	38v	36r		44v	57v	48v	64v	73r		
Chap. 7: Liver	40r	37v		46r	59v	50r	66v	76r		
Chap. 8: Heart	41r	38v	105v	47r	61r	51r	70v	78r		
Part 3										
Chap. on Grains		39v								
Wheat	42r	40r	106v	48r	62v	52v	72v	80v		
Barley	42v		107r	48v	63r	52v	73r			
Millet	43r		107r	49r	63v	53r	73v			
Rice	43r		107v	49r	64r	53v	74r			
Oats (and spelt)	43v		107v	49v	64r	53v	74v			
Sorghum (*rogier*)	43v		108r	49v	64v	53v	75r			
Farro	44r		108r	50r	65r	54r	75r			
Bran	44r		108r	50r	65r	54r	75v			
Chap. on Beverages										
Water	44r	41r	108v	50r	65v	54v	76r	83r		
Wine	44v		108v	50v	65v	54v	76v			
Beer				51r	66v	55r	77r			
Apple wine/cider	45r		109v	51r	66v	55v	77v			
Verjuice	45v		109v							
Vinegar	45v		109v	51v	67r	55v	78r			
Mulberries	46r		110r	51v	67v	56r	78v			
Chap. on Meat		42r	110r					86r		
Pork	46v		110v	52r	68r	56v	79v			
Beef	47r			52v	69r	57r	89v			
Sheep (lamb)				53r	69v	57v	81r			
Mutton	47v			53v	69v	58r	81v			
Billy goat (he-goat)	47v			53v	70r	58r	81v			

Chapter	Sloane 2435	BnF Arsenal 2510	BnF Fr. 12323	Cambridge Ii.V.11	Morgan M.165	Sloane 2401	Ajuda Cod. 52-XIII-26	Leipzig Cod. Haen. 3478	Vatican Reg.lat. 1256	BnF Arsenal 2894*
Goat (she-goat)	48r			54r	70v	58v	82v			
Stag (venison)	48v			54r	71r	58v	82v			
Hare	48v			54v	71r	59r	83r			
Rabbit	48v			54v	71v	59r	83v			
Bear	48v			54v	71v	59r	83v			
Chap. on Birds										
Bird: chicken	49r			54v	71v	59v	84r			
Dove/pigeon	49v			55r	72v	60r	84v			
Geese	49v			55v	72v	60r	85r			
Duck	50r			55v	73r	60v	85v			
Partridge	50r			56r	73v	60v	86r			
Pheasant	50v			56r	73v	61r	86r			
Peacock/heron	50v			56r	74r	61r	86v			
Swan	50v			56v	74r	61r	87r			
Sparrows and small birds	51r			56v	74v	61v	87r			
Quail	51r			56v	74v	61v	87v			
Plovers and blackbirds	51r			57r	75r	61v	87v			
Chap. on Legumes										
Beans	53r	45v	113r	59r	77v	63v	91r	97v		
Chickpea (*chiches*)				59v	78r	64r	92r			
Peas				59v	78v	64v	92v			
Lentils				60r	78v	64v	92v			
String beans				60r	79r	65r	93r			
Lupins				60v	79v	65r	93v			
Spring vetch (*orbe*)					79v		94r			
Chickpea (*cerres*)				60v	80r	65v	94r			
Vetch plant				60v	80r	65v	94v			
Chap. on Fruit:										
Figs	55r	46r	115r	61r	80v		94v	101r		
Grapevine				61v	81r		95v			
Pear tree				62r	82r		97r			
Apple tree				62v	82v		97v			
Pomegranate tree				62v	82v		98r			
Quince tree				62v	83r	66r	98r			
Lemon tree				63r	83r	66r	98v			

Chapter	Sloane 2435	BnF Arsenal 2510	BnF Fr. 12323	Cambridge Ii.V.11	Morgan M.165	Sloane 2401	Ajuda Cod. 52-XIII-26	Leipzig Cod. Haen. 3478	Vatican Reg.lat. 1256	BnF Arsenal 2894*
Date palm tree				63v	84r	66v	99r			
Peach tree				63v	84v	67r	100r			
Gooseberry tree/ currants				64r	84v	67r	100v			
Mulberry tree				64r	85r	67v	100v			
Plum tree				64v	85v	67v	101r			
Walnut tree				65r	86r	68r	102r			
Hazelnut				65v	86v	68v	102v			
Almond				65v	86v	68v	103r			
Pine tree (pine nuts)					87v		103v			
Nettle tree/medlar tree				66r	87v	69v	104r			
Chestnut				66r	88r	69v	104r			
Olive tree				66v	88r	69v	104v			
Strawberries				67r	88v	70r	105v			
Cornel tree				67r	89r	70r	105v			
Sorb apple/hazel tree				67r	89r	70v	106r			
Juniper				67r	89r	70v	106r			
Squash				67v	89v	70v	106v			
Cucumber				67v	89v	71r	107r			
Pumpkin				67v	90r	71r	107r			
Sugarcane				68r	90r	71r	107v			
Chap. on Fish†	66r	47v	125r	74r	99r	77v	119r	121r		
Chap. on Herbs	61v									
Honey		48r		68r	90v	71v	107v			
Cabbage				68v	91r	72r	108v			
Chives				69r	91v	72r	109r			
Onion				69r	92r	72v	109v			
Garlic				69v	92r	72v	110r			
Shallot				69v	92v	73r	110v			
Mustard				70r	93r	73r	110v			
Spinach				70r	93r	73v	111r			
Beets				70r	93r	73v	111r			
Borage				70r	93v	73v	111v			
Mallow				70v	93v	73v	111v			
Turnips				70v	93v	74r	112r			
Skirret (*eschiervies* or *rais*)				70v	94r	74r	112r			

Chapter	Sloane 2435	BnF Arsenal 2510	BnF Fr. 12323	Cambridge Ii.V.11	Morgan M.165	Sloane 2401	Ajuda Cod. 52-XIII-26	Leipzig Cod. Haen. 3478	Vatican Reg.lat. 1256	BnF Arsenal 2894[*]
Parsnip				71r	94v	74r	112v			
Radishes				71r	94v	74v	113r			
Fennel				71r	95r	74v	113r			
Parsley				71v	95r	74v	113v			
Chervil				71v	95v	75r	114r			
Lettuce				71v	95v	75r	114r			
Purslane				72r	96r	75r	114v			
Sorrel					96r		115r			
Sage				72v	96v	75v	115v			
Mint				72v	96v	76r	115v			
Basil				72v	97r	76r	116r			
Rue/rocket				72v	97r	76r	116r			
Mushrooms				73r	97v	76v	116v			
Hyssop				73v	98r	76v	117r			
Cress				73v	98r	77r	117v			
Clary				73v	98v	77r	118r			
Inula (*nula*)				73v	98v	77r	118r			
Pennyroyal (*poulieul*)				74r	98v	77v	118v			
Southernwood plant					99r		118v			
Chap. on Eggs and Dairy										
Eggs	68r	49v (eggs and cheese together)	127r	76r	101v	79v	122r	123v		
Cheese	69r		128r	77r	103r	80v	124r			
Milk	69v		128v	77v	103v	81r	124v			
Chap. on Spices										
Pepper	71r	50v	130r	79r	105v	82v	127v	128v		
Ginger				79v	105v	82v	127v			
Cinnamon				79v	106r	82v	128r			
Clove					106r		128v			
Galangal				80r	107r	83v	129r			
Cumin				80v	107r	83v	129v			
Saffron				80v	107v	84r	130r			
Cubeb				81r	108r	84r	130v			
Cardamom				81r	108r	84v	131r			

Chapter	Sloane 2435	BnF Arsenal 2510	BnF Fr. 12323	Cambridge Ii.V.11	Morgan M.165	Sloane 2401	Ajuda Cod. 52-XIII-26	Leipzig Cod. Haen. 3478	Vatican Reg.lat. 1256	BnF Arsenal 2894*
Anise/aniseed				81v	108v	84v	131v			
Nutmeg				81v	109r	85r	132r			
Zedoary (*citoual*)				82r	109r	85r	132v			
Salt				82r	109v	85r	132v			
Part 4										
Physiognomy	73v	52r	132v	82r	109v	85v	133r	132v		
Total count of images accompanying Régime	72 plus 1 framed scene	37	52	143, plus frontispiece and heraldry	147, plus frontispiece	137	147, plus frontispiece	35 miniatures	22 miniatures	81 miniatures
				5 unfinished		6 unfinished				
L'image du monde	27 diagrams		7 diagrams							
	1 framed explicit		1 framed explicit							
	13 historiated initials		12 historiated initials							
	65 decorated initials		46 decorated initials (plus 1 cutout)							
Misc. medical notes and recipes			1 historiated initial							
Paris faculty on 1348 pestilence			1 historiated initial							
Letter to Caesar by Pseudo-Hippocrates					1 initial	1 initial with line drawing (incomplete)	1 initial			
Book of Galen					1 initial		1 initial			
Astrology chart					1 astrology chart					
De mundo							1 initial			

*BnF Arsenal 2894 contains an amalgamation of different medical treatises, including various pieces of the *Régime du corps* (part 1: chaps. 4–10, 12 and 13; part 2: chaps. 6, 7, and 8; and most of part 3). The components are somewhat mixed up and out of order, as are the images. Additional images (astrological roundels, etc.) that do not correspond to the *Régime du corps* are interspersed.

†The Chapters on Fish and Herbs in Sloane 2435, BnF Fr. 12323, and BnF Arsenal 2510 are reversed in the other manuscripts.

Appendix 3: Known Manuscript Copies of the *Régime du corps*

This list of seventy-five manuscripts has been compiled from a variety of sources, including digitized versions and personal viewing. The manuscripts are organized into three groups: those with programs of illustration, those with minimal illustration, and unillustrated copies (and then alphabetical by city). A note is made when there is a known digital copy and/or additional sources for the manuscript.

The key sources for this list are Fery-Hue, "*Régime du corps*: Tradition manuscrite"; Fery-Hue, "*Régime du corps*: Note"; Fery-Hue, "*Régime du corps*: Complément (1999)"; Fery-Hue, "*Régime du corps*: Complément (2004)"; Landouzy and Pépin, *Régime du corps*; and Nicoud, *Régimes de santé.*

Note that I use *Régime du corps* here for consistency, but, as noted by Nicoud and others, Aldobrandino's text was also referred to as *Livre de Physicke* (or *Physique*) and *Régime de santé* (see Nicoud, *Régimes de santé*, 115, 467, 953–85).

Illustrated (10)

See Appendices 1 and 2 for more details on this group.
The illustrations listed here are only those accompanying the *Régime du corps*.

1. Cambridge, UK: Cambridge University Library, MS Ii.V.11
   Ca. 1450, northern France
   Illustrations: 143 historiated initials, 1 frontispiece, 1 folio with heraldry
   Régime du corps: fols. 71r–85r
   Additional bibliography: Binski and Zutshi, *Western Illuminated Manuscripts*, 312–14; Scott, *Later Gothic Manuscripts*, 2:266

2. Leipzig: Universitätsbibliothek Leipzig, Cod. Haen. 3478
   Ca. 1270–1300, France
   Illustrations: 35 miniatures
   Régime du corps: fols. 2r–138r
   Digitized version available
   Additional bibliography: Fery-Hue, "*Régime du corps*: Complément" (2004)

3. Lisbon: Biblioteca da Ajuda, Cod. 52-XIII-26
   1470s, Bruges
   Illustrations: 147 historiated initials, 1 frontispiece
   Régime du corps: fols. 1–137v
   Digitized version available
   Additional bibliography: Carvalho, "Manuscrit du *Régime du corps*"; Campos Ribeiro, "Picturing Medieval Health"; Campos Ribeiro, "Medicina e dietética medieval"

4. London: British Library, Sloane MS 2435
   Ca. 1265–70, northern France
   Illustrations: 72 historiated initials
   Régime du corps: fols. 1–75v
   Digitized version available
   Additional bibliography: Stones, *Gothic Manuscripts*, pt. 1, vol. 1: 64 and vol. 2: 299–302; P. Jones, "Regime del corpo"

5. London: British Library, Sloane MS 2401
   Fifteenth century
   Illustrations: 137 historiated initials
   Régime du corps: fols. 4r–88r
   Additional bibliography: Tyers, "Rebirth of Fertility"; Tyers, "'In the Merry Month of May'"

6. New York: Morgan Library, MS M.165

Ca. 1440–1450, northern France
Illustrations: 147 historiated initials, 1 frontispiece
Régime du corps: fols. 5r–113r
Digitized version available
Additional bibliography: Fery-Hue, "*Régime du corps*: Complément" (2004)

7. Paris: Bibliothèque nationale de France, Arsenal MS 2510
Ca. 1285, northern France (Cambrai?)
Illustrations: 37 historiated initials
Régime du corps: fols. 1–57r
Digitized version available
Additional bibliography: Stones, *Gothic Manuscripts*, pt. 1, vol. 2: 299–302; Stones, "Stylistic Associations"

8. Paris: Bibliothèque nationale de France, Arsenal MS 2894
Fifteenth century
Illustrations: 81 miniatures
Digitized version available

9. Paris: Bibliothèque nationale de France, Fr. 12323
Ca. 1350, France
Illustrations: 52 historiated initials
Régime du corps: fols. 71r–135r
Digitized version available

10. Rome: Biblioteca Apostolica Vaticana, Reg.lat.1256
Fifteenth century
Illustrations: 22 miniatures
Régime du corps: fols. 1r–101v
Digitized version available

Copies with Frontispiece or Single Initial (13)

The illustrations listed here are only those accompanying the *Régime du corps*.

11. Besançon: Bibliothèque municipale, MS 463
Fifteenth century
Illustration: fol. 1r (apothecary scene)
Régime du corps: fols. 1r–121r

12. London: British Library, Royal MS 16 F VIII
Late fifteenth century, Flanders
Illustration: fol. 1r, half-page frontispiece
Régime du corps: fols. 1r–175v

13. London: British Library, Royal MS 19 A V
Ca. 1494–96, Flanders
Illustration: fol. 1v, frontispiece (French knight Jean Chabot giving book to King Henry VII)
Régime du corps: fols. 1r–110v
Additional bibliography: McKendrick, Lowden, and Doyle, *Royal Manuscripts*, 307

14. London: British Library, Royal MS 19 B X
Late fifteenth century, Flanders
Illustration: fol. 2r, frontispiece
Régime du corps: fols. 1–150

15. London: British Library, Royal MS 20 B IX
Late fifteenth century, Flanders
Illustration: fol. 1r, frontispiece
Régime du corps: fols. 1r–115v

16. London: Wellcome Library, MS.31
Ca. 1390, Paris
Written for Hugues de Salve by Jehan Quatredens
Illustration: fol. 2v, 1 historiated initial
Régime du corps: fols. 1–89v
Digitized version available

17. Manchester, UK: John Rylands Library, MS French 027
Late fifteenth century
Illustration: fol. 1, presentation image and heraldry
Régime du corps: fols. 1–94
Additional bibliography: Fery-Hue, "*Régime du corps*: Note"

18. New York: Morgan Library MS M.459
Ca. 1300, Lombardy(?)
Illustration: fol. 30r, 1 historiated initial
Régime du corps: fol. 30 (fragment)

19. Paris: Bibliothèque nationale de France, Fr. 1109
Ca. 1310, France(?)
Sixteenth-century owner: Marie de Luxembourg (d. 1547)
Illustration: 1 historiated initial (physician looking at urine)
Régime du corps: fols. 242r–281v
Digitized version available

20. Paris: Bibliothèque nationale de France, NAF 6539

Second half of fourteenth century, England(?)
Illustration: 1 historiated initial
Régime du corps: fols. 1r–88r
Digitized version available

21. Oxford: Bodleian Library, MS Bodley 179
Ca. 1459, France
Made for John Falstof (1377–1459)
Illustration: fol. 1r, initial with arms and embellished border
Régime du corps: fols. 1r–110v

22. Oxford: St. John's College, MS 68
Late fifteenth century, Flanders(?)
Illustration: fol. 1, quarter-page frontispiece with embellished border
Régime du corps: fols. 1r–69v
Additional bibliography: Hanna and Griffiths, *Descriptive Catalogue*, 90–91

23. Rome: Biblioteca Apostolica Vaticana, MS Pal.lat.1990
Late fifteenth century, Flanders
Illustrations: fols. 7r, 74r, 85v (3 full-page scenes, at the beginning of parts 1, 2, and 3)
Régime du corps: fols. 1r–127v
Digitized version available

Unillustrated (52)

24. Berlin: Staatsbibliothek, MS Hamilton 407
Ca. 1400
Régime du corps: fols. 147r–185v

25. Bern: Burgerbibliothek, MS 385
Thirteenth century

26. Bordeaux: Bibliothèque municipale, MS 531
Mid-fifteenth century
Régime du corps: fols. 49r–53v, 128r–147r

27. Brussels: Bibliothèque Royale Albert I, MS 11004-11017
Late fifteenth century
Régime du corps: fols. 52r–68v
Additional bibliography: Fery-Hue, "*Régime du corps*: Complément" (1999)

28. Brussels: Bibliothèque Royale Albert I, MS 11130-32
End of fourteenth century
Régime du corps: fols. 1r–110v

29. Chantilly: Musée Condé, MS 331
Fifteenth century
Régime du corps: fols. 1r–132

30. Chantilly: Musée Condé, MS 476
Thirteenth century
Régime du corps: fols. 56ra–58ra (short excerpt of part 4)
Also includes *L'image du monde*
Additional bibliography: Fery-Hue, "*Régime du corps*: Complément" (1999)

31. Florence: Biblioteca Medicea Laurenziana, MS Ashburnham 1076
Fourteenth century, France
Régime du corps: fols. 1r–61v (incomplete)

32. Florence: Biblioteca Medicea Laurenziana, Edili 187
Early fourteenth century(?)
Régime du corps: fols. 29–32 (2 chapters)
Additional bibliography: Fery-Hue, "*Régime du corps*: Complément" (2004)

33. The Hague: Museum Meermanno-Westreenianum, MS 10. E. 40
Thirteenth century, France (Paris region)

34. Kassel: Landesbibliothek, 40 MS Med. 1
Fifteenth century (1430–1475), northern France
Régime du corps: fols. 78r–163v (incomplete)
Additional bibliography: Tyers, "Rebirth of Fertility"; Tyers, "Family, Feud, and Fertility"

35. Leiden: Bibliotheek der Rijksuniversiteit, MS Voss. Lat. Q. 93
Late thirteenth century, Tournai(?)
Régime du corps: fols. 25r–100r
Additional bibliography: De Meyier, "Manuscript de Leyde"

36. Lille: Bibliothèque de l'Université, MS 204 (1180)
Late fourteenth century

37. London: British Library, MS Add. 8863
Fifteenth century (1472–1493), northern France or Flanders
Régime du corps: fols. 1r–82r

38. London: British Library MS Lansdowne 380
Late fifteenth or early sixteenth century
Régime du corps: fols. 263r–268v (excerpt)
Additional bibliography: Sewright, "Introduction to British Library MS Lansdowne 380"; Tyers, "'In the Merry Month of May'"

39. London: British Library, Sloane MS 1611
Thirteenth century, France or England
Régime du corps: fols. 69r–142v
Additional bibliography: Meyer, "Notice du ms. Sloane 1611"

40. London: British Library, Sloane MS 2806
Late thirteenth or fourteenth century
Régime du corps: fols. 1–45 (incomplete)

41. London: British Library, Sloane MS 2986
Late thirteenth or early fourteenth century
Régime du corps: fols. 1–60 (damaged at beginning and end)

42. London: British Library, Sloane MS 3152
Fifteenth century (ca. 1492), Mechelen
Régime du corps: fols. 1r–68v

43. London: British Library, Sloane MS 3525
Late thirteenth or fourteenth century
Régime du corps: fols. 24r–81r
Additional bibliography: Meyer, "Manuscrits médicaux en français," 196–98; Hunt, *Anglo-Norman Medicine*, 2:59–67

44. London: Wellcome Library, MS.32
Mid-fourteenth century, France
Régime du corps: fols. 1–80v

45. London: Wellcome Library, MS.546
Mid-fourteenth century, southern France
Régime du corps: fols. 1r–21r
Digitized version available
Additional bibliography:
Hunt, *Old French Medical Texts*; Tyers, "Rebirth of Fertility"

46. Lyon: Bibliothèque municipale, MS 976
Thirteenth century
Régime du corps: fols. 1–113

47. Munich: Bayerische Staatsbibliothek, MS Gall. 60
Late fourteenth or early fifteenth century

48. Niort: Bibliothèque municipale, MS 70
Fourteenth century
Régime du corps: fols. 1r–117r

49. Paris: Bibliothèque nationale de France, Fr. 625
Fifteenth century, Flanders
Régime du corps: fols. 1r–258r
Digitized version available

50. Paris: Bibliothèque nationale de France, Fr. 1288
Fifteenth century, France
Régime du corps: fols. 135r–184v
Digitized version available

51. Paris: Bibliothèque nationale de France, Fr. 1444
Second half of thirteenth century
Régime du corps: fols. 78r–115r
Digitized version available

52. Paris: Bibliothèque nationale de France, Fr. 2001
Fourteenth century
Régime du corps: fols. 61r–92v
Digitized version available

53. Paris: Bibliothèque nationale de France, Fr. 2021
Second half of thirteenth century (earliest surviving copy)
Régime du corps: fols. 5r–76v
Digitized version available

54. Paris: Bibliothèque nationale de France, Fr. 2022
Fifteenth century
Régime du corps: fols. 1r–109r

55. Paris: Bibliothèque nationale de France, Fr. 2039
Fourteenth century
Régime du corps: fols. 9v–12r (excerpt, physiognomy)

56. Paris: Bibliothèque nationale de France, Fr. 14822
Thirteenth century
Régime du corps: fols. 5r–138v

57. Paris: Bibliothèque nationale de France, Fr. 25247
Thirteenth century, France
Régime du corps: fols. 50v–57v (excerpt, physiognomy)

58. Paris: Bibliothèque nationale de France, NAF 1104
Thirteenth century
Régime du corps: fols. 84r–85r (fragment)
Digitized version available

59. Paris: Bibliothèque nationale de France, Arsenal MS 2059
Fourteenth century, northern France
Régime du corps: fols. 179r–208r (excerpt)

60. Paris: Bibliothèque nationale de France, Arsenal MS 2511
Fourteenth century, northern Italy
Régime du corps: fols. 4r–87r

61. Paris: Bibliothèque nationale de France, Arsenal MS 2814
Fourteenth century
Régime du corps: fols. 1r–174r

62. Paris: Bibliothèque nationale de France, Arsenal MS 2872
End of fourteenth century
Régime du corps: fols. 342r–394r
Digitized version available

63. Paris: Bibliothèque nationale de France, Arsenal MS 2895
Fifteenth century (after 1477)
Régime du corps: fols. 252r–284r (excerpts, chaps. 1–8, part 3)

64. Paris: Bibliothèque nationale de France, Arsenal MS 3174
Fifteenth century
Régime du corps: fols. 62r–64r (excerpt; only part 4, physiognomy)

65. Paris: Bibliothèque nationale de France, Arsenal MS 3190
Fifteenth century
Régime du corps: fols. 21r–109v

66. Philadelphia: Kislak Center for Special Collections, Rare Books and Manuscripts, University of Pennsylvania, Ms. Coll. 591, Folder 19
Late fourteenth century
Régime du corps: 1 leaf (fragment)
Digitized version available

67. Philadelphia: Kislak Center for Special Collections, Rare Books and Manuscripts, University of Pennsylvania, UPenn LJS 55
Late thirteenth century, France (Lorraine?)
Régime du corps: fols. 52r–52v (excerpt, chaps. 18 and 19 on pregnancy and newborn care)
Digitized version available
Additional bibliography: Lacarrière, "Compilation, Collation and Correction"

68. Reims: Bibliothèque municipale, MS 265
Thirteenth century (with twelfth-century content)
Régime du corps: fragment

69. Rome: Biblioteca Apostolica Vaticana, Reg.lat.1334
Fifteenth century, France
Régime du corps: fols. 1r–77r

70. Rome: Biblioteca Apostolica Vaticana, Reg.lat.1451
Thirteenth and fourteenth centuries, France
Régime du corps: fols. 2v–3r (fragment)

71. Rome: Biblioteca Apostolica Vaticana, Pal. lat.1967
First half of fourteenth century
Régime du corps: fols. 1r–38v

72. Turin: Biblioteca nazionale, MS M.IV.11
Fifteenth century (ca. 1463), Namur (lost in fire, 1904)
Régime du corps: fols. 10r–117v

73. Valenciennes: Bibliothèque municipale, MS 329
Fifteenth century
Régime du corps: fols. 1r–118r

74. Venice: Biblioteca nazionale Marciana, MS Gall. App. X
Fourteenth century
Régime du corps: fols. 1r–91v

75. Zagreb: National and University Library, MS MR 92
Thirteenth century (after 1274), northern Italy
Régime du corps: fols. 1r–55r

Notes

Introduction

1. Gil-Sotres, "Derivation and Revulsion."
2. Scholars have most commonly referred to the text as the *Régime du corps*, which appears in earlier copies but becomes predominant in later copies. Some versions refer to the text as *Livre de Physicke* (or *Physique*), and *Régime de santé* is also sometimes used. Marilyn Nicoud states a preference for *Livre de Physique* and cites other titles as well in her inventory; see Nicoud, *Régimes de santé*, 1:115, 467, 2:953–85.
3. The prologue is contained in only some copies of the text, including several of the earliest surviving manuscripts of the *Régime*. A representative version is available in the primary edition of the *Régime du corps*: see Landouzy and Pépin, *Régime du corps*, 3. While some scholars, including Fery-Hue and Theresa L. Tyers, have noted that this prologue may present an apocryphal story (in part because there is no documentary evidence of the commission), several others have taken it as a likely scenario.
4. Landouzy and Pépin, *Régime du corps*.
5. Landouzy and Pépin identify Bibliothèque nationale de France Fr. 2021 as "ms. A." Their transcription contains notes throughout with textual variations between ms. A and ms. B (Bibliothèque nationale de France Fr. 14822), ms. C (Bibliothèque nationale de France Arsenal MS 2510), and ms. D (Bibliothèque nationale de France Fr. 12323); Landouzy and Pépin, *Régime du corps*, lxix. In addition to thirty-five copies in French, they also provide a list of eight copies in Italian (xlviii–xlix).
6. Fery-Hue, "*Régime du corps*: Tradition manuscrite"; Fery-Hue, "*Régime du corps*: Note"; Fery-Hue, "*Régime du corps*: Complément" (1999); Fery-Hue, "*Régime du corps*: Complément" (2004); Nicoud, *Régimes de santé*; and Bisson, "Le témoin gênant."
7. Meyer, "Notice du ms. Sloane 1611"; Sewright, "Introduction to British Library MS Lansdowne 380"; Tyers, "'In the Merry Month of May'"; Tyers, "Family, Feud, and Fertility"; Tyers, "Rebirth of Fertility"; Campos Ribeiro, "Medicina e dietética medieval"; Campos Ribeiro, "Picturing Medieval Health"; M. Green, "Possibilities of Literacy"; P. Jones, *Medieval Medicine*, 95–107; and P. Jones, "Regime del corpo."
8. A preliminary essay takes this approach; see Borland, "Female Networks."
9. Some prominent examples include Bell, "Medieval Women Book Owners"; Sheingorn, "Wise Mother"; Smith and Taylor, *Women and the Book*; Stanton, *Queen Mary Psalter*; Holladay, "Fourteenth-Century French Queens"; Nolan, *Capetian Women*; L'Estrange, *Holy Motherhood*; Hamilton and Proctor-Tiffany, *Moving Women*; Proctor-Tiffany, *Medieval Art in Motion*; and Hamilton, *Pleasure and Politics*. In 2017, on the thirty-fifth anniversary of Bell's essay, Elizabeth L'Estrange and Sherry Lindquist organized a conference session, "Revisiting Susan Groag Bell: New Directions for 'Medieval Women Book Owners'" (Association of Art Historians Conference, Loughborough, England, April 2017); see also the online research project overseen by L'Estrange and Emily Wingfield, "Women and the Book," at https://womenandthebook.wordpress.com (last accessed August 22, 2020).
10. Landouzy and Pépin, *Régime du corps*, lvi–lviii.
11. Landouzy and Pépin cite Bibliothèque nationale de France Fr. 2022, in which Aldobrandino is referred to as a "medecin du roy du France": *Régime du corps*, lix; see also Thomas, "L'identité du médecin Aldebrandin de Sienne." A few fifteenth-century copies refer to Frederick II (1194–1250) as the patron of Aldobrandino's

text, which most scholars view as a far less probable scenario; see Landouzy and Pépin, *Régime du corps*, lv; Fery-Hue, "*Régime du corps*: Tradition manuscrite," 117; and Meyer, "De l'expansion de la langue française," 79–80.

12. The *Régime du corps* is discussed alongside the *Image du monde* and Latini's *Tresor* in Landouzy and Pépin, *Régime du corps*, xv–xvi.
13. Landouzy and Pépin, *Régime du corps*, lxxv. All three early illustrated copies of the *Régime* (British Library Sloane MS 2435, Bibliothèque nationale de France Arsenal MS 2510, and Bibliothèque nationale de France Fr. 12323) are written in Walloon: lx. See also Fery-Hue, "*Régime du corps*: Tradition manuscrite."
14. Wallis, *Medieval Medicine*, 493.
15. Hamilton and Proctor-Tiffany, *Moving Women*; for my contribution to that volume, see Borland, "Female Networks."
16. Joyce and Gillespie, *Things in Motion*; Merleau-Ponty, *Phenomenology of Perception*; Bennett, *Vibrant Matter*; and Kopytoff, "Cultural Biography of Things." For earlier work in which I engage with phenomenology and related concepts, see Borland, "Unruly Reading"; Borland, "Audience and Spatial Experience"; Borland, "Encountering the Inauthentic"; Borland, "Moved by Medicine"; and Overbey and Borland, "Diagnostic Performance and Diagrammatic Manipulation."
17. Joyce, "Things in Motion," 29.
18. Kopytoff, "Cultural Biography of Things."
19. Summarized in Appadurai, "Introduction," 17.
20. Joyce and Gillespie, "Making Things," 4, 11.
21. Joyce, "Things in Motion," 21.
22. Joyce and Gillespie, "Making Things," 12.
23. Joyce, "Things in Motion," 29.
24. Hamilton and Proctor-Tiffany, *Moving Women*; Borland, "Female Networks"; Proctor-Tiffany, *Medieval Art in Motion*; and Hamilton, *Pleasure and Politics*.
25. Examples of unillustrated manuscripts that present the *Régime* alongside academic medical texts include BnF Fr. 1288, Sloane 3525, and Wellcome MS.546; see appendix 3.
26. Sloane 1611 is one example of an unillustrated manuscript that presents the *Régime* alongside religious and devotional texts; see appendix 3. For a study that recovers traces of caregiving by religious women, see Ritchey, *Acts of Care*.
27. M. Green, *Making Women's Medicine Masculine*, and M. Green, "Books as a Source." Green's extensive and groundbreaking scholarship is fundamental to the field of medieval women's medicine, often grappling specifically with questions related to the role of women in their own medical treatment and health. See also M. Green, *Women's Healthcare in the Medieval West* and *Trotula*, in addition to many other publications.
28. M. Green, "Possibilities of Literacy," 45.
29. Monica Green supports this perspective on the *Régime*; see "Possibilities of Literacy," 26–32.
30. Cabré, "Women or Healers?" Cabré has also argued for lay women's use and likely commission of a health guide in "From a Master to a Laywoman."
31. Tyers, "Family, Feud, and Fertility," 391. See also Tyers, "'In the Merry Month of May.'"
32. Leong, *Recipes and Everyday Knowledge*.
33. Leipzig Cod. Haen. 3478 library records. For information and the fully digitized manuscript, see https://digital.ub.uni-leipzig.de/mirador (last accessed September 2, 2020).
34. The digitized manuscript of Biblioteca Apostolica Vaticana Reg.lat.1256 is available at https://digi.vatlib.it (last accessed September 2, 2020).
35. Bibliothèque nationale de France Arsenal MS 2894 is a fifteenth-century copy on paper; see Nicoud, *Régimes de santé*, 2:973. The full manuscript is also available on the Bibliothèque nationale de France's Gallica website: https://gallica.bnf.fr (last accessed September 2, 2020).
36. Fery-Hue notes that the *Régime* text is close to complete in forty-four of the sixty-eight manuscripts she discusses in "*Régime du corps*: Tradition manuscrite," 114.
37. These differences, to be explored more fully in chapter 2, may be a result of the place or date in which the manuscripts were made but also indicate details that may reflect the designers, artists, or patrons involved in the original commissions.
38. For more on my approach to the unique qualities of the historiated initial as a form, see Borland, "Freeze-Framed."

Chapter 1

1. Weitzmann, *Illustrations in Roll and Codex*. See also Whatling, "Narrative Art in Northern Europe"; and Wolf, "Narrative and Narrativity," 190–93. General studies on narrative theory include the 1980 special issue of the journal *Critical Inquiry* edited by W. J. T. Mitchell, republished as Mitchell, *On Narrative*; Mitchell, *Picture Theory*; and Bal, *Narratology*.
2. Borland, "Freeze-Framed," 238. Thompson and Bordell explain this cinematic technique through a well-known example: "the famous ending of *The 400 Blows* made the freeze-frame technique a favored device for expressing an unresolved situation"; Thompson and Bordell, *Film History*, 445.
3. Riddy, "Looking Closely," 225.
4. Landouzy and Pépin, *Régime du corps*, lxix; and Fery-Hue, "*Régime du corps*: Tradition manuscrite," 114. See also Fery-Hue, "*Régime du corps*: Note"; Fery-Hue, "*Régime du corps*: Complément" (1999); and Fery-Hue, "*Régime du corps*: Complément" (2004). Nicoud discusses the various redactions and versions in her discussion of the text's dissemination over time; see Nicoud, *Régimes de santé*, 1:410–18.
5. Fery-Hue, "*Régime du corps*: Tradition manuscrite," 117.
6. Landouzy and Pépin, *Régime du corps*, 28–30; and Camille, "Manuscript Illumination and the Art of Copulation," 63.
7. Cadden, *Meanings of Sex Difference*, 117–30; see also Jacquart and Thomasset, *Sexuality and Medicine*.
8. Landouzy and Pépin, *Régime du corps*, 30; Rhazes is also mentioned in some copies.
9. Ibid., 79–82; and Wallis, *Medieval Medicine*, 499–500.
10. Landouzy and Pépin, *Régime du corps*, 71–73; and Wallis, *Medieval Medicine*, 493–95.
11. Landouzy and Pépin, *Régime du corps*, 72; and Wallis, *Medieval Medicine*, 494.
12. Landouzy and Pépin, *Régime du corps*, 74–78; and Wallis, *Medieval Medicine*, 495–99.
13. Landouzy and Pépin, *Régime du corps*, 179–80; and Scully and Scully, *Early French Cookery*, 231.
14. Baxter, *Bestiaries and Their Users*; Clark and McMunn, *Beasts and Birds*; McCulloch, *Mediaeval French and Latin Bestiaries*; and Hassig, *Medieval Bestiaries*.
15. Dyer, *Standards of Living*, 63; and Landouzy and Pépin, *Régime du corps*, 184–87.
16. Landouzy and Pépin, *Régime du corps*, lxviii.
17. Wallis, *Medieval Medicine*, 493.
18. Stones, "Stylistic Associations," 11. See also Stones, *Gothic Manuscripts*, and Leson, "Pathways of Salvation."
19. The library's curatorial description can be found on the Morgan Library's entry for the manuscript at http://corsair.morganlibrary.org/ (last accessed September 2, 2020).
20. Kren and McKendrick, *Illuminating the Renaissance*, 276; Campos Ribeiro, "Picturing Medieval Health," 13–88; and Campos Ribeiro, "Medicina e dietética medieval."
21. Camille, "Manuscript Illumination and the Art of Copulation," provides examples from a wide range of manuscripts, including images from the *Roman de la Rose* at the Morgan Library, MS M.132, fol. 137r, and several copies of *De generatione*: Biblioteca Apostolica Vaticana MS Barb. lat.165, fol. 234; Bibliothèque nationale de Paris MS lat. 12953, fol. 166; and Bibliothèque nationale de Paris MS lat. 6323, fol. 71v.
22. Whittington, "Picturing Christ as Surgeon and Patient." For a transcription of British Library Sloane MS 1977 as well as an extensive discussion of the manuscript, see Valls, "Studies on Roger Frugardi's *Chirurgia*;" and Stones, *Gothic Manuscripts*, pt. 1, vol. 2: 497–501.
23. For catalogues and analyses of bestiaries, see Baxter, *Bestiaries and Their Users*; Clark and McMunn, *Beasts and Birds*; McCulloch, *Mediaeval French and Latin Bestiaries*; Hassig, *Medieval Bestiaries*; and Hassig, *Mark of the Beast*. Many editions and translations have been published, including T. White, *Book of Beasts*; Barber, *Bestiary*; and Mermier, *Medieval Book of Beasts*.
24. Before 1300, herbals were based on two earlier traditions: Dioscorides's text known as *De materia medica*, and the *Herbarius* by Apuleius Platonicus; after 1300, a new herbal treatise was created, the *Tractatus de herbis*. See Collins, *Medieval Herbals*, 25–26. The

earliest surviving illustrated herbal is the Juliana Anicia Codex, probably created around 515 (Vienna, Österreichische Nationalbibliothek, Cod. Med. Gr. I).

25. Bodleian Library MS Ashmole 1462.

26. Collins, *Medieval Herbals*, 25–28, 307–10; Givens, *Observation and Image-Making*, especially 82–105; and Givens, "Reading and Writing," 117.

27. Collins, *Medieval Herbals*, 307–8; Givens, *Observation and Image-Making*, 128–33; and Kyle, *Medicine and Humanism*.

28. Valls, "Illustrations as Abstracts," 76.

29. Sandler, *Omne Bonum*, 1:98.

30. P. Jones, "Image, Word, and Medicine," 7. Jones focuses on the Paneth Codex as an example of this phenomenon (Yale University, Medical Library MS 28), which he explores more fully in "Picturing Medicine."

31. P. Jones, "Picturing Medicine," 199.

32. Lewis, *Rhetoric of Power*; Lewis, *Reading Images*; Lewis, "Narrative"; Lewis, "Beyond the Frame"; Maekawa, *Narrative and Experience*; Pächt, *Rise of Pictorial Narrative*; and Whatling, "Narrative Art in Northern Europe." For an excellent discussion of continuous narration in several medieval examples, or multiple, sequential events depicted within the same framed space, see Schmitt, "Continuous Narration." See also Chatman, "What Novels Can Do"; Evans, "Episodes in Analysis"; Haidu, "Episode and Semiotic Module"; Martínez Pizarro, *Rhetoric of the Scene*; and Wittig, *Stylistic and Narrative Structures*.

33. Whittington, "Picturing Christ as Surgeon and Patient," 103; see also Valls, "Studies on Roger Frugardi's *Chirurgia*," 129–31.

34. Valls, "Illustrations as Abstracts," which focuses on Montpellier Bibliothèque interuniversitaire, MS H 089.

35. Additional examples of scenes depicting breast examinations in surgical manuscripts can be found in Montpellier Bibliothèque interuniversitaire, MS H 089, fol. 22r, and Besançon Bibliothèque municipale MS 457, fol. 191. See also M. Green, *Making Women's Medicine Masculine*, 91–97.

36. Peter Murray Jones points this out in relation to the Paneth Codex. See P. Jones, "Image, Word, and Medicine," 7–9.

37. Borland, "Freeze-Framed." In that essay I address the surprising lack of scholarship on the historiated initial as a form.

38. An extensive body of scholarship demonstrates this shift. Some key publications include Stones, *Gothic Manuscripts*; Rouse and Rouse, *Manuscripts and Their Makers*; and Branner, *Manuscript Painting in Paris*.

39. Kemp, "Narrative," 68; H. White, "Value of Narrativity," 10; and Valls, "Illustrations as Abstracts," 78.

40. Landouzy and Pépin, *Régime du corps*, 74–82. This section of the *Régime* is translated into English in Wallis, *Medieval Medicine*, 493–500.

41. L'Estrange, *Holy Motherhood*, 76–109.

42. Lewis, *Rhetoric of Power*, 31; Sturges, *Medieval Interpretation*; Ricoeur, "Narrative Time"; Ricoeur, *Temps et récit*; Harris, "Narrative," 54; and Kemp, "Narrative," 67–68.

43. Klapisch-Zuber, "Blood Parents and Milk Parents"; Otis, "Municipal Wet Nurses"; Winer, "Conscripting the Breast"; Winer, "The Mother and the *Dida*"; Blumenthal, "'*With My Daughter's Milk*'"; Miles, *Complex Delight*; Yalom, *History of the Breast*; Winer, "Enslaved Wet Nurse as Nanny"; and van der Lugt, "Nature as Norm."

44. Winer, "Conscripting the Breast," 166. See also van der Lugt, "Nature as Norm."

45. Klapisch-Zuber, "Blood Parents and Milk Parents," 162.

46. Landouzy and Pépin, *Régime du corps*, 74–78, and Wallis, *Medieval Medicine*, 495–99.

47. Winer, "Conscripting the Breast," 176; Landouzy and Pépin, *Régime du corps*, 77. Interestingly, peasant families did not worry about this belief; see Klapisch-Zuber, "Blood Parents and Milk Parents," 160–61.

48. Winer, "Conscripting the Breast," 177.

49. Klapisch-Zuber, "Blood Parents and Milk Parents," 158–59.

50. Howell, *Eleanor of Provence*, 27–30.

51. Ibid., 27, 101–2, and Sivéry, *Marguerite de Provence*, 72. See also Howell, "Royal Women of England and France," 169–70.

52. Tyers, "'In the Merry Month of May'"; Tyers, "Family, Feud, and Fertility"; Tyers, "Rebirth of Fertility"; and Sewright, "Introduction to British Library MS Lansdowne 380."

53. Winer, "Conscripting the Breast," 166–68. See also Klapisch-Zuber, "Blood Parents and Milk Parents," 140–41; and Winer, "Enslaved Wet Nurse as Nanny."

54. Klapisch-Zuber, "Blood Parents and Milk Parents," 140.

55. Winer, "Conscripting the Breast," 176, and Klapisch-Zuber, "Blood Parents and Milk Parents," 135–36.
56. Landouzy and Pépin, *Régime du corps*, 76, and Wallis, *Medieval Medicine*, 497.
57. Klapisch-Zuber, "Blood Parents and Milk Parents," 158–59. See also Otis, "Municipal Wet Nurses"; Winer, "Conscripting the Breast," 176–77.
58. Landouzy and Pépin, *Régime du corps*, 76–77, and Wallis, *Medieval Medicine*, 497–98. Klapisch-Zuber also discusses the role of nurses and infant mortality rates in "Blood Parents and Milk Parents," 146–53.
59. Klapisch-Zuber, "Blood Parents and Milk Parents," 137–38, 140.
60. For example, see Lewis, *Rhetoric of Power*.
61. Camille, *Image on the Edge*.
62. Siraisi, *Medieval and Early Renaissance Medicine*, 135. See also Valls, "Illustrations as Abstracts," 78.
63. Klapisch-Zuber, "Blood Parents and Milk Parents," 143–44, 159–62. See also Winer, "Conscripting the Breast," 169.
64. Winer, "The Mother and the *Dida*," 57, and Blumenthal, "'*With My Daughter's Milk*,'" 103–4.
65. L'Estrange, *Holy Motherhood*, 79.
66. Ibid., 86. For more on churching, see Rieder, *On the Purification of Women*. See also Bleeke, *Motherhood and Meaning*, 30–38.
67. L'Estrange, *Holy Motherhood*, 102; see also Davis, "Women on Top."
68. Fresco, "Gendered Household Spaces," 193.
69. L'Estrange, *Holy Motherhood*, 82–88.
70. Ibid., 1–21.
71. British Library Sloane MS 1977 and Bodleian Library MS Ashmole 399 are two examples of other medical manuscripts that seem to reflect the taboo against male practitioners touching women (see fig. 23). Green discusses these two manuscripts and others in *Making Women's Medicine Masculine*, 91–111.
72. Camille, "Manuscript Illumination and the Art of Copulation," 62–63.
73. Cadden, *Meanings of Sex Difference*, 117–30.
74. For more on theories about defacement in medieval manuscripts, see Camille, "Obscenity Under Erasure." I explore another instance of manuscript defacement in Borland, "Unruly Reading."
75. M. Green, "Possibilities of Literacy," 22–23.
76. For a preliminary study of academic physicians and gesture, see O'Boyle, "Gesturing in the Early Universities."
77. Wallis, "Signs and Senses," and Wallis, *Medieval Medicine*, 389–92 (sample of such text).
78. Valls, "Illustrations as Abstracts," 81–82.
79. McVaugh, "Bedside Manners," 212.
80. Ibid., 215. This specific quote comes from William of Saliceto's *Summa conservationis*.
81. Meyer, "Manuscrits médicaux en français," 196–98; the text on physician behavior is on folios 209–19 in Sloane 3525. See also T. Hunt, *Anglo-Norman Medicine*, 2:17–32.
82. M. Green, *Making Women's Medicine Masculine*, 108–17.
83. Several scholars mention problems with waste in urban environments, to the point where civil authorities had to intervene with penalties for failing to dispose of blood in the appropriate manner; Rawcliffe, *Urban Bodies*, 197; Pouchelle, *Body and Surgery*, 74; and Gil-Sotres, "Derivation and Revulsion," 120.
84. Harris, "Narrative."

Chapter 2

1. I explore the role of female networks in the dissemination of the illustrated *Régime* more fully in Borland, "Female Networks."
2. Landouzy and Pépin, *Régime du corps*, 180, and Scully and Scully, *Early French Cookery*, 86.
3. Fresh cheese is also recommended in the *Tacuinum sanitatis*, which is discussed further in chapter 4. See Scully and Scully, *Early French Cookery*, 86.
4. Dyer, *Standards of Living*, 63; Freedman, *Out of the East*, 40–41; and Freedman, *Images of the Medieval Peasant*, 149.
5. M. Green, "Possibilities of Literacy," 26.
6. Landouzy and Pépin, *Régime du corps*, lii–liii. The language of the prologue is somewhat ambiguous; another interpretation is that she was asking for the text because she was unable to visit them herself at that time.

7. The full prologue is not included in all copies of the text; in addition to being absent in many copies, it is also sometimes a shortened colophon or explicit instead (for instance, on Bibliothèque nationale de France Arsenal MS 2510, fol. 57r, and Biblioteca da Ajuda Cod. 52-XIII-26, fol. 176r). The most representative version is published in the primary edition of the *Régime du corps*, Landouzy and Pépin, *Régime du corps*, 3 (based on the earliest copy of the text, BnF Fr. 2021, which is unillustrated):

> Au commencement de che livre, si dirons pour coi fu fais, et là où il fu prins, et quant il fu fais à le requeste le contesse de Prouvenche ki est mere le roine de France, le roine d'Engletiere, et le roine de Alemaigne, et la contesse d'Anjou. Et si fist maistres Alebrans de Florence, en l'an de l'incarnation Jhesu Crist .m.cc.lvi. ans, quant ele dut venir veir ses filles si com ele fist, et li fist cest livre por che k'il ne pooit aler avoec li, car ele ne vaut mie k'il laissast les marcheans d'outre les mons k'il avoit en cure, et ele tenoit plus de lui ke d'un autre. Si li fist faire che livre por porter avoec li et por garder.

A handful of later copies include a reference to Emperor Frederick II instead of Beatrice.

8. Fery-Hue and Tyers both point to the challenges of relying on the prologue: Fery-Hue, "*Régime du corps*: Tradition manuscrite," 114–15; Tyers, "'In the Merry Month of May,'" 278; and Tyers, "Rebirth of Fertility," 14.
9. Landouzy and Pépin, *Régime du corps*; Howell, *Eleanor of Provence*; and Cox, *Eagles of Savoy*.
10. Howell, *Eleanor of Provence*; Sivéry, *Marguerite de Provence*; Gil, *Marguerite de Provence*; Cox, *Eagles of Savoy*; and Goldstone, *Four Queens*.
11. Beatrice's original copy does not appear to survive; Landouzy and Pépin consider Bibliothèque nationale de France Fr. 2021 to be the earliest extant copy of the text, which has been dated to between 1257 and 1261 and is unillustrated. Landouzy and Pépin, *Régime du corps*, xxiii–xxvii, lii–lxi, lxxv. See also Fery-Hue, "*Régime du corps*: Tradition manuscrite," 114.
12. Speaking about all *Régime* manuscripts (not just the illustrated copies), Fery-Hue states that certain copies were executed on the Continent, brought to England, and completed there with short English texts; Fery-Hue, "*Régime du corps*: Tradition manuscrite," 128. This was one way the text spread throughout western Europe.
13. Howell, *Eleanor of Provence*, 80–92.
14. Bodleian Library MS Bodley 270b; Paris, Bibliothèque nationale MS Lat. 11560; and British Library Harley MS 1526 and Harley MS 1527; see Lowden, *Making of the "Bibles Moralisées,"* 1:2.
15. Lowden, *Making of the "Bibles Moralisées,"* 1:185–86. See also Howell, *Eleanor of Provence*, 136–38; Sivéry, *Marguerite de Provence*; and Gil, *Marguerite de Provence*.
16. Howell, *Eleanor of Provence*, 136–38; see Luard, *Matthaei Parisiensis*, 5:481, and Richard, *Saint Louis*, 68.
17. Lowden, *Making of the "Bibles Moralisées,"* 1:183–87; Howell, *Eleanor of Provence*; Sivéry, *Marguerite de Provence*; and Gil, *Marguerite de Provence*. Howell points to at least one letter from Margaret to Eleanor, written in 1252 while Margaret was in the Holy Land; Howell, *Eleanor of Provence*, 60.
18. For an excellent example that explores the political function of manuscripts for French queen Jeanne de Navarre (1273–1305), see Luyster, "Place of a Queen."
19. Lowden, *Making of the "Bibles Moralisées,"* 1:52. Hamilton argues that it was made for Blanche in "Queenship and Kinship."
20. Stanton, *Queen Mary Psalter*.
21. Hamilton, *Pleasure and Politics*.
22. Ibid., 159, and Proctor-Tiffany, *Medieval Art in Motion*, 92.
23. E. Hunt, *Illuminating the Borders*, 18.
24. Stones, *Gothic Manuscripts*, pt. 1, vol. 2: 299–302. The British Library dates it a little later, to around 1285; Landouzy and Pépin date it to the late thirteenth century; *Régime du corps*, xxxviii. See also P. Jones, "Regime del corpo."
25. The text was composed in verse in 1245 and prose in 1265. See Cassagnes-Brouquet, *L'image du monde*, 12; Prior, *L'image du monde*; Stones, "Stylistic Associations," 22; and Connochie-Bourgne, "Pourquoi et comment réécrire un encyclopédie?"
26. Stones, *Gothic Manuscripts*, pt. 1, vol. 2: 301–2.
27. Ibid., pt. 1, vol. 1: 64 and vol. 2: 299–302. Stones identifies two Bibles (Cambrai, Médiathèque municipale MS 354 and Paris, Bibliothèque Mazarine MS 13) and a missal, Cambrai, Médiathèque municipale MS 183.

28. Stones, *Gothic Manuscripts*, pt. 1, vol. 1: xxxviii, lvi, 64, and vol. 2: 299–302.
29. Stones points out this conundrum as well; ibid., pt. 1, vol. 2: 301–2.
30. Lowden, *Making of the "Bibles Moralisées,"* 1:132–34, 216–18.
31. Stones, "Stylistic Associations"; see also Stones, *Gothic Manuscripts*, pt. 1, vol. 2: 293–96.
32. The text is on fol. 57r: "Ichi endroit fine li livres qui doit iestre apielés la flours et la rose de toute medicine de fisique; et le fist maistre Aldebrandins de Sciane pour le bone contesse de Prouvence, laquele fu mere as iiij. roines, l'une de France, l'autre d'Alemagne, d'Engleterre et de Sezile." See also Landouzy and Pépin, *Régime du corps*, xxxiii–xxxiv, and Nicoud, *Régimes de santé*, 2:971–72. I am grateful to Theresa Tyers for pointing out the nuance of the phrasing here.
33. Beatrice of Provence's husband, Charles of Anjou, invaded Sicily and became king in 1266. Landouzy and Pépin point out that the earliest textual copy of the *Régime*, BnF Fr. 2021, which they also refer to as Redaction A, describes the younger Beatrice as "la contesse d'Anjou," and this and other information leads them to suggest that BnF Fr. 2021 was written sometime between 1257 and 1261, reinforcing the significance of the textual change found in Bibliothèque nationale de France Arsenal MS 2510; Landouzy and Pépin, *Régime du corps*, xxv–xxvi, xxxiii, nos. 1 and 2 on liv.
34. Landouzy and Pépin, *Régime du corps*, xxxiii–xxxiv, no. 1 on xxxiv. For a full record for Arsenal 2510 on BnF's Gallica website, see https://gallica.bnf.fr/ (last accessed September 13, 2020). Folios 33 and 34 of Arsenal 2510 are later copies of the chapters on ears and teeth that apparently went missing. The statement that Jehan Neriot received it from the House of Madame of Vendôme, and that it was lent by Maris Jouris, the mother of a woman named Jacqueline, is on an interleaf now located in front of fol. 1.
35. Stones, "Stylistic Associations," 11.
36. Ibid. See also Stones, *Gothic Manuscripts*, pt. 1, vol. 1, 63–64; pt. 1, vol. 2, 289–93; and Leson, "Pathways of Salvation."
37. Stones, "Stylistic Associations"; Stones, *Gothic Manuscripts*, pt. 1, vol. 2: 299–302; and Leson, "Pathways of Salvation." See the full manuscript at http://www.getty.edu/art/collection (last accessed September 13, 2020).
38. Stones, "Stylistic Associations," 11, 24. She suggests that "his activities were based in a town or city that had a distinguished tradition of making fine illuminated books and where several artists were active at the same time" (24).
39. Ibid., 20–22. These lay audiences included Guillaume of Termonde, son of Guy de Dampierre, count of Flanders (ca. 1226–1305), or possibly Marie de Réthel, wife of Gautier I d'Enghien, brother of the bishop of Tournai and Liège. Guy de Dampierre was among the most prolific book patrons in this northern region in the late thirteenth and very early fourteenth centuries, as reflected in the naming of the Dampierre group of illuminators; see E. Hunt, *Illuminating the Borders*, 45–78.
40. Among the possible patrons Stones proposes for the Bute Psalter is a family member of the counts or dukes of Juliers, perhaps Imagina von Westerburg, wife of Waleran II. Alternatively, it may have come to the Juliers family through a later marriage of a lady of the Hainaut court, such as Jeanne, daughter of the count of Hainaut and sister of Philippa, wife of Edward III of England. See Stones, "Stylistic Associations," 25. Richard Leson also assumes a female recipient: Leson, "Pathways of Salvation," 130, no. 4. The Bute Psalter is one of six psalters known as "the fully illustrated Psalter group"; the three earliest manuscripts in this group were made in Paris around 1220 to 1230 and have been associated with the Parisian *Bibles moralisées* atelier; see Leson, "Pathways of Salvation," 140.
41. These copies of the *Image du monde* include Bibliothèque nationale de France Fr. 14964 (dated 1265), "which was illustrated by one of the painters who worked with the Bute Painter on the pontifical of Cambrai," and possibly Bibliothèque nationale de France Fr. 14970 as well, which contains what appears to be the first image from an otherwise removed copy of the *Image du monde*; Stones, "Stylistic Associations," 22.
42. Nicoud, *Régimes de santé*, 2:978. For an English translation of the plague text, see Horrox, *The Black Death*, 158–63. This plague text also appears in several other copies (unillustrated) of the *Régime*.

43. "Tres noble et poissant prince mons. Charle, conte de Valoys, de Chartres, d'Alenchon et d'Anjou, fist faire cest livret, qui est bon et profitable pour gairir [gairer] toutes manieres de plaies vielles et nouvelles, et pour aucunes autres maladies aussi." For a full record for BnF Fr. 12323, see BnF's Gallica website: https://gallica.bnf.fr (last accessed September 5, 2020).
44. Wallis, *Medieval Medicine*, 414–19.
45. Thomas, "Jean Pitart, chirurgien et poète"; Prioreschi, *History of Medicine*, 462–63. Pitart was friend and master of Henri de Mondeville (ca. 1270–1325), another well-known surgeon who spent part of his life in Paris and was connected with early translations of surgical texts into French; McVaugh, *Rational Surgery*, 43–44, 50, and 230; see also Jacquart, "Medical Practice in Paris," and O'Boyle, *Art of Medicine*.
46. Thomas, "Jean Pitart, chirurgien et poète," 107–8, and Prioreschi, *History of Medicine*, 462–63.
47. Beyond these three illustrated manuscripts of the *Régime du corps*, additional copies of the *Régime* text were also thought to have been moving between the Continent and England; see Fery-Hue, "*Régime du corps*: Tradition manuscrite," 128.
48. These include Sloane 2435, BnF Fr. 12323, BnF Fr. 2021, BnF Fr. 1444, Chantilly Musée Condé MS 476, and UPenn LJS 55; see appendix 3.
49. Lacarrière, "Compilation, Collation and Correction."
50. See also Cassagnes-Brouquet, *L'image du monde*, and Prior, *Caxton's Mirrour of the World*.
51. All of the *Image du monde* images in Sloane 2435 are in rectangular frames; in the case of BnF Fr. 12323, eight images are rectangular (diagrams), and eleven are historiated initials (the latter primarily natural materials and phenomena).
52. This manuscript contains numerous other texts, including the *Livres dou Trésor* by Brunetto Latini; see Cassagnes-Brouquet, *L'image du monde*, 8–10, 110–17, and Rouse and Rouse, *Manuscripts and Their Makers*, 1:173–202.
53. Proctor-Tiffany, *Medieval Art in Motion*, 91–94; see also Rouse and Rouse, *Manuscripts and Their Makers*, 2:178–79. This identification is supported by the inventory that describes the manuscript as having seventeen texts, naming *L'Almanach aux Juifs* as the first text.
54. Hamilton, *Pleasure and Politics*, 159, and Proctor-Tiffany, *Medieval Art in Motion*, 92.
55. Cassagnes-Brouquet, *L'image du monde*, 16–17. In her discussion of UPenn LJS 55, a manuscript with a newly identified *Régime* excerpt that also includes *L'image du monde*, Lacarrière speaks to the appeal of such encyclopedic texts: Lacarrière, "Compilation, Collation and Correction."
56. Landouzy and Pépin, *Régime du corps*, xxix, and Fery-Hue, "*Régime du corps*: Tradition manuscrite," 116. Two other *Régime* manuscripts, British Library Royal MS 19 B X and St. John's College Oxford MS 68, each contain a similar excerpt from Brunetto's *Trésor*, which is focused on birds of prey.
57. Bates and Curry, *England and Normandy*; Curry, *Hundred Years War*; Curry and Hughes, *Arms, Armies and Fortifications*; D. Green, *Hundred Years War*; Allmand, *Lancastrian Normandy*; and Driver, "'Me Fault Faire.'"
58. The folio also includes the inscription "Roy Henry VII, a qui dieu doint bonne vie et paradis" (King Henry VII, may God give him a good life and paradise); *Catalogue of the Manuscripts*, 3:482–83. The nineteenth-century catalogue dates this manuscript to late in the fifteenth century; the more recent catalogue suggests mid-fifteenth century: Binski and Zutshi, *Western Illuminated Manuscripts*, 312–14. See also K. Scott, *Later Gothic Manuscripts*, 2:266.
59. On books collected by Henry VII, see K. Scott, "Manuscripts for Henry VII"; K. Scott, *Later Gothic Manuscripts*, 2:266; Backhouse, "Founders of the Royal Library"; Backhouse, "Illuminated Manuscripts Associated with Henry VII"; and Binski and Zutshi, *Western Illuminated Manuscripts*, 312–14.
60. K. Scott, "Manuscripts for Henry VII," 283. Janet Backhouse also distinguishes between Edward's patronage of original manuscripts and Henry's acquisition primarily through gifts, inheritance, and purchasing of secondhand books: Backhouse, "Illuminated Manuscripts Associated with Henry VII," 266; Backhouse, "Founders of the Royal Library"; Kipling, "Henry VII,"; and Binski and Zutshi, *Western Illuminated Manuscripts*, 312–14.
61. Kipling, "Henry VII," 122, 127. See also Alexander, "Foreign Illuminators and

Illuminated Manuscripts," 54, and K. Scott, *Later Gothic Manuscripts*, 2:365–67.

62. As Kathleen Scott points out, "[o]therwise, why bother to purchase a text in French produced some fifty years earlier?" Scott, "Manuscripts for Henry VII," 283.

63. Ibid., 280–81.

64. Morgan Library online database and documents: http://corsair.themorgan.org (last accessed September 13, 2020).

65. The manuscript also includes a table of contents on fols. 2–4. See Landouzy and Pépin, *Régime du corps*, and Morgan Library online database and catalogue documents. In the nineteenth century it was owned by William Morris; it was then in Richard Bennett's collection (purchased in 1897) before going to Morgan (who bought it from Bennett in 1902).

66. Reynolds, "English Patrons and French Artists," 311–13. See also Driver, "'Me Fault Faire,'" and Alexander, "Foreign Illuminators and Illuminated Manuscripts."

67. Curatorial notes, Morgan Library, citing Weale, *Bookbindings and Rubbings of Bindings*, 1:xxxix and 2:115.

68. Sixteenth-century inscription "John Thwayte" (British Library Harley MS 1527, fol. 2v). See also Lowden, *Making of the "Bibles Moralisées,"* 1:187, and James and Gale, *Western Manuscripts*, 186. Thanks to Kathleen E. Kennedy for her help in proposing a possible identity for Thwayte. Possibly a relation, Thomas Thwaytes (ca. 1435–1503) was an official in Henry VII's court whom Backhouse links to several manuscripts in Henry's collection: Backhouse, "Founders of the Royal Library," 30, 38.

69. The major episodes and events that took place in France in the fifteenth century include an English attack led by Henry V in 1415; the seizure of Rouen by the English in 1419 and Paris in 1420; and the Treaty of Troyes in 1420. The French recaptured Paris in 1436 and, led by King Charles VII, reclaimed Rouen in 1449, after thirty years of English occupation; the French effectively ended the war and English presence in 1453. See Allmand, *Lancastrian Normandy*; Curry and Hughes, *Arms, Armies and Fortifications*; D. Green, *Hundred Years War*; Reynolds, "English Patrons and French Artists"; and Driver, "'Me Fault Faire.'"

70. These included the Masters of the Munich Golden Legend, of Sir John Fastolf, of Lord Talbot, and of Lord Hoo; Reynolds, "English Patrons and French Artists," 312. See also Driver, "'Me Fault Faire,'" and Alexander, "Foreign Illuminators and Illuminated Manuscripts."

71. Reynolds, "English Patrons and French Artists," 310.

72. Tyers, "Rebirth of Fertility," 83. She highlights the similarities between this manuscript and the unillustrated Kassel manuscript (which also includes some of the *Trotula*).

73. These include "a tract on medicinal waters, herbal recipes, and recipes of 'domestic economy'"; see Tyers, "Rebirth of Fertility," 83, and Tyers, "'In the Merry Month of May,'" 271.

74. Tyers, "'In the Merry Month of May,'" 271. See also Tyers, "Rebirth of Fertility," 276–80; a translation of the manuscript's ownership statement on fol. 1v can be found on 276–77.

75. Tyers, "Rebirth of Fertility," 276–80. For more on Rowland Brydges (also seen as Brugys, or Brugge), see Bindoff, *History of Parliament*. Two other medically related printed books may also have been owned by Rowland Brydges, as is suggested by inscriptions: Johannes Jacobi, *Regimen contra Pestilentiam* (1486/91, British Library IA.49872) and *Herbarius Latinus* (ca. 1486, British Library IA.39860); See Baker, *Men of Court*, 391–93.

76. Tyers, "Rebirth of Fertility," 278.

77. Carvalho, "Manuscrit du *Régime du corps*"; Campos Ribeiro, "Picturing Medieval Health," 8–9; and Campos Ribeiro, "Medicina e dietética medieval." This copy has been linked to several others that have only a frontispiece (see appendix 3); McKendrick, Lowden, and Doyle, *Royal Manuscripts*, 307.

78. Cassagnes-Brouquet, *L'image du monde*, 15.

79. Campos Ribeiro proposes that Cambridge was the basis for Sloane 2401 and Morgan, and that Morgan was the model for Ajuda; see Campos Ribeiro, "Picturing Medieval Health," 155–58.

80. Kren and McKendrick, *Illuminating the Renaissance*, 276; Campos Ribeiro, "Picturing Medieval Health," 14, 56; and Campos Ribeiro, "Medicina e dietética medieval."

81. Campos Ribeiro explores the provenance, suggesting the manuscript left England between 1542 and 1666, was rebound

by a Dutch bookseller in the eighteenth century, and was sold to the Portuguese king soon thereafter; "Picturing Medieval Health," 159–66.

82. Backhouse, "Founders of the Royal Library"; McKendrick, "Manuscripts of Edward IV"; Campos Ribeiro, "Picturing Medieval Health," 159–60; and McKendrick, Lowden, and Doyle, *Royal Manuscripts*, 69, 307.

83. Kren and McKendrick, *Illuminating the Renaissance*, 276; Campos Ribeiro, "Picturing Medieval Health," 13–88; and Campos Ribeiro, "Medicina e dietética medieval."

84. Campos Ribeiro, "Picturing Medieval Health," 81.

85. Sandler, *Gothic Manuscripts*, 1:51. Stanton has also pointed to the crossovers between English royalty and French collecting practices in the fourteenth century in her discussion of Isabelle of France; Stanton, *Queen Mary Psalter*, 10.

86. Rouse and Rouse, *Manuscripts and Their Makers*, 1:96–97; Overty, "Cost of Doing Scribal Business."

87. Rouse and Rouse, *Manuscripts and Their Makers*, 1:11, and see Stones, *Gothic Manuscripts*, pt. 1, vol. 1, 34–35.

88. Rouse and Rouse, *Manuscripts and Their Makers*, 1:14.

89. Ibid.

90. For more on rental pecias, see ibid., 1:85–97.

91. Stones, *Gothic Manuscripts*, pt. 1, vol. 1, 36–44, and map on p. 15.

92. Stones points to additional centers of artistic production in Arras, Douai, Thérouanne, Courtrai, Ypres, and Valenciennes; see Stones, "Stylistic Associations," 24–42.

93. Kren and McKendrick, *Illuminating the Renaissance*, 276; Campos Ribeiro, "Picturing Medieval Health," 13–88; and Campos Ribeiro, "Medicina e dietética medieval."

94. Proctor-Tiffany, *Medieval Art in Motion*, 94–103.

95. Sandler, *Survey of Manuscripts*, 1:50. Oxford and Cambridge, as university towns, had robust book production, but most of those manuscripts would have been unillustrated.

96. Ibid., 1:49–50.

97. Rouse and Rouse, *Manuscripts and Their Makers*, 1:96–97, 285–302; Reynolds, "English Patrons and French Artists," 311–13; Driver, "'Me Fault Faire'"; and Alexander, "Foreign Illuminators and Illuminated Manuscripts."

98. Reynolds, "English Patrons and French Artists," 311; see also Rouse and Rouse, *Manuscripts and Their Makers*, 1:285–302.

99. Reynolds, "English Patrons and French Artists," 312–13; Alexander, "Foreign Illuminators and Illuminated Manuscripts," 49; K. Scott, *Later Gothic Manuscripts*, 1:62–64; and Driver, "'Me Fault Faire.'"

100. Driver, "'Me Fault Faire,'" 420, 438.

101. For example, the medical manuscript Bibliothèque nationale de France Fr. 24246 was made for the Duke of Bedford in Rouen around 1430; it contains several historiated initials and embellished marginal decoration. And, although we do not know the content of the commissions, William Bradwardine, an English surgeon who was in Rouen from at least 1415 through 1421, financed the scribe Jacquet le Caron in 1420 in a trade agreement to produce manuscripts and market them, possibly in England. See Reynolds, "English Patrons and French Artists," 309, 311; see also Talbot and Hammond, *Medical Practitioners in Medieval England*.

102. M. Green, *Making Women's Medicine Masculine*, 161–62.

Chapter 3

1. Park, "Medical Practice," 620–21; O'Boyle, "Surgical Texts and Social Contexts," 179–84, esp. 182; and McVaugh, "Bedside Manners," 208–9.

2. Significant discrepancies existed between university towns and other places in terms of medical practice; Jacquart, "Medical Practice in Paris," 200.

3. Park, "Medical Practice," 617–24; O'Boyle, "Surgical Texts and Social Contexts," 182; Rawcliffe, *Medicine and Society*, 134 (outside London, physicians were "relatively thin on the ground"); and Rawcliffe, *Urban Bodies*, 299–312.

4. Rawcliffe, *Medicine and Society*, 134, and O'Boyle, "Surgical Texts and Social Contexts."

5. Around 1335 in Paris, practical training was required alongside learned medicine, suggesting an awareness that physicians

needed hands-on training, too; Jacquart, "Medical Practice in Paris," 198–99.

6. Mustain, "Rural Medical Practitioner," 471; Voigts, "Fifteenth-Century English Banns," 259; P. Jones, "Thomas Fayreford"; and Talbert, "Notebook of a Fifteenth-Century Practicing Physician."

7. Park, "Medical Practice," 619–20; Rawcliffe, *Medicine and Society*, 106–8; McVaugh, *Medicine Before the Plague*, 78–87; O'Boyle, *Art of Medicine*, 9–32; and Bullough, "Medieval Medicine." In some larger university towns like Paris, the university faculty of medicine did oversee such things; see Jacquart, "Medical Practice in Paris," 199–201.

8. O'Boyle, "Surgical Texts and Social Contexts," 182.

9. Temkin, *Galenism*; Nutton, "Early Medieval Medicine and Natural Science"; Jacquart, "Anatomy, Physiology, and Medical Theory"; and García-Ballester, "On the Origin."

10. Siraisi, *Medieval and Early Renaissance Medicine*, 101; Burns, "The Nonnaturals," 203; García-Ballester, "On the Origin"; Jacquart, "Anatomy, Physiology, and Medical Theory," 602; Gil-Sotres, "Regimens of Health"; Nicoud, *Régimes de santé*, 1:153–60; and Gil-Sotres, "Derivation and Revulsion."

11. Landouzy and Pépin, *Régime du corps*, 3–4, lxi. This list is not quite accurate, however, because Aldobrandino does not actually cite some of these authors; he also leaves Haly Abbas, a key source for him, off this list (see ibid., lxi–lxix).

12. Ibid., lxvi. Landouzy and Pépin provide several examples of direct citations from the Latin sources used by the *Régime*'s author, including work by Avicenna, Isaac, Rhazes, and Johannitius (lx–lxix); they also list which texts, down to the precise sections or chapters of those sources, are used in specific chapters of the *Régime*.

13. Ibid., 71; translation in Wallis, *Medieval Medicine*, 493.

14. Landouzy and Pépin, *Régime du corps*, 73; translation in Wallis, *Medieval Medicine*, 495.

15. M. Green, *Making Women's Medicine Masculine*, 169–70.

16. Siraisi, *Medieval and Early Renaissance Medicine*, 4; Nutton, "Early Medieval Medicine and Natural Science," 327, 329; and Temkin, *Galenism*.

17. Nutton, "Early Medieval Medicine and Natural Science," 327, and Temkin, *Galenism*.

18. Savage-Smith, "Medicine in Medieval Islam," 144–45, and Pormann and Savage-Smith, *Medieval Islamic Medicine*, 23–37.

19. Savage-Smith, "Medicine in Medieval Islam," 146.

20. Pormann and Savage-Smith, *Medieval Islamic Medicine*, 89–93, 115–19.

21. Ibid., 55–56, 166. See also Burnett and Jacquart, *Constantine the African*.

22. Pormann and Savage-Smith, *Medieval Islamic Medicine*, 61–64, 166, and Savage-Smith, "Medicine in Medieval Islam," 146.

23. Pormann and Savage-Smith, *Medieval Islamic Medicine*, 41, 50–51, 164–66. See Ibn Sīnā (Avicenna), *Canon of Medicine*, and Abu-Asab, Amri, and Micozzi, *Avicenna's Medicine*.

24. Wallis, *Medieval Medicine*, 493, and Landouzy and Pépin, *Régime du Corps*, lxi–lxix.

25. Park, "Medical Practice"; Park, *Doctors and Medicine*; McVaugh, *Medicine Before the Plague*; Shatzmiller, *Jews, Medicine, and Medieval Society*; O'Boyle, "Surgical Texts and Social Contexts"; Jacquart, "Medical Practice in Paris"; Jacquart, *Médecine médiévale*; O'Boyle, *Art of Medicine*; Bullough, *Universities, Medicine and Science*; and Burnett, "Translation and Transmission."

26. Jacquart, "Anatomy, Physiology, and Medical Theory," 596; Gil-Sotres, "Derivation and Revulsion," 110; Ibn Sīnā (Avicenna), *Canon of Medicine*; and Abu-Asab, Amri, and Micozzi, *Avicenna's Medicine*.

27. Gil-Sotres, "Regimens of Health," 296–97, and Jacquart, "Anatomy, Physiology, and Medical Theory," 590–93. See also Burnett and Jacquart, *Constantine the African*.

28. Burnett, "Translation and Transmission," 342–43. See also Burnett and Jacquart, *Constantine the African*.

29. Burnett, "Translation and Transmission," 343.

30. The astronomical tables that were the standard used throughout the Middle Ages are known as "Alfonsine Tables," in part because they were created under Alfonso's patronage; ibid., 344. See also Chabás and Goldstein, *Alfonsine Tables of Toledo*; García-Ballester, "On the Origin"; and Samsó, *Islamic Astronomy and Medieval Spain*.

31. Burnett, "Translation and Transmission," 345, and Jacquart, "Anatomy, Physiology, and Medical Theory," 592–94.
32. Wallis, *Medieval Medicine*, 485–510, specifically at 485–86.
33. Gil-Sotres, "Regimens of Health," 299. See also Gil-Sotres, Paniagua, and García-Ballester, *Regimen sanitatis ad regem Aragonum*; Ibn Buṭlān, *Taqwīm al-ṣiḥḥa (Tacuini sanitatis)*; Hoeniger, "Illuminated *Tacuinum sanitatis* Manuscripts"; Bertiz, "Picturing Health"; and Arano, *Tacuinum sanitatis*.
34. Hoeniger, "Illuminated *Tacuinum sanitatis* Manuscripts," 66–68. Hoeniger notes that the workshop of Giovannino de' Grassi, which is connected to several illuminated copies of the *Tacuinum*, also produced a number of illustrated herbals.
35. Nicoud, *Régimes de santé*, 1:87–145; Gil-Sotres, "Regimens of Health," 301; Gil-Sotres, Paniagua, and García-Ballester, *Regimen sanitatis ad regem Aragonum*, 535–43; Demaitre, *Doctor Bernard de Gordon*; and Wallis, *Medieval Medicine*, 485–86.
36. Nicoud, *Régimes de santé*, 1:87–145.
37. The title suggests a connection to the medical school of Salerno, but the text was likely written too late to have any real connection to the school, which was most active as a center in the twelfth century. A version circulated with Arnau de Vilanova's *Regimen for the King of Aragon*, which gave the *Regimen sanitatis salernitanum* some additional legitimacy despite its lack of an author. Wallis points out that "the career of the Salerno Regimen illustrates the ironic truth that health advice for the masses always sells best when packaged as health advice for the elite"; Wallis, *Medieval Medicine*, 487. See also García-Ballester and McVaugh, *Regimen sanitatis ad regem Aragonum*.
38. Gil-Sotres, "Regimens of Health," 301, and Gil-Sotres, Paniagua, and García-Ballester, *Regimen sanitatis ad regem Aragonum*, especially 517–20 on Juan of Toledo.
39. McVaugh, *Medicine Before the Plague*, 7–10, 144. See also Gil-Sotres, Paniagua, and García-Ballester, *Regimen sanitatis ad regem Aragonum*, 528–34; the Latin transcription of the *Regimen sanitatis ad regem Aragonum* can be found in the same volume, edited by García-Ballester and McVaugh, 417–70. Also see McVaugh, "Arnald of Villanova's *Regimen Almarie*," and Nicoud, *Régimes de santé*, 1:153–84.
40. "Arnau seems deliberately to have adopted a homely, non-technical language for the king"; McVaugh, *Medicine Before the Plague*, 145; see also 115. For translations, see the table in García-Ballester and McVaugh, *Regimen sanitatis ad regem Aragonum*, 559–62, 563.
41. McVaugh, "Experience-Based Medicine," 109; Demaitre, *Doctor Bernard de Gordon*, 51–70; Nicoud, *Régimes de santé*, 1:185–228, 229–79. Gil-Sotres, Paniagua, and García-Ballester, *Regimen sanitatis ad regem Aragonum*, 528–43; and Jacquart, "Medical Practice in Paris," 202. Maynus de Mayneriis (Maino de Mainieri) was at the faculty of medicine in Paris and master regent from 1326 to 1331; he wrote his *Regimen sanitatis* during a stay in France between 1331 and 1333 and was in Bernabò Visconti's service in Milan from 1346.
42. Gil-Sotres, "Regimens of Health," 301, and Gil-Sotres, Paniagua, and García-Ballester, *Regimen sanitatis ad regem Aragonum*.
43. M. Green, "Possibilities of Literacy," 44, and M. Green, *Making Women's Medicine Masculine*, 12–13, 163–64.
44. Brown, "Vernacular Universe." For example, Brown mentions the description of a fountain scene as similar to a version of Chrétien de Troyes's *Chevalier au lion* (154).
45. Lacarrière, "Compilation, Collation and Correction"; Tyers, "'In the Merry Month of May,'" 269; Tyers, "Family, Feud, and Fertility"; and C. Jones, "Assortment of Doctors."
46. Surveys of medieval medical imagery include MacKinney, *Medical Illustrations*, and P. Jones, *Medieval Medicine*. For a broader survey up to ca. 1600, see Herrlinger, *History of Medical Illustration*.
47. Park, *Secrets of Women*, and Jacquart, "Anatomy, Physiology, and Medical Theory," 591.
48. McCall, "Illuminating the Interior." See also Sudhoff, "Anatomische Zeichnungen"; Sudhoff, *Beitrag zur Geschichte der Anatomie*; Sudhoff, *Beiträge zur Geschichte der Chirurgie*; Hill, "*Fünfbilderserie* and Medieval Anatomy"; and P. Jones, *Medieval Medicine*, 30–31. Prominent examples include Bodleian Library MS Ashmole 399 (ca. 1292) and Wellcome Library MS.49 (1420). For more on Ashmole 399, see M. Green, *Making Women's Medicine Masculine*,

91–111, and Whittington, "Cruciform Womb."

49. O'Boyle, *Art of Medicine*, and Wallis, *Medieval Medicine*, 139–74.

50. Another example is an illustrated copy of Avicenna, Besançon Bibliothèque municipale MS 457, thought to have been made around 1260 in Paris. See Stones, *Gothic Manuscripts*, pt. 1, vol. 2, 11–13, and M. Green, *Making Women's Medicine Masculine*, 104.

51. McVaugh, *Medicine Before the Plague*, 139.

52. Talbot, "Mediaeval Physician's Vade Mecum"; Hartnell, "Medicine's Image," 328–29; and P. Jones, *Medieval Medicine*, 43–54. A transcription and English translation of the diagram's text, based on Bodleian Library MS Ashmole 391, can be found in Tavormina, *Dome of Uryne*, 45–57.

53. Tavormina, *Dome of Uryne*, 45–57.

54. McVaugh, *Medicine Before the Plague*, 139–44.

55. McVaugh, *Rational Surgery*; Gil-Sotres, "Derivation and Revulsion"; T. Hunt, *Medieval Surgery*; Kirkham and Warr, *Wounds in the Middle Ages*; and Tracy and DeVries, *Wounds and Wound Repair*. For more on the visual culture of medieval surgery, see P. Jones, *Medieval Medicine*, 76–94; Hartnell, "Tools of the Puncture"; and Valls, "Illustrations as Abstracts."

56. Rawcliffe, *Medicine and Society*, 72.

57. McVaugh, "Royal Surgeons," 224, and O'Boyle, "Surgical Texts and Social Contexts," 175–79.

58. For discussions of types of medical practitioners (physician, barber, surgeon, apothecary, leech) and their various training and practices, as well as more on the role of the barber, see Bullough, "Medical Practice," 280–83; Rawcliffe, "Profits of Practice"; Rawcliffe, *Medicine and Society*, 62–63, 105–215; McVaugh, *Medicine Before the Plague*, 38–40, 123–27; Gil-Sotres, "Derivation and Revulsion," 120–22, 140–48; O'Boyle, "Surgical Texts and Social Contexts," 157–60, 179–85; and Park, "Medical Practice," 611–29.

59. O'Boyle, "Surgical Texts and Social Contexts," 175–85; McVaugh, *Rational Surgery*; and Jacquart, "Medical Practice in Paris," 189–94.

60. On Roger's *Chirurgia*, see Whittington, "Picturing Christ as Surgeon and Patient"; Valls, "Studies on Roger Frugardi's *Chirurgia*"; Sudhoff, *Beiträge zur Geschichte der Chirurgie*, 2:148–236 (for a Latin transcription); and T. Hunt, *Anglo-Norman Medicine*, vol. 1.

61. Valls, "Studies on Roger Frugardi's *Chirurgia*," 137, 253, and Whittington, "Picturing Christ as Surgeon and Patient," 86–87.

62. Valls makes this point about another illustrated copy of *Chirurgia*, Montpellier Bibliothèque Interuniversitaire, Section Médecine MS H089 (see fig. 39); see Valls, "Illustrations as Abstracts," 76.

63. Whittington, "Picturing Christ as Surgeon and Patient," 85. See also Valls, "Illustrations as Abstracts," 69; Valls, "Studies on Roger Frugardi's *Chirurgia*"; and P. Jones, *Medieval Medicine*, 82–86.

64. Hartnell, "Tools of the Puncture," 32–34; P. Jones, *Medieval Medicine*, 89–91; P. Jones, "*Sicut hic depingitur . . .*"; and P. Jones, "Staying with the Programme."

65. P. Jones, "Staying with the Programme"; P. Jones, "*Sicut hic depingitur . . .*"; and P. Jones, *Medieval Medicine*, 89–91.

66. I discuss recipes further in chapter 4; some sources on medieval recipes include T. Hunt, *Popular Medicine*; Cabré, "Women or Healers?"; Riddy, "Looking Closely"; Tyers, "Family, Feud, and Fertility"; Tyers, "'In the Merry Month of May'"; and Skemer, *Binding Words*.

67. Siraisi, *Medieval and Early Renaissance Medicine*, 141, and Rawcliffe, *Medicine and Society*, 149.

68. Tyers, "Family, Feud, and Fertility," n. 53. She points out that one of the recipe collections in Kassel is also in Sloane 2401.

69. Rawcliffe, *Medicine and Society*, 150–51; Matthews, *Royal Apothecaries*; Trease, "Spicers and Apothecaries"; and T. Hunt, *Popular Medicine*.

70. Rawcliffe, *Medicine and Society*, 148–69, and McVaugh, *Medicine Before the Plague*, 108–35, 153–58.

71. Kyle, *Medicine and Humanism*, 30–42, and Collins, *Medieval Herbals*. See also Riddle, *Dioscorides on Pharmacy and Medicine*.

72. Rawcliffe, *Medicine and Society*, 54, 148–69; McVaugh, *Medicine Before the Plague*, 150–58; and Cabré, "Women or Healers?"

73. P. Jones, "Image, Word, and Medicine," 9.

74. Williams, *Secret of Secrets*, and Tyers, "Rebirth of Fertility," 145, 189. For an example of a medical collection that includes both the *Secret of Secrets* and the *Lettre d'Hippocrate* and has been tied to household health management and female readers, see the discussion of

the Trinity College Library Cambridge manuscript CTC O.2.5 in McAvoy, Skinner, and Tyers, "Family, Feud, and Fertility." The Old French version of the *Lettre d'Hippocrate* included in Wellcome MS.546, a manuscript that also includes a short section of the *Régime*, is transcribed in T. Hunt, *Old French Medical Texts*, 41–102.

75. Richard de Fournival, *Bestiaires d'amours*; Richard de Fournival, *Master Richard's "Bestiary of Love"*; and Beer, *Beasts of Love*.
76. Park, "Medical Practice," 614; McVaugh, *Medicine Before the Plague*, 138.
77. Cooper, "Approaches to the Critical Days"; Jacquart, "Medical Practice in Paris," 201–5; and Siraisi, *Medieval and Early Renaissance Medicine*, 135–36.
78. Folding almanacs are good examples of manuscripts with astronomical content that may have required relatively little expertise to use. For more on such folding almanacs, see Overbey and Borland, "Diagnostic Performance and Diagrammatic Manipulation"; Borland, "Moved by Medicine"; Carey, "What Is the Folded Almanac?"; Carey, "Astrological Medicine"; and Silva, "Opening the Medieval Folding Almanac." For useful diagrams of various types, see Gumbert, *Bat Books*, 8–9, 121–206.
79. Tyers, "Family, Feud, and Fertility."
80. McAvoy, Skinner, and Tyers, "Family, Feud, and Fertility."
81. The *Circa instans* was later translated into French as *Le livre des simples médecines*; Matthaeus Platearius, *Livre des simples médecines*. See also Horrox, *The Black Death*, 158–63; Givens "Reading and Writing"; Demaitre, *Doctor Bernard de Gordon*; M. Green, *Trotula*; Tyers, "Rebirth of Fertility."
82. For the transcriptions of several texts in Wellcome MS.546, see T. Hunt, *Old French Medical Texts*; see also Tyers, "Rebirth of Fertility," 99.
83. Tyers, "Rebirth of Fertility," 99–107, and Tyers, "'In the Merry Month of May,'" 271.
84. Tyers, "'In the Merry Month of May,'" 272–73, and Sewright, "Introduction to British Library MS Lansdowne 380," 637–38; for a detailed inventory of contents, see 675–736.
85. Tyers, "'In the Merry Month of May,'" 268.
86. Sewright, "Introduction to British Library MS Lansdowne 380."
87. Tyers, "'In the Merry Month of May,'" 272.
88. Tyers, "Family, Feud, and Fertility."
89. Meyer, "Notice du ms. Sloane 1611;" and Ritchey, *Acts of Care* 195–96.
90. I noted the condition of the manuscript when I looked at it in 2019 and 2020. See also Ritchey, *Acts of Care*, 195–96.
91. Borland, "Violence on Vellum," and Borland, "Unruly Reading." For studies on Saint Margaret in England, see Clayton and Magennis, *Old English Lives of St. Margaret*; Dresvina, *Maid with a Dragon*; and Heyes, *Margaret's Monsters*.
92. Rawcliffe, *Medicine and Society*, 106.
93. Ibid., 144. For such elite audiences, "eating well and healthily was their privilege"; Hoeniger, "Illuminated *Tacuinum sanitatis* Manuscripts," 81. McVaugh categorizes the royal family of Aragon as "indefatigable consumers of learned medicine"; McVaugh, *Medicine Before the Plague*, 111.
94. Ingram, "'Pottes of Tryacle,'" 761–62. See especially Table 3 in Ingram's essay, which demonstrates the instances of use of medical professionals versus home remedies.
95. Park, "Medical Practice," 611–12.
96. Rawcliffe, *Medicine and Society*, 118; Park, "Medical Practice," 612; and McVaugh, "Bedside Manners."
97. Rawcliffe, *Medicine and Society*, 105–24, and McVaugh, *Medicine Before the Plague*, 4–34.
98. Howell, *Eleanor of Provence*, 99–102.
99. M. Green, *Making Women's Medicine Masculine*, 73; see also 264–70.
100. M. Green, "Possibilities of Literacy," 22–24, 45.
101. Ingram, "'Pottes of Tryacle.'"
102. Sometimes charms were written directly on the body. One charm was to be written on the cheek: P. Jones, "Amulets," 95. Others were written on consumables and ingested: Olsan, "Charms and Prayers," 358, and appendix. See also Voigts, "What's the Word?"; Olsan, "Corpus of Charms"; Olsan, "Marginality of Charms"; Park, "Medical Practice," 614, 629; Park, *Doctors and Medicine*, 51; Rawcliffe, *Medicine and Society*, 94–95, 218; T. Hunt, *Popular Medicine*; and Skemer, *Binding Words*.
103. Ingram, "'Pottes of Tryacle,'" 717–19. See also Whitaker, "Reading the Paston Letters Medically"; Watt, *Paston Women*; and Barwell, "Healing Arts and Social Capital."

104. Rawcliffe, *Medicine and Society*, 72, 144. See also Cabré, "Women or Healers?"; Ingram, "'Pottes of Tryacle'"; and Park, "Medical Practice," 621.

105. Park, "Medical Practice," 621–22. A similar point has been made about the role of folding almanacs in demonstrating a practitioner's knowledge, and thus reinforcing their authority; see Overbey and Borland, "Diagnostic Performance and Diagrammatic Manipulation."

106. Rawcliffe, *Medicine and Society*, 218–19.

107. Ingram, "'Pottes of Tryacle.'"

Chapter 4

1. Cabré, "Women or Healers?," 23; see also her observation that "household recipes attest to the basic everyday management of the six non-naturals as well as close attention to the body and its well-being" (36).

2. But these activities were not completely unrecorded, as the letters of several fifteenth-century gentry families demonstrate; see Ingram, "'Pottes of Tryacle.'" For an excellent study of later household-based health knowledge, focused on seventeenth-century England, see Leong, *Recipes and Everyday Knowledge*. See also Ritchey, *Acts of Care*; Ritchey and Strocchia, *Gender, Health, and Healing*.

3. Even some of the early printed works from the fifteenth century may be relevant here, such as *The Book of Courtesy* printed by William Caxton in 1477. Caxton is noteworthy as well for publishing an English translation in 1481 of *L'image du monde*, the text that accompanies the *Régime* in several copies, including two illustrated versions; he also published a print version of Lydgate's "Dietary" in 1489. Many of these texts exist in multiple translations and were popular in both England and France.

4. A recent English translation with an excellent critical introduction can be found in Greco and Rose, *Good Wife's Guide*. See also Crossley-Holland, *Living and Dining in Medieval Paris*.

5. Greco and Rose, "Introduction," *Good Wife's Guide*, 1–43, at 1.

6. Tyers, "Family, Feud, and Fertility," 398.

7. Christine de Pizan, *Medieval Woman's Mirror of Honor*; Brown-Grant, *Christine de Pizan*, especially 175–214; Krueger, "'Nouvelles Choses'"; Davis, "Foreword"; and Ashley, "*Miroir des bonnes femmes*."

8. Christine de Pizan, *Medieval Woman's Mirror of Honor*, and Krueger, "Nouvelles Choses," 66.

9. Brown-Grant, *Christine de Pizan*, 175.

10. Krueger, "'Nouvelles Choses,'" 56.

11. Sponsler, "Eating Lessons," 8–9.

12. Ashley and Clark, *Medieval Conduct*, xiv–xv.

13. Amos, "'For Manners Make Man,'" 26.

14. Krueger, "'Nouvelles Choses,'" 51, 54.

15. Krueger, "'Nouvelles Choses'"; Dufresne, "A Woman of Excellent Character"; and Sponsler, "Narrating the Social Order."

16. Proctor-Tiffany, *Medieval Art in Motion*, 102.

17. M. Green, "Possibilities of Literacy," 4, and M. Green, *Making Women's Medicine Masculine*, 163–203.

18. For a discussion of another health text that was likely intended for and commissioned by lay women readers, see Cabré, "From a Master to a Laywoman."

19. Cabré, "Women or Healers?," 38.

20. McVaugh, *Medicine Before the Plague*, 155–56. The attribution of *De ornatu mulierum* to Arnau, however, is debated.

21. Cabré, "Women or Healers?," 37. She also states that the "open collections of recipes indicate new literate forms of collecting knowledge regarding women's regular health-care activities within the household" (50). Tony Hunt makes a similar point that such miscellaneous recipes that appear individually, rather than in collections, are those "most frequently encountered": Hunt, *Popular Medicine*, 64. Hunt goes on to provide in-depth information about recipes that also appear in collections and that can be found in a number of specific manuscripts; he focuses on Anglo-Norman examples.

22. Cabré, "Women or Healers?," 38.

23. M. Green, "Possibilities of Literacy," 47–48.

24. Cabré, "Women or Healers?," 39.

25. Tyers, "'In the Merry Month of May'"; Tyers, "Family, Feud, and Fertility"; and Tyers, "Rebirth of Fertility."

26. Cabré, "Women or Healers?," 46.

27. Ingram, "'Pottes of Tryacle,'" 703.

28. M. Green, *Making Women's Medicine Masculine*, 308.

29. Vale, *Princely Court*; Beattie, Maslakovic, and Jones, *Medieval Household*; and Kowaleski and Goldberg, *Medieval Domesticity*.
30. Vale, *Princely Court*, and Kipling, "Henry VII."
31. S. Jones, "Preface: The Public Household," 11.
32. Riddy, "Looking Closely," 222.
33. Ibid.
34. Cabré, "Women or Healers?," 23.
35. "The open collections of recipes indicate new literate forms of collecting knowledge regarding women's regular healthcare activities within the household"; ibid., 50.
36. For more on female practitioners, including a discussion of these manuscripts, see M. Green, *Making Women's Medicine Masculine*, 120–34; M. Green, "Possibilities of Literacy"; M. Green, "Documenting Medieval Women's Medical Practice"; Cabré, "Women or Healers?"; Rawcliffe, *Medicine and Society*, 170–215; McVaugh, *Medicine Before the Plague*, 103–7; and Blumenthal, "Domestic Medicine." For more on Laud Misc. 724, see M. Green, "Moving from Philology to Social History."
37. Riddy, "Looking Closely," 213.
38. Ibid.
39. Kowaleski and Goldberg, *Medieval Domesticity*, 2.
40. Ibid. Kowaleski and Goldberg also note that, in the later Middle Ages, the idea of the household "need not mean just people; it could denote possessions."
41. Vale, *Princely Court*, 15–16.
42. Ibid., 23, 34–42. See also Woolgar, *Great Household*.
43. S. Jones, "Preface: The Public Household," 12.
44. Riddy, "'Burgeis' Domesticity," 25.
45. Kowaleski and Goldberg, *Medieval Domesticity*, 4–5.
46. Ibid., 4, and Riddy, "Looking Closely," 216.
47. Kowaleski and Goldberg, *Medieval Domesticity*, 6; see also Gardiner, "Buttery and Pantry," and S. Jones, "Building Domesticity in the City."
48. Riddy, "'Burgeis' Domesticity," 17, and Riddy, "Looking Closely," 222.
49. Howell, *Eleanor of Provence*, 267.
50. Ibid., 99–102.
51. The "bourgeois ethos" of such household management is explored in Riddy, "Mother Knows Best."
52. Vale, *Princely Court*, 326 (table 16), 336–38 (table 21). Vale focuses on the kings of England and France, the German emperor, the counts of Flanders, dukes of Brabant, counts of Hainault, counts of Artois, and counts of Holland and Zeeland.
53. Dyer, *Standards of Living*, 50.
54. Ibid.
55. Howell, *Eleanor of Provence*, 71–75.
56. Stanton, "Personal Geography."
57. Howell, *Eleanor of Provence*, 71–108.
58. Ibid., 266–67.
59. Dyer, *Standards of Living*, table on p. 36. Eleanor of Provence's household (just for the queen, not including the king's household) showed receipts of 3,360 pounds over two years in 1250–52; Howell, *Eleanor of Provence*, 267–68.
60. Dyer, *Standards of Living*, 55–57.
61. Vale, *Princely Court*, 81.
62. Howell, *Eleanor of Provence*, 267–68.
63. Dyer, *Standards of Living*, 77–79. For a summary of the vastness of one queen's clothes, jewelry, and related expenses, see Howell, *Eleanor of Provence*, 75–79. Building was also a significant expense. At the same time, metalwork was often a major component of one's wealth; as Mariah Proctor-Tiffany demonstrates, Clémence of Hungary's inventory shows that precious metalwork made up 55 percent of the value of her belongings; Proctor-Tiffany, *Medieval Art in Motion*, 57–58.
64. Howell, *Eleanor of Provence*, 83–92.
65. Sponsler, "Narrating the Social Order," deals with the English statutes: 1337 (11 Edward III), 1363 (37 Edward III), 1463 (3 Edward IV), and 1483 (22 Edward IV). Piponnier and Mane discuss the Statutes of Savoy, created for the Duchy of Savoy under Duke Amadeus VIII in 1430; Piponnier and Mane, *Dress in the Middle Ages*, 83–86.
66. Krueger, "'Nouvelles Choses,'" 50.
67. Piponnier and Mane, *Dress in the Middle Ages*, 78–81, and Owen-Crocker, Coatsworth, and Hayward, *Encyclopedia of Medieval Dress and Textiles*, 74–75.
68. Owen-Crocker, Coatsworth, and Hayward, *Encyclopedia of Medieval Dress and Textiles*, 261–62, 329. Such headdresses are also discussed in M. Scott, *Medieval Dress and Fashion*, 64; she uses the term *gebende*.
69. M. Scott, *Medieval Dress and Fashion*, 72. Piponnier and Mane describe a

"geography of styles" in *Dress in the Middle Ages*, 89–95. See also Houston, *Medieval Costume in England and France*. France and England shared much in terms of fashion in this period.

70. This beret of a physician is discussed further in Houston, *Medieval Costume in England and France*, 46–47.
71. "From the 14th century gloves were worn as a fashion accessory" and often made of leather: see Owen-Crocker, Coatsworth, and Hayward, *Encyclopedia of Medieval Dress and Textiles*, 236–37.
72. Krueger, "'Nouvelles Choses,'" 49–51; Piponnier and Mane, *Dress in the Middle Ages*, 65–86; Dyer, *Standards of Living*, 20–26; and Amos, "'For Manners Make Man,'" 24–25.
73. Kreuger, "Nouvelles Choses," 51; M. Scott, *Medieval Dress and Fashion*, 97, 100, 112–16; Dyer, *Standards of Living*, 176; and Houston, *Medieval Costume in England and France*.
74. The houppelande replaced various sleeved outer garments. Piponnier and Mane, *Dress in the Middle Ages*, 68–70, 79; and Owen-Crocker, Coatsworth and Hayward, *Encyclopedia of Medieval Dress and Textiles*, 272, 275.
75. M. Scott, *Medieval Dress and Fashion*, 117.
76. Piponnier and Mane point out that the houppelande is abandoned by women in the mid-fifteenth century, as elite women "rediscovered gowns with close-fitting sleeves and bodices whose V-necklines were edged with fur"; see their *Dress in the Middle Ages*, 80; and M. Scott, *Medieval Dress and Fashion*, 85.
77. Piponnier and Mane, *Dress in the Middle Ages*, 79.
78. Kreuger, "Nouvelles Choses," 80.
79. Gil-Sotres, "Regimens of Health," 299. See also Hoeniger, "Illuminated *Tacuinum sanitatis* Manuscripts," 52–54; Ibn Buṭlān, *Taqwīm al-ṣiḥḥa (Tacuini sanitatis)*; Bertiz, "Picturing Health"; Arano, *Tacuinum sanitatis*; and Bovey, *Tacuinum sanitatis*.
80. Hoeniger, "Illuminated *Tacuinum sanitatis* Manuscripts," 54. Three copies can be associated with the Visconti court and the artist Giovannino de' Grassi: Bibliothèque nationale de France MS Nouv. acq. lat. 1673; Vienna Österreichische Nationalbibliothek, MS series nova 2644; and Rome, Biblioteca Casanatense, MS 4182.
81. Hoeniger, "Illuminated *Tacuinum sanitatis* Manuscripts," 57. Included in that library was, coincidentally, a (presumably unillustrated) copy of the *Régime du corps*, suggesting that the *Régime* was considered, at least in this context, to be have been worthwhile enough to contribute to the library's robust collection. From the 1426 inventory: Galen, Rhazes, Averroes, Albucasis, Mesue of Bagdad, Avicenna's *Canon*, Serapion, Constantine the African and Johannitius, Arnau de Vilanova, Aldobrandino, the *Circa instans*, Dioscorides, and Macer; for details on the inventory, see Pellegrin, *Bibliothèque des Visconti et des Sforza*, 75–289.
82. A handful of copies of the *Régime* contain full-page or half-page frontispieces; usually that image depicts not medical content, but rather the handing of the manuscript to the owner; see appendix 3.
83. Hoeniger, "Illuminated *Tacuinum sanitatis* Manuscripts," 66–81.
84. Ibid., 76.
85. Frabbri, "Treating Medieval Plague," 248.
86. For more on apothecaries and pharmacists, see Rawcliffe, *Medicine and Society*, 148–69.
87. The *Régime* does happen to contain a reference to garlic as "the peasant's theriac": see Scully and Scully, *Early French Cookery*, 114, and Landouzy and Pépin, *Régime du corps*, 162–63.
88. Tyers, "Rebirth of Fertility," 214, 239; this statement is in Sloane 2401, fol. 93r.
89. Some of the copies have a physician or author-type portrait, in which a man is sitting at a podium; interestingly, in the vomiting scene of some of the *Tacuinum* copies, there are two attendants who both appear to be women (BnF Lat. 9333, fol. 89; Casanatense MS 4182, fol. CXCII); see Arano, *Tacuinum sanitatis*, 144.
90. Borland, "Freeze-Framed."
91. Riddy, "Looking Closely," 222.
92. Ibid.
93. Dyer, *Standards of Living*, 53–55.
94. Rawcliffe, *Urban Bodies*, 232.
95. Sponsler, "Eating Lessons," 19.
96. Greco and Rose, "Introduction," *Good Wife's Guide*, 1–43.
97. Dyer, *Standards of Living*, 61.
98. Ibid., 63; Freedman, "Spices," 1209–27; and Freedman, *Out of the East*.
99. Freedman, *Out of the East*, 35. See also Dyer, *Standards of Living*, 55–70; Howell, *Eleanor of Provence*; and Vale, *Princely Court*.

100. Greco and Rose, *Good Wife's Guide*, 9.
101. Riddy, "Looking Closely," 223.
102. Ibid., 222.
103. Camille, *Image on the Edge*, 111–12.
104. Ibid., 111.
105. M. Green, "Possibilities of Literacy," 23, 32.
106. Riddy, "Looking Closely," 225. See also Tyers, "'In the Merry Month of May'"; Tyers, "Family, Feud, and Fertility"; Tyers, "Rebirth of Fertility"; and Ingram, "'Pottes of Tryacle.'"
107. M. Green, "Possibilities of Literacy," 26–27.
108. Tyers, "'In the Merry Month of May'"; Tyers, "Family, Feud, and Fertility"; Tyers, "Rebirth of Fertility"; and Sewright, "Introduction to British Library MS Lansdowne 380."

Conclusion

1. Riddy, "Looking Closely"; Joyce and Gillespie, *Things in Motion*; and Hamilton and Proctor-Tiffany, *Moving Women*.

Bibliography

Abu-Asab, Mones, Hakima Amri, and Marc S. Micozzi. *Avicenna's Medicine: A New Translation of the 11th-Century Canon with Practical Applications for Integrative Health Care*. Rochester, VT: Healing Arts Press, 2013.

Alexander, J. J. G. "Foreign Illuminators and Illuminated Manuscripts." In *The Cambridge History of the Book in Britain*, edited by Lotte Hellinga and J. B. Trapp, 45–64. Cambridge: Cambridge University Press, 1999.

Allmand, C. T. *Lancastrian Normandy, 1415–1450: The History of a Medieval Occupation*. Oxford: Clarendon Press/ Oxford University Press, 1983.

Amos, Mark Addison. "'For Manners Make Man': Bourdieu, de Certeau, and the Common Appropriation of Noble Manners in the Book of Courtesy." In Ashley and Clark, *Medieval Conduct*, 23–48.

Appadurai, Arjun. "Introduction: Commodities and the Politics of Value." In *The Social Life of Things: Commodities in Cultural Perspective*, edited by Arjun Appadurai, 3–63. Cambridge: Cambridge University Press, 1986.

Arano, Luisa Cogliati. *Tacuinum sanitatis: The Medieval Health Handbook*. New York: Braziller, 1976.

Ashley, Kathleen. "The *Miroir des bonnes femmes*: Not for Women Only?" In Ashley and Clark, *Medieval Conduct*, 86–105.

Ashley, Kathleen, and Robert L. A. Clark, eds. *Medieval Conduct*. Minneapolis: University of Minnesota Press, 2001.

Backhouse, Janet. "Founders of the Royal Library: Edward IV and Henry VII as Collectors of Illuminated Manuscripts." In *England in the Fifteenth Century: Proceedings of the 1986 Harlaxton Symposium*, edited by David Williams, 23–41. Woodbridge, UK: Boydell Press, 1987.

———. "Illuminated Manuscripts Associated with Henry VII and Members of His Immediate Family." In *The Reign of Henry VII: Proceedings of the 1993 Harlaxton Symposium*, edited by Benjamin Thompson, 75–87. Stamford, UK: Paul Watkins, 1995.

Baker, John H. *The Men of Court, 1440 to 1550: A Prosopography of the Inns of Court and Chancery and the Courts of Law*. London: Selden Society, 2012.

Bal, Mieke. *Narratology: Introduction to the Theory of Narrative*. Toronto: University of Toronto Press, 1985.

Barber, Richard W., trans. *Bestiary: An English Version of the Bodleian Library, Oxford MS Bodley 764*. Woodbridge, UK: Boydell Press, 1993.

Barwell, Ashlee. "The Healing Arts and Social Capital: The Paston Women of Fifteenth-Century England." *Canadian Bulletin of Medical History* 35, no. 1 (2018): 137–59.

Bates, David, and Anne Curry, eds. *England and Normandy in the Middle Ages*. London: Hambledon Press, 1994.

Baxter, Ron. *Bestiaries and Their Users in the Middle Ages*. Stroud, UK: Sutton Publishing in association with the Courtauld Institute, 1998.

Beattie, Cordelia, Anna Maslakovic, and Sarah Rees Jones, eds. *The Medieval Household in Christian Europe, c. 850–c. 1550: Managing Power, Wealth, and the Body*. Turnhout, Belgium: Brepols, 2003.

Beer, Jeanette. *Beasts of Love: Richard de Fournival's "Bestiaire d'amour" and a Woman's "Response."* Toronto: University of Toronto Press, 2003.

Bell, Susan Groag. "Medieval Women Book Owners: Arbiters of Lay Piety and Ambassadors of Culture." *Signs* 7, no. 4 (1982): 742–68.

Bertiz, Agnes A. "Picturing Health: The Garden and Courtiers at Play in the Late Fourteenth-Century Illuminated *Tacuinum sanitatis*." PhD diss.,

University of Southern California, 2003.
Bindoff, S. T. *The History of Parliament: The House of Commons, 1509–1558*. 3 vols. London: Secker and Warburg, 1982.
Binski, Paul, and Patrick Zutshi. *Western Illuminated Manuscripts: A Catalogue of the Collection in Cambridge University Library*. Cambridge: Cambridge University Press, 2011.
Bisson, Sebastiano. "Le témoin gênant: Une version latine du *Régime du corps* d'Aldebrandin de Sienne." *Médiévales* 42 (2002): 117–30.
Bleeke, Marian. *Motherhood and Meaning in Medieval Sculpture: Representations from France, c. 1100–1500*. Woodbridge, UK: Boydell and Brewer, 2017.
Blumenthal, Debra. "Domestic Medicine: Slaves, Servants and Female Medical Expertise in Late Medieval Valencia." *Renaissance Studies* 28, no. 4 (2014): 515–32.
———. "'*With My Daughter's Milk*': Wet Nurses and the Rhetoric of Lactation in Valencian Court Records." In *Medieval and Renaissance Lactations: Images, Rhetorics, Practices*, edited by Jutta Gisela Sperling, 101–14. Farnham, UK: Ashgate, 2013.
Borland, Jennifer. "Audience and Spatial Experience in the Nuns' Church at Clonmacnoise." *Different Visions: A Journal of New Perspectives in Medieval Art* 3 (2011): 1–45.
———. "Encountering the Inauthentic." In *Transparent Things: A Cabinet*, edited by Karen Eileen Overbey and Maggie M. Williams, 17–38. New York: Punctum Books, 2013.
———. "Female Networks and the Circulation of a Late Medieval Illustrated Health Guide." In Hamilton and Proctor-Tiffany, *Moving Women, Moving Objects (400–1500)*, 108–36.
———. "Freeze-Framed: Theorizing the Historiated Initials of the *Régime du corps*." *Word and Image: A Journal of Verbal/Visual Inquiry* 32, no. 2 (2016): 235–50.
———. "Moved by Medicine: The Controlled Experience of Handling Folding Almanacs." In *Sensory Reflections: Traces of Experience in Medieval Artifacts*, edited by Fiona Griffiths and Kathryn Starkey, 203–24, plates 280–82. Berlin: De Gruyter, 2018.
———. "Unruly Reading: The Consuming Role of Touch in the Experience of a Medieval Manuscript." In *Scraped, Stroked, and Bound: Materially Engaged Readings of Medieval Manuscripts*, edited by Jonathan Wilcox, 97–114, plates 225–30. Turnhout, Belgium: Brepols, 2013.
———. "Violence on Vellum: Saint Margaret's Transgressive Body and Its Audience." In *Representing Medieval Genders and Sexualities in Europe: Construction, Transformation, and Subversion, 600–1530*, edited by Elizabeth L'Estrange and Alison More, 67–88. Aldershot, UK: Ashgate, 2011.
Bovey, Alixe. *Tacuinum sanitatis: An Early Renaissance Guide to Health*. London: Sam Fogg, 2005.
Branner, Robert. *Manuscript Painting in Paris During the Reign of Saint Louis: A Study of Styles*. Berkeley: University of California Press, 1977.
Brown, Katherine A. "The Vernacular Universe: Gossuin de Metz's *Image du monde, Translatio studii*, and Vernacular Narrative." *Viator* 44, no. 2 (2013): 137–58.
Brown-Grant, Rosalind. *Christine de Pizan and the Moral Defense of Women: Reading Beyond Gender*. Cambridge: Cambridge University Press, 1999.
Bullough, Vern L. "Medical Practice in the Middle Ages, or Who Treated Whom." In *Universities, Medicine and Science in the Medieval West*, 277–88.
———. "Medieval Medicine and the Search for Status." In *Universities, Medicine and Science in the Medieval West*, 151–59.
———. *Universities, Medicine and Science in the Medieval West*. Variorum Collected Studies Series. Aldershot, UK: Ashgate, 2004.
Burnett, Charles. "Translation and Transmission of Greek and Islamic Science to Latin Christendom." In Lindberg and Shank, *Medieval Science*, 341–64.
Burnett, Charles, and Danielle Jacquart, eds. *Constantine the African and ʿAlī ibn al-ʿAbbās al-Mağūsī: The "Pantegni" and Related Texts*. Leiden: Brill, 1994.
Burns, Chester R. "The Nonnaturals: A Paradox in the Western Concept of Health." *Journal of Medicine and Philosophy* 1, no. 3 (1976): 202–11.

Cabré, Montserrat. "From a Master to a Laywoman: A Feminine Manual of Self-Help." *Dynamis: Acta Hispanica ad Medicinae Scientiarumque Historiam Illustrandam* 20 (2000): 371–93.

———. "Women or Healers? Household Practices and the Categories of Healthcare in Late Medieval Iberia." *Bulletin of the History of Medicine* 82, no. 1 (2008): 18–51.

Cadden, Joan. *The Meanings of Sex Difference in the Middle Ages: Medicine, Science, and Culture*. Cambridge: Cambridge University Press, 1993.

Camille, Michael. *Image on the Edge: The Margins of Medieval Art*. Cambridge: Harvard University Press, 1992.

———. "Manuscript Illumination and the Art of Copulation." In *Constructing Medieval Sexuality*, edited by Karma Lochrie, Peggy McCracken, and James Alfred Schultz, 58–90. Minneapolis: University of Minnesota Press, 1997.

———. "Obscenity Under Erasure: Censorship in Medieval Illuminated Manuscripts." In *Obscenity: Social Control and Artistic Creation in the European Middle Ages*, edited by Jan M. Ziolkowski, 139–54 (and figs. 1–13). Leiden: Brill, 1998.

Campos Ribeiro, Luís. "Medicina e dietética medieval o *Le régime du corps* de Aldobrandino de Siena." In *Luz, cor e ouro: Estudos sobre manuscritos iluminados*, edited by Catarina F. Barreira, 249–58. Lisbon: Biblioteca Nacional de Portugal, 2016.

———. "Picturing Medieval Health: Artistic Production and Visual Discourse in *Le Régime du corps* of the Ajuda Library (COD 52-XIII-26)." Master's thesis, Universidade Nova de Lisboa, 2016.

Carey, Hilary M. "Astrological Medicine and the Medieval English Folded Almanac." *Social History of Medicine* 17, no. 3 (2004): 345–63.

———. "What Is the Folded Almanac? The Form and Function of a Key Manuscript Source for Astro-Medical Practice in Later Medieval England." *Social History of Medicine* 16, no. 3 (2003): 481–509.

Carvalho, Augusto da Silva. "Le manuscrit du *Régime du corps* d'Aldebrandino, de La Bibliothèque d'Ajuda, à Lisbonne." In *Essays in the History of Medicine*, 318–24. Baltimore: Johns Hopkins University Press, 1944.

Cassagnes-Brouquet, Sophie. *L'image du monde: Un trésor enluminé de la Bibliothèque de Rennes*. Rennes: Presses Universitaires de Rennes/ Bibliothèque de Rennes Métropole, 2003.

A Catalogue of the Manuscripts Preserved in the Library of the University of Cambridge. 5 vols. Cambridge: Cambridge University Press, 1856–67.

Chabás, José, and Bernard R. Goldstein. *The Alfonsine Tables of Toledo*. Dordrecht: Kluwer Academic Publishers, 2003.

Chatman, Seymour. "What Novels Can Do That Films Can't (and Vice Versa)." In "On Narrative," special issue, *Critical Inquiry* 7, no. 1 (1980): 121–40.

Christine de Pizan. *The Book of the City of Ladies*. Translated by Earl Jeffrey Richards. Foreword by Natalie Zemon Davis. Rev. ed. New York: Persea Books, 1998.

———. *A Medieval Woman's Mirror of Honor: The Treasury of the City of Ladies*. Translated by Charity Cannon Willard. Edited by Madeleine Pelner Cosman. Tenafly, NJ: Bard Hall Press, 1989.

Clark, Willene B., and Meradith T. McMunn, eds. *Beasts and Birds of the Middle Ages: The Bestiary and Its Legacy*. Philadelphia: University of Pennsylvania Press, 1989.

Clayton, Mary, and Hugh Magennis. *The Old English Lives of St. Margaret*. Cambridge: Cambridge University Press, 1994.

Collins, Minta. *Medieval Herbals: The Illustrative Traditions*. London: British Library; Toronto: University of Toronto Press, 2000.

Connochie-Bourgne, Chantal. "Pourquoi et comment réécrire un encyclopédie? Deux rédactions de l'Image du monde." In *Discours et savoirs: Encyclopédies médiévales*, edited by Bernard Baillaud, Jérôme de Gramont, and Denis Hüe, 143–54. Cahiers Diderot no. 10. Rennes: Presses Universitaires de Rennes, 1998.

Cooper, Glen M. "Approaches to the Critical Days in Late Medieval and Renaissance Thinkers." *Early Science and Medicine* 18, no. 6 (2013): 536–65.

Cox, Eugene L. *The Eagles of Savoy*. Princeton: Princeton University Press, 1974.
Crossley-Holland, Nicole. *Living and Dining in Medieval Paris: The Household of a Fourteenth-Century Knight*. Cardiff: University of Wales Press, 1996.
Curry, Anne. *The Hundred Years War*. 2nd ed. New York: Palgrave Macmillan, 2003.
Curry, Anne, and Michael Hughes. *Arms, Armies and Fortifications in the Hundred Years War*. Woodbridge, UK: Boydell Press, 1994.
Davis, Natalie Zemon. "Foreword." In *The Book of the City of Ladies*, by Christine de Pisan, translated by Earl Jeffrey Richard, xv–xxii. Rev. ed. New York: Persea Books, 1998.
———. "Women on Top." In *Society and Culture in Early Modern France: Eight Essays*, 124–51. Palo Alto: Stanford University Press, 1975.
Demaitre, Luke E. *Doctor Bernard de Gordon: Professor and Practitioner*. Toronto: Pontifical Institute of Mediaeval Studies, 1980.
De Meyier, K. A. "Un manuscrit de Leyde contenant le *Régime du corps* d'Aldebrandin de Sienne." *Scriptorium* 15, no. 1 (1961): 112–14.
Dresvina, Juliana. *A Maid with a Dragon: The Cult of St Margaret of Antioch in Medieval England*. Oxford: Oxford University Press, 2016.
Driver, Martha W. "'Me Fault Faire': French Makers of Manuscripts for English Patrons." In *Language and Culture in Medieval Britain: The French of England, c. 1100–c. 1500*, edited by Jocelyn Wogan-Browne, 420–43. Woodbridge, UK: York Medieval, 2009.
Dufresne, Laura Rinaldi. "A Woman of Excellent Character: A Case Study of Dress, Reputation and the Changing Costume of Christine de Pizan in the Fifteenth Century." *Dress* 17 (1990): 104–17.
Dyer, Christopher. *Standards of Living in the Later Middle Ages: Social Change in England, c. 1200–1520*. Cambridge: Cambridge University Press, 1989.
Evans, Jonathan. "Episodes in Analysis of Medieval Narrative." *Style* 20, no. 2 (1986): 126–41.
Fery-Hue, Françoise. "Le *Régime du corps* d'Aldebrandin de Sienne: Complément à la tradition manuscrite." *Romania* 117 (1999): 51–77.
———. "Le *Régime du corps* d'Aldebrandin de Sienne: Complément à la tradition manuscrite (suite)." *Scriptorium* 58, no. 1 (2004): 99–108.
———. "Le *Régime du corps* d'Aldebrandin de Sienne: Note sur une version française récrite." *Romania* 110 (1989): 253–64.
———. "Le *Régime du corps* d'Aldebrandin de Sienne: Tradition manuscrite et diffusion." In *Santé, médecine et assistance au Moyen Âge: Actes du 110e Congrès National des Sociétés Savantes, Montpelier, 1985, Section d'Histoire Médiévale et de Philologie*, 113–34. Paris: Editions du C.T.H.S., 1987.
Frabbri, Christiane Nockels. "Treating Medieval Plague: The Wonderful Virtues of Theriac." *Early Science and Medicine* 12, no. 3 (2007): 247–83.
Freedman, Paul. *Images of the Medieval Peasant*. Stanford: Stanford University Press, 1999.
———. *Out of the East: Spices and the Medieval Imagination*. New Haven: Yale University Press, 2008.
———. "Spices and Late Medieval European Ideas of Scarcity and Value." *Speculum* 80, no. 4 (2005): 1209–27.
Fresco, Karen L. "Gendered Household Spaces in Christine de Pizan's *Livre des trois vertus*." In *The Medieval Household in Christian Europe, c. 850–1550: Managing Power, Wealth, and the Body*, edited by Cordelia Beattie, Anna Maslakovic, and Sarah Rees Jones, 187–97. Turnhout, Belgium: Brepols, 2003.
García-Ballester, Luis. "On the Origin of the 'Six Non-natural Things' in Galen." In *Galen und das hellenistische Erbe: Verhandlungen des IV. Internationalen Galen-Symposiums, 18.–20. September 1989*, edited by Jutta Kollesch, 105–15. Stuttgart: Franz Steiner Verlag, 1993.
García-Ballester, Luis, Roger French, Jon Arrizabalaga, and Andrew Cunningham, eds. *Practical Medicine from Salerno to the Black Death*. Cambridge: Cambridge University Press, 1994.
García-Ballester, Luis, and Michael R. McVaugh, eds. *Regimen sanitatis ad regem Aragonum*, vol. 10.1 of *Arnaldi de Villanova Opera medica omnia*. Barcelona: Seminarium Historiae Scientiae Barchinone,

Fundació Noguera and Universitat de Barcelona, 1996.
Gardiner, Mark. "Buttery and Pantry and Their Antecedents: Idea and Architecture in the English Medieval House." In Kowaleski and Goldberg, *Medieval Domesticity*, 37–65.
Gil, Christiane. *Marguerite de Provence: Épouse de Saint Louis, mère de Philippe III*. Histoire des Reines de France. Paris: Pygmalion, 2006.
Gil-Sotres, Pedro. "Derivation and Revulsion: The Theory and Practice of Medieval Phlebotomy." In García-Ballester et al., *Practical Medicine*, 110–55.
———. "Regimens of Health." In *Western Medical Thought from Antiquity to the Middle Ages*, edited by Mirko D. Grmek and Bernardino Fantini; translated by Antony Shugaar, 291–318, 395–99. Cambridge: Harvard University Press, 1998.
Gil-Sotres, Pedro, in collaboration with Juan A. Paniagua and Luis García-Ballester. *Regimen sanitatis ad regem Aragonum*. Vol. 10.1 of *Arnaldi de Villanova Opera medica omnia*, edited by Luis García-Ballester and Michael R. McVaugh. Barcelona: Seminarium Historiae Scientiae Barchinone, Fundació Noguera and Universitat de Barcelona, 1996.
Givens, Jean A. *Observation and Image-Making in Gothic Art*. Cambridge: Cambridge University Press, 2005.
———. "Reading and Writing the Illustrated *Tractatus de herbis*, 1280–1526." In Givens, Reeds, and Touwaide, *Visualizing Medieval Medicine and Natural History*, 115–45.
Givens, Jean A., Karen M. Reeds, and Alain Touwaide, eds. *Visualizing Medieval Medicine and Natural History, 1200–1550*. Aldershot, UK: Ashgate, 2006.
Greco, Gina L., and Christine M. Rose, eds. and trans. *The Good Wife's Guide/Le menagier de Paris: A Medieval Household Book*. Ithaca: Cornell University Press, 2009.
Green, David. *The Hundred Years War: A People's History*. New Haven: Yale University Press, 2014.
Green, Monica H. "Books as a Source of Medical Education for Women in the Middle Ages." *Dynamis: Acta Hispanica ad Medicinae Scientiarumque Historiam Illustrandam* 20 (2000): 331–69.
———. "Documenting Medieval Women's Medical Practice." In García-Ballester et al., *Practical Medicine*, 322–52.
———. *Making Women's Medicine Masculine: The Rise of Male Authority in Pre-Modern Gynaecology*. Oxford: Oxford University Press, 2008.
———. "Moving from Philology to Social History: The Circulation and Uses of Albucasis's Latin Surgery in the Middle Ages." In *Between Text and Patient: The Medical Enterprise in Medieval and Early Modern Europe*, edited by Florence Eliza Glaze and Brian K. Nance, 331–72. Florence: SISMEL, Edizioni del Galluzzo, 2011.
———. "The Possibilities of Literacy and the Limits of Reading: Women and the Gendering of Medical Literacy." In *Women's Healthcare in the Medieval West: Texts and Contexts*, essay 7. Aldershot, UK: Ashgate, 2000.
———. *The Trotula: A Medieval Compendium of Women's Medicine*. Philadelphia: University of Pennsylvania Press, 2001.
———. *Women's Healthcare in the Medieval West: Texts and Contexts*. Variorum Collected Studies Series. Aldershot, UK: Ashgate, 2000.
Gumbert, J. P. *Bat Books: A Catalogue of Folded Manuscripts Containing Almanacs or Other Texts*. Turnhout, Belgium: Brepols, 2016.
Haidu, Peter. "The Episode and Semiotic Module in Twelfth-Century Romance." *Poetics Today* 4, no. 4 (1983): 655–81.
Hamilton, Tracy Chapman. *Pleasure and Politics at the Court of France: The Artistic Patronage of Queen Marie of Brabant (1260–1321)*. Turnhout, Belgium: Brepols, 2019.
———. "Queenship and Kinship in the French *Bible moralisée*: The Example of Blanche of Castile and Vienna ÖNB 2554." In *Capetian Women*, edited by Kathleen Nolan, 177–208. New York: Palgrave Macmillan, 2003.
Hamilton, Tracy Chapman, and Mariah Proctor-Tiffany, eds. *Moving Women, Moving Objects (400–1500)*. Leiden: Brill, 2019.
Hanna, Ralph, with Jeremy Griffiths. *A Descriptive Catalogue of the Western Medieval Manuscripts of St. John's College, Oxford*. Oxford: Oxford University Press, 2002.

Harris, Anne. "Narrative." *Studies in Iconography* 33 (2012): 47–60.

Hartnell, Jack. "Medicine's Image." In *The Routledge Companion to Medieval Iconography*, edited by Colum Hourihane, 322–39. New York: Routledge, 2017.

———. "Tools of the Puncture: Skin, Knife, Bone, Hand." In *Flaying in the Pre-Modern World: Practice and Representation*, edited by Larissa Tracy, 20–50. Woodbridge: Boydell and Brewer, 2017.

Hassig, Debra. *The Mark of the Beast: The Medieval Bestiary in Art, Life, and Literature*. New York: Garland, 1999.

———. *Medieval Bestiaries: Text, Image, Ideology*. Cambridge: Cambridge University Press, 1995.

Herrlinger, Robert. *History of Medical Illustration from Antiquity to A.D. 1600*. London: Pittman Medical and Scientific Publishing, 1970.

Heyes, Michael E. *Margaret's Monsters: Women, Identity, and the "Life of St. Margaret" in Medieval England*. London: Routledge, 2020.

Hill, Boyd H., Jr. "The *Fünfbilderserie* and Medieval Anatomy." PhD diss., University of North Carolina at Chapel Hill, 1963.

Hoeniger, Cathleen. "The Illuminated *Tacuinum sanitatis* Manuscripts from Northern Italy, ca. 1380–1400: Sources, Patrons, and the Creation of a New Pictorial Genre." In Givens, Reeds, and Touwaide, *Visualizing Medieval Medicine and Natural History*, 51–81.

Holladay, Joan. "Fourteenth-Century French Queens as Collectors and Readers of Books: Jeanne d'Evreux and Her Contemporaries." *Journal of Medieval History* 32 (2006): 69–100.

Horrox, Rosemary, ed. *The Black Death*. Manchester: Manchester University Press, 1994.

Houston, Mary G. *Medieval Costume in England and France: The 13th, 14th, and 15th Centuries*. London: Adam and Charles Black, 1979. Originally published in 1939.

Howell, Margaret. *Eleanor of Provence: Queenship in Thirteenth-Century England*. Oxford: Blackwell, 1998.

———. "Royal Women of England and France in the Mid-Thirteenth Century: A Gendered Perspective." In *England and Europe in the Age of Henry III (1216–1272)*, edited by Björn K. U. Weiler and Ifor W. Rowlands, 163–81. Aldershot, UK: Ashgate, 2002.

Hunt, Elizabeth Moore. *Illuminating the Borders of Northern French and Flemish Manuscripts, 1270–1310*. New York: Routledge, 2007.

Hunt, Tony. *Anglo-Norman Medicine*. Vol. 1. Rochester: Boydell and Brewer, 1994.

———. *Anglo-Norman Medicine*. Vol. 2. Rochester: Boydell and Brewer, 1997.

———. *Medieval Surgery*. Woodbridge, UK: Boydell Press, 1992.

———. *Old French Medical Texts*. Paris: Classiques Garnier, 2011.

———. *Popular Medicine in Thirteenth-Century England: Introduction and Texts*. Cambridge: D. S. Brewer, 1990.

Ibn Buṭlān. *Le Taqwīm al-ṣiḥḥa (Tacuini sanitatis) d'Ibn Buṭlān: Un traité médical du XIe siècle*. Translated and edited by Hosam Elkhadem. Leuven: Peeters, 1990.

Ibn Sīnā (Avicenna). *The Canon of Medicine (al-Qānūn fī'l-ṭibb)*. Vol. 1. Adapted by Laleh Bakhtiar. Translated by Oskar Cameron Gruner and Mazhar H. Shah. Chicago: Great Books of the Islamic World, 1999.

Ingram, Hannah. "'Pottes of Tryacle' and 'Bokes of Phisyke': The Fifteenth-Century Disease Management Practices of Three Gentry Families." *Social History of Medicine* 32, no. 4 (2018): 751–72.

Jacquart, Danielle. "Anatomy, Physiology, and Medical Theory." In Lindberg and Shank, *Medieval Science*, 590–610.

———. *La médecine médiévale dans le cadre parisien (XIVe–XVe siècle)*. Paris: Fayard, 1998.

———. "Medical Practice in Paris in the First Half of the Fourteenth Century." In García-Ballester et al., *Practical Medicine*, 186–210.

Jacquart, Danielle, and Claude Alexandre Thomasset. *Sexuality and Medicine in the Middle Ages*. Princeton: Princeton University Press, 1988.

James, M. R., and Roger Gale. *The Western Manuscripts in the Library of Trinity College, Cambridge*. 4 vols. Cambridge: Cambridge University Press, 1900.

Jones, Carol. "An Assortment of Doctors: The Readers of Medical Books in Late Medieval England." *Journal of the Early Book Society* 3 (2000): 135–51.

Jones, Peter Murray. "Amulets: Prescriptions and Surviving Objects from Late Medieval England." In *Beyond Pilgrimage Souvenirs and Secular Badges*, edited by Sarah Blick, 92–107. Oxford: Oxbow, 2007.

———. "Image, Word, and Medicine in the Middle Ages." In Givens, Reeds, and Touwaide, *Visualizing Medieval Medicine and Natural History*, 1–24.

———. *Medieval Medicine in Illuminated Manuscripts*. London: British Library, 1998. Originally published as *Medieval Medical Miniatures*, 1984.

———. "Picturing Medicine in the Age of Petrarch." In *Petrarca e la medicina: Atti del convegno di Capo d'Orlando, 27–28 giugno 2003*, edited by Monica Berté, Vicenzo Fera, and Tiziana Pesenti Marangon, 179–200. Messina: Centro Interdipartimentale di Studi Umanistici, 2006.

———. "Il regime del corpo." Translated by Davide Panzieri. *Kos: Rivista di cultura e storia delle scienze mediche, naturali e umane* 2 (1985): 42–53.

———. "*Sicut hic depingitur . . . :* John of Arderne and English Medical Illustration in the 14th and 15th Centuries." In *Die Kunst und das Studium der Nature vom 14. zum 16. Jahrhundert*, edited by Wolfram Prinz and Andreas Beyer, 103–26. Weinheim: VCH: Acta Humaniora, 1987.

———. "Staying with the Programme: Illustrated Manuscripts of John of Arderne, c. 1380–c. 1550." In *Decoration and Illustration in Medieval English Manuscripts*, edited by A. S. G. Edwards, 204–27. London: British Library, 2002.

———. "Thomas Fayreford: An English Fifteenth-Century Medical Practitioner." In *Medicine from the Black Death to the French Disease*, edited by Roger French, 156–83. Aldershot, UK: Ashgate, 1998.

Jones, Sarah Rees. "Building Domesticity in the City: English Urban Housing Before the Black Death." In Kowaleski and Goldberg, *Medieval Domesticity*, 66–91.

———. "Preface: The Public Household and Political Power." In *The Medieval Household in Christian Europe, c. 850–1550: Managing Power, Wealth, and the Body*, edited by Cordelia Beattie, Anna Maslakovic, and Sarah Rees Jones, 11–18. Turnhout, Belgium: Brepols, 2003.

Joyce, Rosemary A. "Things in Motion: Itineraries of Ulua Marble Vases." In *Things in Motion: Object Itineraries in Anthropological Practice*, edited by Rosemary A. Joyce and Susan D. Gillespie, 21–39. Santa Fe: School for Advanced Research Press, 2015.

Joyce, Rosemary A., and Susan D. Gillespie. "Making Things Out of Objects That Move." In *Things in Motion: Object Itineraries in Anthropological Practice*, edited by Rosemary A. Joyce and Susan D. Gillespie, 3–20. Santa Fe: School for Advanced Research Press, 2015.

Joyce, Rosemary A., and Susan D. Gillespie, eds. *Things in Motion: Object Itineraries in Anthropological Practice*. Santa Fe: School for Advanced Research Press, 2015.

Kemp, Wolfgang. "Narrative." In *Critical Terms for Art History*, edited by Robert S. Nelson and Richard Shiff, 58–69. Chicago: University of Chicago Press, 1996.

Kipling, Gordon. "Henry VII and the Origins of Tudor Patronage." In *Patronage in the Renaissance*, edited by Guy Fitch Lytle and Stephen Orgel, 117–64. Princeton: Princeton University Press, 1981.

Kirkham, Anne, and Cordelia Warr, eds. *Wounds in the Middle Ages*. Farnham, UK: Ashgate, 2014.

Klapisch-Zuber, Christiane. "Blood Parents and Milk Parents: Wet Nursing in Florence, 1300–1530." In *Women, Family, and Ritual in Renaissance Italy*, 132–64. Chicago: University of Chicago Press, 1985.

Kopytoff, Igor. "The Cultural Biography of Things: Commoditization as Process." In *The Social Life of Things: Commodities in Cultural Perspective*, edited by Arjun Appadurai, 64–91. Cambridge: Cambridge University Press, 1986.

Kowaleski, Maryanne, and P. J. P. Goldberg, eds. *Medieval Domesticity: Home, Housing and Household in Medieval England*. Cambridge: Cambridge University Press, 2008.

Kren, Thomas, and Scot McKendrick. *Illuminating the Renaissance: The Triumph of Flemish Manuscript*

Painting in Europe. Los Angeles: J. Paul Getty Museum, 2003.
Krueger, Roberta L. "'Nouvelles Choses': Social Instability and the Problem of Fashion in the *Livre du Chevalier de la Tour Landry*, the *Ménagier de Paris*, and Christine de Pizan's *Le livre des trois vertus*." In Ashley and Clark, *Medieval Conduct*, 49–85.
Kyle, Sarah R. *Medicine and Humanism in Late Medieval Italy: The Carrara Herbal in Padua*. Abingdon, UK: Routledge, 2017.
Lacarrière, Nathalie. "Compilation, Collation and Correction in the Time of Encyclopedism: The Case of UPenn LJS 55." *Manuscript Studies* 3, no. 1 (2019): 238–48.
Landouzy, Louis, and Roger Pépin, eds. *Le Régime du corps de Maître Aldebrandin de Sienne*. Paris: H. Champion, 1911.
Leong, Elaine. *Recipes and Everyday Knowledge: Medicine, Science, and the Household in Early Modern England*. Chicago: University of Chicago Press, 2018.
Leson, Richard. "The Pathways of Salvation: Spatiality and Devotion in the Bute Psalter." *Gesta* 53, no. 2 (2014): 129–54.
L'Estrange, Elizabeth. *Holy Motherhood: Gender, Dynasty and Visual Culture in the Later Middle Ages*. Manchester and New York: Manchester University Press and Palgrave, 2008.
Lewis, Suzanne. "Beyond the Frame: Marginal Figures and Historiated Initials in the Getty Apocalypse." *The J. Paul Getty Museum Journal* 20 (1992): 53–76.
———. "Narrative." In *A Companion to Medieval Art: Romanesque and Gothic in Northern Europe*, edited by Conrad Rudolph, 86–105. Malden, MA: Blackwell, 2006.
———. *Reading Images: Narrative Discourse and Reception in the Thirteenth-Century Illuminated Apocalypse*. Cambridge: Cambridge University Press, 1995.
———. *The Rhetoric of Power in the Bayeux Tapestry*. Cambridge: Cambridge University Press, 1999.
Lindberg, David C., and Michael H. Shank, eds. *Medieval Science*. Vol. 2 of *The Cambridge History of Science*. Cambridge: Cambridge University Press, 2013.
Lowden, John. *The Making of the "Bibles Moralisées."* 2 vols. University Park: Pennsylvania State University Press, 2000.
Luard, Henry Richards, ed. *Matthaei Parisiensis, Monachi Sancti Albani, Chronica Majora*. 7 vols. Rerum Britannicarum Medii Ævi Scriptores. London: Longman, 1872.
Luyster, Amanda. "The Place of a Queen/A Queen and Her Places: Jeanne of Navarre's *Kalila and Dimna* as a Political Manuscript in Early Fourteenth-Century France." In Hamilton and Proctor-Tiffany, *Moving Women, Moving Objects (400–1500)*, 160–80.
MacKinney, Loren. *Medical Illustrations in Medieval Manuscripts*. Berkeley: University of California Press, 1965.
Maekawa, Kumiko. *Narrative and Experience: Innovations in Thirteenth-Century Picture Books*. Frankfurt am Main: Peter Lang, 2000.
Martínez Pizarro, Joaquín. *A Rhetoric of the Scene: Dramatic Narrative in the Early Middle Ages*. Toronto: University of Toronto Press, 1989.
Matthaeus Platearius. *Le livre des simples médecines: D'après le manuscrit français 12322 de la Bibliothèque nationale de Paris*. Translated and edited by Ghislaine Malandin, François Avril, and Pierre Lieutaghi. Paris: Editions Ozalid et Textes Cardinaux, 1986.
Matthews, Leslie G. *The Royal Apothecaries*. London: Wellcome Historical Medical Library, 1967.
McAvoy, Liz Herbert, Patricia Skinner, and Theresa Tyers. "Family, Feud, and Fertility at Manorbier Castle, Pembs., 1200–1400." *Transactions of the Honourable Society of Cymmrodorion* 22 (2016): 8–25.
McCall, Taylor Jane. "Illuminating the Interior: The Illustrations of the Nine Systems of the Body and Anatomical Knowledge in Medieval Europe." PhD diss., Pembroke College, Cambridge, 2017.
McCulloch, Florence. *Mediaeval French and Latin Bestiaries*. Chapel Hill: University of North Carolina Press, 1962.
McKendrick, Scot. "The Manuscripts of Edward IV: The Documentary Evidence." In *1000 Years of Royal Books and Manuscripts*, edited by Kathleen Doyle and Scot McKendrick,

149–77. London: The British Library, 2013.

McKendrick, Scot, John Lowden, and Kathleen Doyle. *Royal Manuscripts: The Genius of Illumination*. London: The British Library, 2011.

McVaugh, Michael R. "Arnald of Villanova's *Regimen Almarie* (*Regimen castra sequentium*) and Medieval Military Medicine." *Viator* 23 (1992): 201–14.

———. "Bedside Manners in the Middle Ages." *Journal of the History of Medicine* 71, no. 2 (1997): 201–23.

———. "The Experience-Based Medicine of the Thirteenth Century." *Early Science and Medicine* 14 (2009): 105–30.

———. *Medicine Before the Plague: Practitioners and Their Patients in the Crown of Aragon, 1285–1345*. Cambridge: Cambridge University Press, 1993.

———. *The Rational Surgery of the Middle Ages*. Florence: SISMEL Edizioni del Galluzzo, 2006.

———. "Royal Surgeons and the Value of Medical Learning: The Crown of Aragon, 1300–1350." In García-Ballester et al., *Practical Medicine*, 211–36.

Mermier, Guy R., trans. *A Medieval Book of Beasts: Pierre de Beauvais' Bestiary*. Lewiston, NY: The Edwin Mellen Press, 1992.

Meyer, Paul. "De l'expansion de la langue française en Italie pendant le moyen-âge." In *Atti del Congresso Internazionale di Scienze Storiche (Roma, 1–9 Aprile 1903)*, vol. 4 of 12, 61–104. Rome: Tipografia della R. Accademia dei Lincei, 1904.

———. "Manuscrits médicaux en français." *Romania* 44, no. 174 (1915–17): 161–214.

———. "Notice du ms. Sloane 1611 du Musée britannique: Une poésie de Nicole Bozon.—Traités français de médecine.—Vie de sainte Marguerite." *Romania* 40, no. 160 (1911): 532–58.

Miles, Margaret R. *A Complex Delight: The Secularization of the Breast, 1350–1750*. Berkeley: University of California Press, 2008.

Mitchell, W. J. T., ed. *On Narrative*. Chicago: University of Chicago Press, 1981.

———. *Picture Theory: Essays on Verbal and Visual Representation*. Chicago: University of Chicago Press, 1994.

Moulinier-Brogi, Laurence. *L'uroscopie au Moyen Âge: "Lire dans un verre la nature de l'homme."* Paris: H. Champion, 2012.

Mustain, James K. "A Rural Medical Practitioner in Fifteenth-Century England." *Bulletin of the History of Medicine* 46 (1972): 469–76.

Nicoud, Marilyn. *Les Régimes de santé au Moyen Âge: Naissance et diffusion d'une écriture médicale, Xiiie–Xve siècle*. 2 vols. Rome: École française de Rome, 2007.

Nolan, Kathleen. *Capetian Women*. New York: Palgrave Macmillan, 2003.

Nutton, Vivian. "Early Medieval Medicine and Natural Science." In Lindberg and Shank, *Medieval Science*, 323–40.

O'Boyle, Cornelius. *The Art of Medicine: Medical Teaching at the University of Paris, 1250–1400*. Education and Society in the Middle Ages and Renaissance. Leiden: Brill, 1998.

———. "Gesturing in the Early Universities." *Dynamis: Acta Hispanica ad Medicinae Scientiarumque Historiam Illustrandam* 20 (2000): 249–81.

———. "Surgical Texts and Social Contexts: Physicians and Surgeons in Paris, c. 1270 to 1430." In García-Ballester et al., *Practical Medicine*, 156–85.

Olsan, Lea T. "Charms and Prayers in Medieval Medical Theory and Practice." *Social History of Medicine* 16, no. 3 (2003): 343–66 (and appendix).

———. "The Corpus of Charms in the Middle English Leechcraft Remedy Books." In *Charms, Charmers and Charming: International Research on Verbal Magic*, edited by Jonathan Roper, 214–37. New York: Palgrave Macmillan, 2009.

———. "The Marginality of Charms in Medieval England." In *The Power of Words: Studies on Charms and Charming in Europe*, edited by James Kapaló, Éva Pócs, and William Ryan, 135–64. Budapest: Central European University Press, 2013.

Otis, Leah L. "Municipal Wet Nurses in Fifteenth-Century Montpelier." In *Women and Work in Preindustrial Europe*, edited by Barbara Hanawalt, 83–93. Bloomington: Indiana University Press, 1986.

Overbey, Karen Eileen, and Jennifer Borland. "Diagnostic Performance and Diagrammatic Manipulation in the

Physician's Folding Almanacs." In *The Agency of Things in Medieval and Early Modern Art: Materials, Power and Manipulation*, edited by Grażyna Jurkowlaniec, Ika Matyjaszkiewicz, and Zuzanna Sarnecka, 130–42. New York: Routledge, 2018.

Overty, Joanne Filippone. "The Cost of Doing Scribal Business: Prices of Manuscript Books in England, 1300–1483." *Book History* 11 (2008): 1–32.

Owen-Crocker, Gale R., Elizabeth Coatsworth, and Maria Hayward, eds. *Encyclopedia of Medieval Dress and Textiles in the British Isles, c. 450–1450*. Leiden: Brill, 2012.

Pächt, Otto. *The Rise of Pictorial Narrative in Twelfth-Century England*. Oxford: Clarendon Press, 1962.

Park, Katharine. *Doctors and Medicine in Early Renaissance Florence*. Princeton: Princeton University Press, 1985.

———. "Medical Practice." In Lindberg and Shank, *Medieval Science*, 611–29.

———. *Secrets of Women: Gender, Generation, and the Origins of Human Dissection*. New York: Zone Books, 2006.

Pellegrin, Elisabeth. *La bibliothèque des Visconti et des Sforza, ducs de Milan, au XVe siècle*. Paris: Vente au Service des publications du C.N.R.S., 1955.

Piponnier, Françoise, and Perrine Mane, eds. *Dress in the Middle Ages*. Translated by Caroline Beamish. New Haven: Yale University Press, 1997.

Pormann, Peter E., and Emilie Savage-Smith. *Medieval Islamic Medicine*. Washington, DC: Georgetown University Press, 2007.

Pouchelle, Marie-Christine. *The Body and Surgery in the Middle Ages*. Translated by Rosemary Morris. New Brunswick: Rutgers University Press, 1990.

Prior, Oliver H., ed. *Caxton's Mirrour of the World*. London: For the Early English Text Society by Kegan Paul, Trench, Trübner and Co., and by H. Milford, Oxford University Press, 1913.

———, ed. *L'image du monde de Maitre Gossouin: Rédaction en prose*. Lausanne and Paris: Payot, 1913.

Prioreschi, Plinio. *A History of Medicine*. Vol. 5 of *Medieval Medicine*. 2nd ed. Omaha: Horatius Press, 2003.

Proctor-Tiffany, Mariah. *Medieval Art in Motion: The Inventory of Gift Giving of Queen Clémence de Hongrie*. University Park: Pennsylvania State University Press, 2019.

Rawcliffe, Carole. *Medicine and Society in Later Medieval England*. Stroud, England: Alan Sutton Publishing, 1995.

———. "The Profits of Practice: The Wealth and Status of Medical Men in Later Medieval England." *Social History of Medicine* 1 (1988): 61–78.

———. *Urban Bodies: Communal Health in Late Medieval English Towns and Cities*. Woodbridge, Suffolk: The Boydell Press, 2013.

Reynolds, Catherine. "English Patrons and French Artists in Fifteenth-Century Normandy." In *England and Normandy in the Middle Ages*, edited by David Bates and Anne Curry, 299–313. London: Hambledon Press, 1994.

Richard, Jean. *Saint Louis: Crusader King of France*. Edited and abridged by Simon Lloyd. Translated by Jean Birrell. Cambridge: Cambridge University Press, 1992.

Richard de Fournival. *Li Bestiaires d'amours di Maistre Richart de Fornival e li Response du Bestiaire*. Translated by Cesare Segre. Milan: R. Ricciardi, 1957.

———. *Master Richard's "Bestiary of Love" and "Response."* Translated by Jeanette Beer. Berkeley: University of California Press, 1986.

Ricoeur, Paul. "Narrative Time." In *On Narrative*, edited by W. J. T. Mitchell, 165–86. Chicago: University of Chicago Press, 1981.

———. *Temps et récit*. Paris: Seuil, 1983–85.

Riddle, John M. *Dioscorides on Pharmacy and Medicine*. Austin: University of Texas Press, 1985.

Riddy, Felicity. "'Burgeis' Domesticity in Late-Medieval England." In Kowaleski and Goldberg, *Medieval Domesticity*, 14–36.

———. "Looking Closely: Authority and Intimacy in the Late Medieval Urban Home." In *Gendering the Master Narrative: Women and Power in the Middle Ages*. Edited by Mary C. Erler and Maryanne Kowaleski, 212–28. Ithaca: Cornell University Press, 2003.

———. "Mother Knows Best: Reading Social Change in a Courtesy Text." *Speculum* 71, no. 1 (1996): 66–86.

Rieder, Paula M. *On the Purification of Women: Churching in Northern France,*

1100–1500. Basingstoke: Palgrave Macmillan, 2006.
Ritchey, Sara. *Acts of Care: Recovering Women in Late Medieval Health*. Ithaca and London: Cornell University Press, 2021.
Ritchey, Sara, and Sharon Strocchia, eds. *Gender, Health, and Healing, 1250–1550*. Amsterdam: Amsterdam University Press, 2020.
Rouse, Richard H., and Mary A. Rouse. *Manuscripts and Their Makers: Commercial Book Producers in Medieval Paris, 1200–1500*. 2 vols. Turnhout, Belgium: Harvey Miller, 2000.
Samsó, Julio. *Islamic Astronomy and Medieval Spain*. Aldershot, UK: Ashgate Variorum, 1994.
Sandler, Lucy Freeman. *Gothic Manuscripts, 1285–1385*. 2 vols. A Survey of Manuscripts in the British Isles. London: Harvey Miller, 1986.
———. *Omne Bonum: A Fourteenth-Century Encyclopedia of Universal Knowledge: British Library MSS Royal 6 E VI–6 E VII*. 2 vols. London: Harvey Miller, 1996.
Savage-Smith, Emilie. "Medicine in Medieval Islam." In Lindberg and Shank, *Medieval Science*, 139–67.
Schmitt, Natalie Crohn. "Continuous Narration in the *Holkham Bible Picture Book* and *Queen Mary Psalter*." *Word and Image: A Journal of Verbal/Visual Inquiry* 20, no. 2 (2004): 123–37.
Scott, Kathleen L. *Later Gothic Manuscripts, 1390–1490*. 2 vols. A Survey of Manuscripts Illuminated in the British Isles. London: Harvey Miller, 1996.
———. "Manuscripts for Henry VII, His Household and Family." In *The Cambridge Illuminations: The Conference Papers*, edited by Stella Panayotova, 279–86. London: Harvey Miller, 2007.
Scott, Margaret. *Fashion in the Middle Ages*. Los Angeles: J. Paul Getty Museum, 2011.
———. *Medieval Dress and Fashion*. London: British Library, 2007.
Scully, D. Eleanor, and Terence Scully. *Early French Cookery: Sources, History, Original Recipes, and Modern Adaptations*. Ann Arbor: University of Michigan Press, 1995.
Sewright, Kathleen. "An Introduction to British Library MS Lansdowne 380." *Notes*, 2nd ser., 65, no. 4 (2009): 633–736.
Shatzmiller, Joseph. *Jews, Medicine, and Medieval Society*. Berkeley: University of California Press, 1994.
Sheingorn, Pamela. "The Wise Mother: The Image of St. Anne Teaching the Virgin Mary." *Gesta* 32, no. 1 (1993): 69–80.
Silva, Chelsea. "Opening the Medieval Folding Almanac." *Exemplaria* 30, no. 1 (2018): 49–65.
Siraisi, Nancy. *Medieval and Early Renaissance Medicine: An Introduction to Knowledge and Practice*. Chicago: University of Chicago Press, 1990.
Sivéry, Gérard. *Marguerite de Provence: Une reine au temps des cathédrales*. Paris: Librarie Arthème Fayard, 1987.
Skemer, Don C. *Binding Words: Textual Amulets in the Middle Ages*. University Park: Pennsylvania State University Press, 2006.
Smith, Lesley, and Jane H. M. Taylor, eds. *Women and the Book: Assessing the Visual Evidence*. London: British Library; Toronto: University of Toronto Press, 1997.
Sponsler, Claire. "Eating Lessons: Lydgate's 'Dietary' and Consumer Conduct." In Ashley and Clark, *Medieval Conduct*, 1–22.
———. "Narrating the Social Order: Medieval Clothing Laws." *Clio* 21 (1992): 265–83.
Stanton, Anne Rudloff. "The Personal Geography of a Dowager Queen: Isabella of France and Her Inventory." In Hamilton and Proctor-Tiffany, *Moving Women, Moving Objects (400–1500)*, 205–27.
———. *The Queen Mary Psalter: A Study of Affect and Audience*. Philadelphia: American Philosophical Society, 2001.
Stones, Alison. *Gothic Manuscripts: 1260–1320*. 2 parts, 4 vols. A Survey of Manuscripts Illuminated in France. London and Turnhout, Belgium: Harvey Miller/Brepols, 2013, 2015.
———. "Stylistic Associations, Evolution, and Collaboration: Charting the Bute Painter's Career." *J. Paul Getty Museum Journal* 23 (1995): 11–29.
Sturges, Robert Stuart. *Medieval Interpretation: Models of Reading in Literary Narrative, 1100–1500*. Carbondale: Southern Illinois University Press, 1991.

Sudhoff, Karl. "Anatomische Zeichnungen (Schemata) aus dem 12. und 13. Jahrhundert und eine Skelettzeichnung des 14. Jahrhunderts." *Studien zur Geschichte der Medizin* 1 (1907): 49–65.
———. *Ein Beitrag zur Geschichte der Anatomie im Mittelalter, speziell der anatomischen Graphik nach Handschriften des 9. bis 15. Jahrhunderts*. Studien zur Geschichte der Medizin 4. Leipzig: Barth, 1908. Reprint, Hildesheim: G. Olms, 1964.
———. *Beiträge zur Geschichte der Chirurgie im Mittelalter*. 2 vols. Leipzig: J. A. Barth, 1914/1918.
Talbert, E. W. "The Notebook of a Fifteenth-Century Practicing Physician." *Studies in English* 22 (1942): 5–30.
Talbot, C. H. "A Mediaeval Physician's Vade Mecum," *Journal of the History of Medicine and Allied Sciences* 16, no. 3 (1961): 213–33.
Talbot, C. H., and Eugene Ashby Hammond. *The Medical Practitioners in Medieval England: A Biographical Register*. London: Wellcome Historical Medical Library, 1965.
Tavormina, M. Teresa. *The Dome of Uryne: A Reading Edition of Nine Middle English Uroscopies*. Oxford: Oxford University Press, 2019.
Temkin, Owsei. *Galenism: Rise and Decline of a Medical Philosophy*. Ithaca: Cornell University Press, 1973.
Thomas, Antoine. "L'identité du médecin Aldebrandin de Sienne." *Romania* 35 (1906): 454–56.
———. "Jean Pitart, chirurgien et poète." *Comptes rendus des séances de l'Académie des Inscriptions et Belles-Lettres* 60, no. 1 (1916): 107–8.
Thompson, Kristen, and David Bordell. *Film History: An Introduction*. 2nd ed. New York: McGraw-Hill, 2002.
Tracy, Larissa, and Kelly DeVries. *Wounds and Wound Repair in Medieval Culture*. Leiden: Brill, 2015.
Trease, G. E. "The Spicers and Apothecaries of the Royal Household in the Reigns of Henry III, Edward I and Edward II." *Nottingham Medieval Studies* 3 (1959): 19–52.
Tyers, Theresa L. "Family, Feud, and Fertility in Late Medieval Artois and Flanders." *Dynamis: Acta Hispanica ad Medicinae Scientiarumque Historiam Illustrandam* 38, no. 2 (2018): 389–406.
———. "'In the Merry Month of May': Instructions for Ensuring Fertility in MS British Library, Lansdowne 380." *Social History of Medicine* 29, no. 2 (2016): 267–89.
———. "The Rebirth of Fertility: The *Trotula* and Her Travelling Companions, c. 1200–1450." PhD diss., University of Nottingham, 2012.
Vale, Malcolm. *The Princely Court: Medieval Courts and Culture in North-West Europe, 1270–1380*. Oxford: Oxford University Press, 2001.
Valls, Helen. "Illustrations as Abstracts: The Illustrative Programme in a Montpellier Manuscript of Roger Frugardi's *Chirurgia*." In *Medicina nei Secoli—Arte e Scienza: Journal of History of Medicine* 8 (1996): 67–83.
———. "Studies on Roger Frugardi's *Chirurgia*." PhD diss., University of Toronto, 1995.
van der Lugt, Maaike. "Nature as Norm in Medieval Medical Discussions of Maternal Breastfeeding and Wet-Nursing." *Journal of Medieval and Early Modern Studies* 49, no. 3 (2019): 563–88.
Voigts, Linda Ehrsam. "Fifteenth-Century English Banns Advertising the Services of an Itinerant Doctor." In *Between Text and Patient: The Medical Enterprise in Medieval and Early Modern Europe*, edited by Florence Eliza Glaze and Brian K. Nance, 245–77. Florence: SISMEL, Edizioni del Galluzzo, 2011.
———. "What's the Word? Bilingualism in Late-Medieval England." *Speculum* 71, no. 4 (1996): 813–26.
Wallis, Faith, ed. *Medieval Medicine: A Reader*. Toronto: University of Toronto Press, 2010.
———. "Signs and Senses: Diagnosis and Prognosis in Early Medieval Pulse and Urine Texts." *Social History of Medicine* 13, no. 2 (2000): 265–78.
Watt, Diane. *Paston Women: Selected Letters*. Rochester: D. S. Brewer, 2004.
Weale, W. H. James. *Bookbindings and Rubbings of Bindings*. 2 vols. London: Printed for Her Majesty's Stationery Office by Eyre and Spottiswoode, 1894–98.
Weitzmann, Kurt. *Illustrations in Roll and Codex: A Study of the Origin and*

Method of Text Illustration. Princeton: Princeton University Press, 1947.

Whatling, Stuart. "Narrative Art in Northern Europe, c. 1140–1300: A Narratological Re-Appraisal." PhD diss., University of London, 2010.

Whitaker, Elaine E. "Reading the Paston Letters Medically." *English Language Notes* 31, no. 1 (1993): 19–27.

White, Hayden. "The Value of Narrativity in the Representation of Reality." In *On Narrative*, edited by W. J. T. Mitchell, 1–24. Chicago: University of Chicago Press, 1981.

White, T. H., trans. *The Book of Beasts: A Translation from a Latin Bestiary of the Twelfth Century*. New York: G. P. Putnam's Sons, 1954.

Whittington, Karl. "The Cruciform Womb: Process, Symbol and Salvation in Bodleian Library MS. Ashmole 399." *Different Visions: A Journal of New Perspectives on Medieval Art* 1 (September 2008): 1–24.

———. "Picturing Christ as Surgeon and Patient in British Library MS Sloane 1977." *Mediaevalia* 35 (2014): 83–115.

Williams, Steven J. *The Secret of Secrets: The Scholarly Career of a Pseudo-Aristotelian Text in the Latin Middle Ages*. Ann Arbor: University of Michigan Press, 2003.

Winer, Rebecca Lynn. "Conscripting the Breast: Lactation, Slavery and Salvation in the Realms of Aragon and Kingdom of Majorca, c. 1250–1300." *Journal of Medieval History* 34, no. 2 (2008): 164–84.

———. "The Enslaved Wet Nurse as Nanny: The Transition from Free to Slave Labor in Childcare in Barcelona After the Black Death (1348)." *Slavery and Abolition: A Journal of Slave and Post-Slave Studies* 38, no. 2 (2017): 303–319.

———. "The Mother and the *Dida* [Nanny]: Female Employers and Wet Nurses in Fourteenth-Century Barcelona." In *Medieval and Renaissance Lactations: Images, Rhetorics, Practices*, edited by Jutta Gisela Sperling, 55–78. Farnham, UK: Ashgate, 2013.

Wittig, Susan. *Stylistic and Narrative Structures in the Middle English Romances*. Austin: University of Texas Press, 1978.

Wolf, Werner. "Narrative and Narrativity: A Narratological Reconceptualization and Its Applicability to the Visual Arts." *Word and Image: A Journal of Verbal/Visual Inquiry* 19, no. 3 (2003): 180–97.

Woolgar, C. M. *The Great Household in Late Medieval England*. New Haven: Yale University Press, 1999.

Yalom, Marilyn. *A History of the Breast*. New York: Ballantine Books, 1997.

Index

Italicized page numbers indicate illustrations. Endnotes are referenced with "n" followed by the endnote number.

age, and life cycle, 21
air quality, 20, 100
Ajuda Cod. 52-XIII-26 (Biblioteca da Ajuda)
  artists of, 9, 27, 85
  breastfeeding, 40, 47, *48*
  copulation, 53–54, *55*
  dating of, 9, 67
  herbal recipes, 113
  historiated initials in, statistics, 83
  historical context, 78
  illustration style descriptions, 27, 85
  manuscript models for, 182n79
  manuscript summary, 161, 169
  materiality of, 27
  pregnancy, *86*
  production location, 9, 87
  provenance, 9, 79, 85
  scenes depicted in, overview, 163–68
  texts of, 83, 85, 130
Albucasis, 102, 190n81
Aldobrandin Master, 8, 26, 68, 88
Aldobrandino of Siena
  biographical information, 5, 54, 93
  breastfeeding guidance of, 43, 47
  as health guide author, 2, 3
  medical sources used by, 25, 98, 99, 100, 101–3, 104, 105
  patrons of, 5, 25, 47
  physician references, 98
  procreation guidance, 53
Alfonso X, king of Castile, 70, 103
Almanach aux Juifs, L', 181n53
almanacs
  astrological medicine illustrations in, 116, *117*
  folding, 116
  manuscript texts, 181n53
  urine charts and wheels, 108–9, *110*
alternative health practices, 121
amulets, 121, 122
anatomy, 102, 106, *107*, *108*
Anicia Juliana, 114
animals, 11, 23, 29, 31, *32*, *33*
Annunciation, *36*
anxiety representations, 17, 45, *46*, 49, 51
apothecaries (pharmacists)
  in apothecary shops, *36*, *112*, 148, *149*
  clothing styles of, 148, *149*
  as practitioner type, 98, 113, 114, 120
apothecary shops (pharmacies)
  history and development of, 113–14
  as medical treatment, 113
  in surgical texts, *36*, 111, *112*
  theriac scenes in, 148–49, *149*
  women as customers in, *112*, 148–49, *149*, *150*
Apuleius Platonicus, 176n24
Arderne, John, 112, *113*, 134, *135*
Aristotle, 28, 100, 115
Arnau de Vilanova, 105, 130, 185n37, 190n81
Arrangement of Medical Knowledge for One Who Is Not Able to Compile a Book for Himself, The (Albucasis), 102
Arsenal 2510 (Bibliothèque nationale de France)
  artists of, 8, 11, 72
  clothing accessories, 142
  copulation, 53, *53*
  cupping, 133, *133*, 134
  dating of, 8, 65, 67, 70, 72
  grain, *71*
  hair care, 11, *13*, 25
  herbal recipes, 113
  historiated initials in, statistics, 70
  illustration style descriptions, 8, 11, 13, 26–27, 70
  manuscript summary, 161, 170
  materiality of, 72
  newborn care, 39, *41*
  production location, 8, 72, 75
  provenance, 70, 72
  purging, 153, *153*
  scenes depicted in, overview, 163–68
  texts of, 20, 70, 130
  vomiting, 123, *124*
Arsenal 2894 (Bibliothèque nationale de France), 9, 10, *10*, 162, 163–68, 170
Articella (medical text), 107–8, *109*
Ashmole 399 (Bodleian Library, Oxford), 106, *107*, *108*, 178n71
astrology, 21, 75, 81, 85, 116, *117*
astronomy, 68, 75–77, *76*, *77*, 116

Averroes, 102, 190n81
Avicenna (Ibn Sīnā)
in book collections, 190n81
illustrated copies of, 186n50
as medieval medical source, 102, 103, 104
as regimen literature source, 105
as *Régime* source, 2, 100, 102–3, 104
axe-wielding figures, *72*

Bacon, Roger, 103
barbers and barber-surgeons
attributes of, *9*, 142
as bloodletting practitioners, *3*, 4, 97, 97, *97*, 113
clothing styles of, *3*, 4, *9*, 96, 97, *97*
ear examination scenes with, *9*, *97*
as practitioner type, 95, 98, 99
training and roles of, 111
bathing
historiated initials featuring, 38, *69*, 106
as household activity, 132, 158
newborn care featuring, 21, 39–40, *41*, *50*, 51, *52*
for preventative health care, 100, 146
as *Régime* discussion topic, 11, 20, 21, 132
Bathsheba (biblical character), 28, *29*
bears, 31, *33*
Beatrice of Provence
book circulation through family of, 89, 91
death of, 65
family reunions, 66
household management responsibilities, 132
marriage, 65, 180n33
Régime ownership, 65, 70
Beatrice of Savoy
daughters of, 43, 65
family reunion, 66
patronage of, 5
physician relationship with, 119–20
Régime commission, 2, 3, 64, 65
Régime dissemination, 89
social status and authority of, 47
beds, canopy
copulation scenes with, *28*, *29*, 53, *53*, *55*
lying-in scenes with, 39–40, 49, *50*, *52*
symbolism of, 49, 137
bedside manners, 57
beer production, 23, *24*, 134
Bennett, Richard, 182n65
Benoit de Florenche, 68
Bernard de Gordon, 7, 105, 117
Bestiare d'amour (Richard de Fournival), 115
bestiaries
animal composition comparisons, 11, 27–28, 31–32
food representations comparisons, 23
in medicinal herbals, 31
visual traditions of, descriptions, 29, 31, *32*
Bible moralisée, 66, 70, 81, 88
bibles, illustrated
copulation imagery from, 27–28, *29*
historiated initials in, function, 13–14
imagery tradition influences, 29
moralized, 66, 70, 81, 88
biblical characters
copulation models, 28, *29*
lying-in scenes featuring births of, 49
skin care conversation models, 28, *31*
wet nurse selection models, *31*, 39, *42*
Biblioteca Apostolica Vaticana Reg.lat.1256, 9, *10*, 118, 162, 163–68, 172
Biblioteca da Ajuda, Cod. 52-XIII-26. *See* Ajuda Cod. 52-XIII-26 (Biblioteca da Ajuda)
Bibliothèque municipale de Besançon manuscripts
MS 457, 186n50
MS 463, 148, *150* , 170
Bibliothèque municipale de Rennes, MS 593, 77–78, 181n52–53
Bibliothèque nationale de France (BnF) manuscripts
Arsenal MS 2510 (*see* Arsenal 2510)
Arsenal MS 2894, 9, 10, *10*, 162, 163–68, 170
Fr. 1109, 78, 118, 170
Fr. 1288, 101, 117, 172, 175n25
Fr. 2021, 3, 75, 172, 180n33
Fr. 12323 (*see* BnF Fr. 12323)
Fr. 14822, 172, 174n5
Fr. 14964, 68, 77, 180n41
Fr. 14970, 68, 77, 180n41
Fr. 24246, 183n101
Lat. 9333, 148–49, *149*
Nouv. acq. lat. 1673, 146, 147, *147*, *148*, 190n80
Bibliothèque nationale de France Nouv. acq. Fr. 6739, 128
birds, 20, 31, 181n56
Bisson, Sebastiano, 3
Blanche of Castile, 66
Blanche of France, 70
bliaut, 93, 141
bloodletting
illustration composition and style, 1, 4
patient clothing descriptions, *3*, 4
practitioner clothing descriptions, *3*, 4, 97, *97*
practitioner touching during, 58
pregnancy care and, 21
purpose, 100
as *Régime* subject, 20, 101, 112–13
treatment descriptions, 1, *3*, *97*
Bloodletting Man, 116
Blumenthal, Debra, 47
BnF Fr. 1109 (Bibliothèque nationale de France), 78, 118, 170

BnF Fr. 1288 (Bibliothèque nationale de France), 101, 117, 172, 175n25
BnF Fr. 2021 (Bibliothèque nationale de France), 3, 75, 172, 180n33
BnF Fr. 12323 (Bibliothèque nationale de France)
astronomical diagrams, 76, 77
bloodletting, 97, *97*
cheese, 61, *62*
clothing styles in, *42*, *56*, 141, 142, *143*
copulation, 53, *53*
cupping, 97, *97*
dating of, 67, 73
defacement of images, 73
eye treatment, 25, *25*
grain, *71*
heart consultations, *143*
historiated initials in, statistics, 73
illustration style descriptions, 26, 73
manuscript summary, 161, 170
medical texts relationships, 108
pepper, 23, *23*
physicians featured in, 54, *56*, *95* , 96, 142, *143*
practitioner clothing styles in, 97, *97*
pregnancy, 54, *56*
production location, 8
provenance, 73
purging, *74*
scenes depicted in, overview, 163–68
Sloane 2435 manuscript comparisons, 61, 73, 75
teeth, *95*
texts of, 20, 73, 75, 77, 113, 130, 181n51
vomiting, 123, *125*
wet nurse selection, 39, 40, *42*, 51
BnF Fr. 14822 (Bibliothèque nationale de France), 172, 174n5
BnF Fr. 14964 (Bibliothèque nationale de France), 68, 77, 180n41
BnF Fr. 24246 (Bibliothèque nationale de France), 183n101
BnF Lat. 9333 (Bibliothèque nationale de France), 148–49, *149*, 190n89
BnF Nouv. acq. lat. 1673 (Bibliothèque nationale de France), 146, 147, *147*, *148*, 190n80
Bodleian Library, Oxford, manuscripts
Ashmole 399, 106, *107*, *108*, 178n71
Laud Misc. 724, 107, 134, *136*
body care
ears, *9*
eyes, 25, *25*
hair, 11, *13*, 25
human waste and messiness of, 153
as *Régime* section, 20
See also bathing
Boleyn KG, Thomas, 85
Book of Courtesy, The (Caxton), 188n3
Book of Galen, 81, 83, 85
book-sellers/book-contractors, 88
books of hours
astrological medicine illustrations in, 116
defecation scenes in, 153–54, *154*
idealized worlds portrayed in, 147
physicians with urine flasks, *111*
skin care conversation modeling, 28, *31*
botanical pharmacology, 113–14
See also apothecaries; apothecary shops; herbals
bourgeois
household descriptions, 131–32, 137, 138
household management roles, 138–39
social mobility and status markers of, 129, 132, 140–41
bourrelet, 143
Boutemont, Robin, 77
Bradwardine, William, 183n101
bran, *82*
breastfeeding, 40, 43, 47, *48*
See also wet nurses
breasts
disease consultation and examination of, 35, *37*, 45, 52, 54, 55, *57*
wet nurse selection and inspection of, 13, 17, *18*, *46*
British Library manuscripts
Additional MS 18719, 70
Additional MS 29301, 112, *113*, 118
Harley MS 3140, 107–8, *109*
Harley MS 3745, 107–8
Lansdowne MS 380, 106, 118, 155, 159, 172
Royal MS 19 B X, 170, 181n56
Royal MS 12 C XIX, 31, *32*
Sloane MS 6, 107, 112, 134, 135, *135*
Sloane MS 1611, 118–19, 172
Sloane MS 1977 (*see* Sloane 1977)
Sloane MS 2401 (*see* Sloane 2401)
Sloane MS 2435 (*see* Sloane 2435)
Sloane MS 3525, 57, 101, 117, 172
Brown, Katherine A., 105
Brown-Grant, Rosalind, 128
Bruges (Belgium), 88, 89
Brunetto Latini, 5, 78, 181n52, 181n56
Brydges, Elizabeth, 83
Brydges, Margaret, 83
Brydges, Richard, 83
Brydges, Rowland, 83
Bute Painter, The
biographical information, 8
copulation scenes, 53, *53*
cupping scenes, 133, *133*
grain illustrations, *71*
hair care illustrations, 11, *13*, 25
illustration style descriptions, 11, 27, 70

- Bute Painter, The (*continued*)
  - manuscripts illustrated by, 8, 68, 72
  - man with axe, *72*
  - newborn care, *41*
  - patrons of, 72
  - production location, 70, 72, 88
  - purging, *153*
  - vomiting, 11, 13, *124*
- Bute Psalter, The, 70, 72, *72* , 180n40

- Cabré, Monserrat, 7, 130, 131, 132
- Caesar, letters to, 81, 83, 85, 109, 115, 118
- Cambrai (France), 8, 64, 72, 75, 78, 87, 88
- Cambridge University Library, MS Ii.V.II
  - audience of, 79, 89
  - cheese, 63, *64*
  - cider and beer production, 23, *24*
  - coats of arms, 67, 78, 79
  - copulation, 53
  - dating of, 8, 79, 181n58
  - food production and consumption, 151
  - hat styles, 144, *144*
  - herbal recipes, 113
  - historiated initials in, statistics, 79
  - historical context, 78, 81
  - illustration style descriptions, 27
  - as manuscript model, 182n79
  - manuscript summary, 161, 169
  - materiality of, 27
  - millet and rice, *80*
  - Morgan manuscript comparisons, 81
  - newborn care and lying-in scenes, 49, *50*
  - ownership page inserts, 79
  - production location, 8, 72, 79, 87
  - provenance, 9, 79
  - scenes depicted in, overview, 163–68
  - texts of, 79, 130
  - vomiting, *144*
- Camille, Michael, 45, 52–53, 153–54
- Campos Ribeiro, Luís, 3, 85, 182n79
- *Canon of Medicine, The* (Avicenna), 2, 102, 103, 104, 190n81
- Carrara Herbal, 114
- Cassagnes-Brouquet, Sophie, 77
- cauterization, 109, 111
- Caxton, William, 188n3
- chainse (chemise), 58, 141
- chaperons, 97, *98*, 143, 144, *144*
- character of individual, 100
- Charles I of Anjou, 65, 180n33
- Charles of Valois, 73
- charms, 115, 121, 122, 187n102
- cheese, 61–63, *62*, *63*, *64*, 146, *147*
- chemise, 58, 141
- childbirth
  - intimacy in scenes of, 51
  - lying-in rites after, 39–40, 49–51, *50*, *52*
  - patron saints of, 119
  - physicians' touching and anxiety during, 48
  - purification rites after, 49
- childcare, 21, 132
  - *See also* newborn care; wet nurses
- *Chirurgia* (Frugardi)
  - breast disease consultation, 35, *37*, 45, 52, 54, 55, 57, *57*
  - historiated initials in, function of, 32, 112
  - narrative organization, 35, *36*
  - as *Régime* text accompaniment, 7, 117
  - surgical scenes with biblical themes, 35, *36*, 45
- Christ-as-physician (trope), 28
- Christine de Pizan, 125, 128
- churching rites, 49
- cider production, 11, *12*, 23, *24*, 134, 152
- *Circa instans* (Matthaeus Platearius, trans.), 111, 117, 187n81, 190n81
- *Cité des dames* (Christine de Pizan), 128
- Clémence of Hungary, 67, 77, 88, 129
- clothing and accessories
  - of apothecaries, 148, *149*
  - of barber-surgeons, *3*, 4, 97, *97*
  - of cupping practitioners, 97, *97*, *98*
  - fifteenth-century styles, 143–44
  - fourteenth-century styles, 141, 142–43
  - of physicians, 54–55, *55*, *56*, 57, 93, *94*, 96, *96*, *98*, 142, *143*, 143–44
  - practitioners *vs.* patients indicated by, 58
  - practitioner touch and, 58
  - romantic idealizations, 147, *147*
  - as social status markers, 26, 51, 93, 97–98, 127, 140, 142, 144–45
  - sumptuary laws on, 141
  - thirteenth-century styles, 141–42, *142*, *143*
  - of wet nurses, 17, *18*, 40, *42*
  - *See also* gloves, physicians'; hats and headdresses
- coifs
  - of bloodletting patients, *97*
  - of bloodletting practitioners, 1, *3*, 97
  - in copulation scenes, *28*
  - of cupping patients, 58, *59*, 133, *133*
  - of hybrid creatures, *22*, 23
  - of laborers, *23*, 142
  - of physicians, *37*
  - popularity of, 142
  - of practitioners, *36*
  - of purging patients, *153*
- Collins, Minta, 32
- color (pigments)
  - imagery representing mixing of, *34*
  - urine charts and substances representing, 109
  - use of, 16, 38, 83, 158
- *Complete Book of the Medical Art* (Haly Abbas), 102

complexion (*complexio*). *See* humors
complexion (face and skin care), 28, *30*, *142*
Comprehensive Book on Medicine, The (Rhazes), 102
conduct (courtesy) literature, 127–29, 132, 141, 145, 151, 152
Constantine the African, 2, 100, 103, 190n81
consumption and materialism
  dietary guides on, 63, 127, 128–29, 151
  manuscript illustrations and displays of, 127
  public *vs.* private, 151
  as social status marker, 129, 132, 140–41, 151–52
  sumptuary laws for control of, 141
Continens (Rhaze), 102
contra-naturals, 100
copulation
  breastfeeding beliefs and, 43
  defacement of images, 53, *53*
  illustration style descriptions, 11, 28, *29*
  as *Régime* subject, 20–21
  touch and gender status, *28*, 52–54, *53*, *55*
  wet nurses and pregnancy restrictions, 44
cotehardies, 143
courtesy (conduct) literature, 127–29, 132, 141, 145, 151, 152
crespine/crespinette, 141
critical days (illness theory), 116
Crophill, John, 99
Crusader Bible, The, 28, *29*
cucumbers, *148*
"Cultural Biography of Things" (Kopytoff), 5–6
cupping
  practice descriptions and purpose, 13, 100, 111
  practitioner clothing styles, 97, *97*, *98*
  as *Régime* subject, 20, 109
  touching during, 58, *59*
  women as practitioners, 13, *59*, 107, 113, 133, *133*, 134, *135*, *136*

David (biblical character), 28, *29*
De dietis (Isaac Judaeus), 117
defecation, 153–54, *154*
De flebotomia (Bernard de Gordon), 105
De generatione (Aristotle), 28
De materia medica (Dioscorides), 114, 176n24
De mundo, 85
De passionibus mulierum (Trota), 117
De pulsibus (Bernard de Gordon), 105
De urinis (Bernard de Gordon), 105
De urinis (Gilles de Corbeil), 117
diet. *See* food and drink
"Dietary" (Lydgate), 127, 128–29, 151
Dioscorides, 101, 102, 114, 176n24, 190n81
disease theory, 100
dissection, 106
dog-headed beasts, 1, *3*, *142*
domestic geography, 138
Dominicus Gundissalinus, 103
Driver, Martha, 89
Dyer, Christopher, 139

ear treatments, *9*, 97
Edward I, king of England, 139
Edward II, king of England, 66
Edward III, king of England, 72
Edward IV, king of England, 78, 79, 85
eggs, 23
Eleanor of Aquitaine, 66
Eleanor of Provence
  family reunions, 66
  household descriptions, 139
  household expenditures of, 139, 189n59
  household management responsibilities, 132
  manuscript collections, 65, 81, 140
  manuscript commissions, 66
  manuscript dissemination, 89, 91
  marriage, 65
  physicians of, 120
  procreation of, 43
Elizabeth (biblical character), 28, *31*, *36*, 39
Elizabeth of York, 67, 78, 79
emotions, as non-natural, 100, 150
encyclopedias
  audiences of, 106
  historiated initials in, function, 32–34, *33*
  illustrated, 125, 145–49, *147*, *148*, *149*
  medical, 102, 105
  popularity of, 78
  as text accompaniments, 75, 106, 116
  See also herbals; *image du monde, L'* (Gossuin de Metz)
evacuation
  defecation, 153–54, *154*
  household intimacy and, 134, 153
  leeching, 100, 109
  methods of, 100
  for preventative health care, 100, 126
  purpose, 111
  See also bloodletting; cupping; purging; vomiting
eye treatments, 25, *25*

face and skin care, 28, *30*, *142*
farro, *82*
fashion. *See* clothing and accessories; gloves, physicians'; hats and headdresses
Ferdinand de la Cerda, 70
fertility and procreation
  dietary instructions for men, 21
  gender roles and beliefs on, 21, 53
  as health care topic, 20, 43, 91, 117, 118, 119, 130

fertility and procreation (*continued*)
medieval practices of, 43, 44
preventative health care and, 100
See also copulation; pregnancy
Fery-Hue, François, 3, 20, 175n36, 179n12
fillet and barbette, 133, *133*, 141
fish, 10, *10*, 20, 23
fistula-in-ano diagram with tools, 112, *113*
Fitzwilliam Museum MS 261, 79
Flos medicinae Scholae Salerni, 81
food and drink
clean up after, 152–53
consumption advice, 23, 61–63, 127, 128–29, 151, 152
illustration composition traditions, 23
for male fertility, 21
plants, *22*, 23, *23*
pregnancy instructions on, 21
preparation of, 152–53
for preventative health care, 100, 126
production of, 11, *12*, 23, 134, 152
as *Régime* subject, 20, 21, 23, 134, 140, 151–53
royal court expenditures on, 139
as social status markers, 127, 139–40, 151–52
See also specific foods and drinks
Frederick II, Holy Roman Emperor, 103, 175–76n11
freeze-frame scenes, 19
Frugardi, Roger, 7, 111
See also *Chirurgia* (Frugardi)

Galen of Pergamum
astrological medicine treatises by, 116
biographical information, 101–2
collections featuring, 190n81
as health guide text accompaniments, 81, 83, 85
medical manuscripts with texts attributed to, 111
medical treatment theories, 114
as medieval medical source, 99, 101–2, 103
as *Régime* source, 21, 100, 104
Gautier I d'Enghien, 180n39
Gerard of Cremona, 103
gestures
artistic styles for depicting, 26, 27
function of, 45, 51
of patients indicating question or acceptance, 35, *37*, 93, *94*
of physicians indicating authority, 54, 96, *97*
of physicians indicating consultation, 35, *37*, 93, *94*
of physicians indicating seriousness of situation, 57
of purging practitioners indicating command, 153
social status indicated through, 17, *18*, 19, 40, *42*, 51
gift-giving, 6, 13, 65, 66, 88
Gilles de Corbeil, 117
Gillespie, Susan D., 5–6
Giovannino de' Grassi, 185n34
Givens, Jean, 32
gloves, physicians'
patients holding, 142, *142*
removed and holding, 54–55, 57, 95, 96, *96*, 142, *143*
wearing, 142
gold and gilding, 1, 16, 26, 27, 38, 68, 158
Goldberg, P. J. P., 137
Good Wife's Guide, The (*Le ménagier de Paris*) (anonymous), 100, 125, 127–28, 129, 151, 152
Gossuin de Metz. See *image du monde, L'*
grains, *22*, 23, *71*, *80*, *82*, 151
Green, Monica H.
health guide audiences, 101, 120
medical text audiences, 7, 129
physicians touching female patients, 57–58
Régime commission and dissemination, 64
scholarship studies of, 3
women as medical reading communities, 90
women as physicians' patients, 120–21
Grosseteste, Robert, 103
Guillaume of Termonde, 180n39
Guy de Chauliac, 102, 111
Guy de Dampierre, 180n39

hair care, 11, *13*, 25
hairnets, 58, 141
Haly Abbas, 21, 102, 103, 184n11
Hamilton, Tracy Chapman, 5, 77
hares, *33*
Harley MS 3140 (British Library), 107–8, *109*
Harley MS 3745 (British Library), 107–8
hats and headdresses
of barber-surgeons, *3*, 4, 97, *98*
of bloodletting patients, *97*
of bloodletting practitioners, 1, *3*, 97
in copulation scenes, *28*, 53
of cupping patients, 58, *59*, 133, *133*
of cupping practitioners, 58, *59*, 133, *133*
fifteenth-century styles, 144, *144*
fourteenth-century styles, 141, 143
of hybrid creatures, *22*, 23, *69*
of laborers, *23*, 142
lack of, 142
mothers in lying-in scenes, 49, *50*, *52*
of newborn care servants, 49, *50*, *52*

of physicians, *37*, *94*, 96, 142, *143*
popular styles, 142
of purging/vomiting patients, 144, *144*, *153*
of surgeons, *36*
heart consultations, *143*
Henri de Mondeville, 111, 181n45
Henry III, king of England, 65, 66, 72, 81, 83, 85, 118
Henry VII, king of England, 67, 78, 79, 181n58
Henry VIII, king of England, 118
herbal medicine, 113–14
See also apothecaries; apothecary shops; herbals
herbals
bestiary sections in, 31
function of, 32
genre descriptions, 29, 114
plant illustration compositions compared to, 11
regimen genre comparisons, 27, 147
as regimen text accompaniments, 111, 117
traditional sources for, 101, 114, 176n24
Herbarius (Apuleius Platonicus), 176n24
Hippocrates, 99, 100, 107, 111
historiated initials of *Régime du corps*
chronological groupings of extant copies and, 8–9
compositional format, 11, 19, 38
description overview, 11
function of, 4, 8, 10–11, 14, 38, 91–92, 147
historical usage, 38
materiality of, 16, 26
medical illustrations in, 112–13
medical illustration styles, 106
narrative ambiguity of, 14, 17, 18–19, 20, 40
narrative content and scene selection, 37–40
size of, 26, 38
social status associations, 38
statistics in extant copies, 1, 67, 68, 70, 73, 77, 79, 81, 83
style descriptions, 1, 4, 9–10, 18, 26
subjects and themes, 132
text relationships, 20–25, 34
visual content of, 18, 34
visual traditions compared to, 27–37
wealth and consumption displays in, 127
Hoeniger, Cathleen, 146, 147
Honorius Augustodunensis, 85
houppelande, 143
Hours of Jeanne d'Evreux, The (Pucelle), 109, *111*
household health care
defecation, 153–54, *154*
focus of, 132, 150–51
food production and consumption, 134, 151–53
gender and practitioners of, 125, 130–31
illustrations with themes of, 133–34
management of, as medical option, 120
manuscript materiality *vs*. everyday scenes of, 123, 125
medical supply shopping responsibilities, *112*, 148, *149*, *150*
narrative and outcome ambiguity of, 17, 20
preventative practices, 99–100, 126, 132, 150–51
recipes for, 130, 131
as *Régime* theme, 1, 2, 4, 15, 20, 122–23, 132–34, 155–56
social status conventions disregarded for, 19
women's management roles in, 5, 7, 15, 132, 134
household management guides, 100, 127–29
households, medieval
clothing styles, 141–45
descriptions of, 131, 137–38
intimacy in scenes of, 49, 134, 153
management of, 100, 127–29, 132, 139, 154–55
social status markers, 137–38, 139–40
term definitions, 131, 137
See also household health care
human waste, 58, 134, 153–54, 158, 178n83
humors (complexion; *complexio*)
health remedies for moderating, 151
as medical theory, 99–100, 102, 104, 114, 151
as preventative household health care focus, 132, 150
treatments for excess, 111, 114
Hundred Years War, 78, 81, 182n69
Hunt, Tony, 188n21
hybrid creatures
defacement of, 53
dog-faced, 1, *3*, *142*
with hats, *22*, 23, *69*
as historiated initial embellishment, 11

Ibn Buṭlān, 104, 145–46
Ibn Sīnā. *See* Avicenna
image du monde, (Gossuin de Metz)
artists of, 72, 77
astronomical illustrations in, 75, *76*, 77, *77*
audience of, 114, 115
authors of, 75
commission of, 67
content descriptions, 68, 75
dating of, 75
illustration compositional formats, 77
manuscripts with copies of, 68, 73, 75, 77–78, 181n51
as *Régime* accompaniment text, 115, 116
translations of, 188n3
vernacularization of, 105

Imagina von Westerburg, 180n40
Imago mundi (Honorius Augustodenensis), 85
infants
  bathing scenes with, 39, *41*, *50*, 51, *52*
  in breastfeeding imagery, 47, *48*
  in lying-in scenes, 49, *50*, 51, *52*
Ingram, Hannah, 120, 121, 131
inheritance, as book dissemination method, 65, 77, 79, 88
intimacy, household, 49, 134, 153
Isaac Judaeus, 2, 63, 100, 107, 117
Isabella of France, 66, 139
Isagoge (Johannitius), 103

J. Paul Getty Museum
  MS 46 (92.MK.92), 70, 72, *72* , 180n40
  MS Ludwig IX 3 (83.ML.99), 28, 29, *31*
Jacquet le Caron, 183n101
Jaume (James) II, king of Aragon, 105
Jean, Duke of Berry, 147
Jean d'Aunoy, 73
Jean de Chalon, 73
Jean de Meun, 128
Jeanne of Hainaut, 72
Jeanne of Navarre and Champagne, 77
jewelry, 121, 140, 141, 147
Johannes de Toleto, 104
Johannitius, 100, 103, 107, 190n81
John, Duke of Bedford, 78, 183n101
John the Baptist, 49
Jones, Peter Murray, 3, 34, 114
Jones, Sarah Rees, 131
Joyce, Rosemary A., 5–6
Juan of Toledo, 104
Juliana Anicia Codex, 176–77n24

Kassel Landesbibliothek 40 MS Med. I.
  astrological texts featured in, 116
  audience of, 106, 118, 128
  manuscript summary, 171
  provenance, 155
  texts of, 113, 118
Klapisch-Zuber, Christiane, 43, 47
Kopytoff, Igor, 5–6
Kowaleski, Maryanne, 137
Krueger, Roberta L., 129, 141, 142
Kyngstone, Elizabeth de, 118
Kyngstone, Sir William, 118

laborers
  beer production, 23, *24*, 134
  cider production, 11, *12*, 23, *24*, 134, 152
  clothing styles of, *23*, 97, 142
  food production, 23, *23*
  foods associated with, 63
  as household demographic, 131, 138
  idealized portrayals of, 147–48
  rice sifting, *80*, 152

Lacarrière, Nathalie, 106
Landouzy, Louis, 3, 20, 25, 101
Lansdowne 380 (British Library), 106, 118, 155, 159, 172
Laud Misc. 724 (Bodleian Library, Oxford), 107, 134, *136*
leeching, 100, 109
Leipzig manuscript. *See* Universitätsbibliothek Leipzig Cod. Haen. 3478
L'Estrange, Elizabeth, 49
Lettre d'Hippocrate á César (Pseudo-Hippocrates), 81, 83, 85, 109, 115, 118
Liber de conservacione vite humane (Bernard de Gordon), 105
Liber de conservanda sanitate (Juan of Toledo/Johannes de Toleto), 104
libraires, 87–88
Life of St. Margaret, 7, 118–19
Lilium medicine (Bernard de Gordon), 105
Lille (France), 8, 72, 88
Limbourg Brothers, 147
literacy, as value, 5, 13, 67, 104, 127
liver, 56
Livre de physique. See *Régime du corps*
livre des simples médecines, Le (Matthaeus Platearius), 187n81
livre des trois vertus, Le (or *The Treasury of the City of Ladies*) (Christine de Pizan), 125, 127, 128, 129
livre du Chevalier de la Tour Landry pour l'enseignement de les filles, Le (Geoffrey Tour de la Landry), 127, 128, 129
Livres dou Trésor (Brunetto Latini), 78, 181n52
Louis de Guyenne, 128
Louis IX, king of France, 6, 65, 66, 70
Lydgate, John, 127, 128–29, 151
lying-in practices, 39–40, 49–51, *50*, *52*

"Making Things" (Joyce and Gillespie), 5, 6
Manfred, king of Sicily, 104
manuscripts (books), overview
  collection practices, 79, 85
  damage/defacement of, 53, 73
  dissemination of, 65, 77, 79, 87–92, 129
  ownership as social status markers, 67
  patronage practices, 66, 88–89
  production of, 87–88, 183n95
  as social status markers, 29, 67, 93, 126, 127, 128, 129, 140, 146, 148, 166
Margaret, Saint, 7, 118–19
Margaret Beaufort, 79
Margaret of Burgundy, 128
Margaret of Provence
  book circulation through family of, 77, 89, 91
  family reunions, 66
  household management responsibilities, 132

manuscript patronage and ownership, 5, 65, 66, 70, 81
marriage, 65
procreation of, 43
margins
anxiety representations in, 45, *46*, 49, 51
defecation scenes in, 153–54, *154*
figures in, purpose, 45
hybrid beasts in, 1, *3*, 11, *22*, 23, 53, *69*
notes written in, 118
physicians with urine flasks in, 109, *111*
recipes written in, 7, 130
Marguerite of Ghistelles, 128
Marie de Brabant, 66–67, 77
Marie de Réthel, 180n39
Maris Jouris, 180n34
Mary, Virgin (biblical character), 28, *31*, *36*, 39, 47, 49
Master of Lord Hoo, 182n70
Master of Lord Talbot, 182n70
Master of Sir John Fastolf, 182n70
Master of the Harley Froissart (Philippe de Mazerolles), 9, 27, 85, 88
Master of the London Wavrin, 9, 27, 85, 88
Master of the Munich Golden Legend, 182n70
Master of Thomas de Maubeuge, 77, *77*
Mattheaus Platearius, 111, 117, 187n81
Matthew Paris, 66
Maynus de Mayneriis, 105, 185n41
McKendrick, Scot, 85
McVaugh, Michael, 57, 108, 109, 120, 130
meat, 20, 23, 31–32, *33*
medical illustrations
anatomical, 106, *107*, *108*
astrological, 116, *117*
diagnostic tools, 108–9, *110*
herbal medicine and apothecary shops, *112*, 113–14
medieval imagery traditions, 106–14
models for, 34
physician attributes, 54, 107, *109*, *111*
of physicians with students, 34, *35*, 96, *96*, 107
of practitioners, 107
surgical, 32, 35, *36*, 109–13, *113*
textual relationship to, 114
women as cupping practitioners, 134, *135*, *136*
medical traditions
astrological theories, 116
dissections, 106
diversity of, 95, 98, 121
literary genres reflecting, 93–94, 126
preventative health care theories, 99–100, 126
textual foundations for, 99, 100, 101–3
universities as developmental influences on, 103
See also apothecary shops; herbal medicine; household health care; medical treatises and texts; medical treatments; physicians; surgeons
medical treatises and texts
on aphorisms, 81
audience of, 121
Christ-as-physician themes, 28
as *Régime* content, 129
Régime du corps comparisons, 27–28
as *Régime* text accompaniment, 117
as *Régime* textual sources, 2, 25, 99, 100
in women's book collections, 129
See also medical illustrations
medical treatments
ear, *9*, 97
eye, 25, *25*
herbal medicine and pharmaceuticals, 113–14
illustration composition descriptions, overview, 20, 25
leeching, 100, 109
practitioner roles in, 110–11
self-, 120, 121, 122
surgery, 28, *36*
touch and social status during, 51–52, 58–59
See also bloodletting; cupping; purging; remedies
ménagier de Paris, Le (anonymous), 100, 125, 127–28, 129, 151, 152
Meyer, Paul, 3, 118
mice, *32*
midwives, 98, 101
millet, *80*
moderation, 63, 128–29, 151
moles, *32*
Montpellier Bibliothèque interuniversitaire, MS H089, 55, *57*, 177n35, 186n62
moon cycle diagrams, 75–77, *76*, *77*, 116
morality, 29, 78, 129
Morgan Library & Museum
MS M.240, 70
MS M.638, 28, *29*
See also Morgan Library & Museum, MS M.165
Morgan Library & Museum, MS M.165
audience of, 89
Cambridge manuscript comparisons, 81
cider and beer production, 23
clothing styles of, 97, *98*, 143, *144*
copulation, 53, *55*
cupping, 97, *98*
dating of, 8, 67, 81
farro and bran, *82*
heart, *143*
historical context, 78, 81, 182n69
illustrations of, statistics, 81

Morgan Library & Museum, MS M.165 (*continued*)
illustration style descriptions, 27
liver, *96*
as manuscript model, 182n79
manuscript models for, 182n79
manuscript summary, 161, 169–70
newborn care and lying-in scenes, 49, *52*
physicians featured in, 96, *96*, 144
pregnancy, *144*
production location, 8, 72, 81, 87
provenance, 9, 81, 182n65
rebinding history, 81
scenes depicted in, overview, 163–68
texts of, 81
vomiting, 123, *126* , 134
Morris, William, 182n65
Moving Women, Moving Objects (Hamilton and Proctor-Tiffany), 5
mulberries, 23, *23*, 97

narrative
ambiguity of, for viewer engagement, 14, 18–19, 40
ambiguity of, health care comparisons, 17, 20
anxiety representations, 45, *46*, 49, 51
childbirth and lying-in scenes as positive outcomes, 51
historiated initial formats and complexity of, 38
invention and originality in, 37
medical illustrations as, 35, *36*, 112
visual traditions for, 34–35
Nativity, *36*
naturals, 100
Neriot, Jehan, 70
newborn care
bathing, 21, 39–40, *41*, 50, 51, *52*
breastfeeding, 40, 43, 47, *48*
content characteristics, 21
lying-in scenes depicting, 39–40, 49–51, *50*, *52*
narrative content and image selection, 39, 40
as *Régime* subject, 20, 21, 47
touch and social status, 51
See also wet nurses
Nicholas of Reggio, 103
Nicoud, Marilyn, 3, 174n2
non-naturals, 100, 104, 126, 132, 150

object biography, 5–6
object itinerary, 5, 6
Omne Bonum, 32–34, *34*
On Crisis (Galen), 116
On Critical Days (Galen), 116
Paneth Codex, 34, *35*
Pantegni (Haly Abbas), 102, 103
Paris (France)
copulation scenes in manuscripts produced in, 28
family reunions in, 66
as manuscript production center, 81, 87–88, 89
manuscripts produced in, 28, 73, 77, 108
medical schools in, 103
patients
gestures of, 35, *37*, 93, *94*
medical care based on social status, 93, 119–21, 122, 127
physician consultations with, breast disease, 35, *37*, 45, 52, 54, 55, *57*, 107
physician consultations with, pregnancy, 54, *56*, 93, *94*
physicians' behavior protocols with, 57–58, 178n71
in *Régime*, 133
self-managed health care of, 120, 121, 122
social status of, 57, 58, 93, 119–20, 127
touching of female, 57–58
See also medical treatments
peasantry, 63, 121, 138
Pépin, Roger, 3, 20, 25, 101
pepper (spice), *23*, 25
Pere II, king of Aragon, 105
pharmacies. *See* apothecary shops
pharmacists. *See* apothecaries
Philippe de Mazerolles (Master of the Harley Froissart), 9, 27, 85, 88
Philip VI, king of France, 73
phlebotomy, 100, 109, 110, 111, 112
See also bloodletting
physicians
alternative medical partnerships, 121–22
attributes of, 54, 107, *109*, *111*
behavior protocols, 57–58, 178n71
breast disease consultations, 35, *37*, 45, 52, 54, 55, *57*
Christ-as-, 28
clothing styles of, 54, *55*, *56*, 93, *93*, 95, 96, *98*, 142, *143*, 143–44
diagnostic tools of, 108–9, *110*
eye treatments, 25, *25*
gender of, 132
heart consultations, *143*
history of, 98–99
household inclusion of, 15
liver consultations, *96*
medical roles of, 109, 120
medical texts and illustrations of, 107
patient access to, as social status marker, 93, 127
patient demographics, 119–21, 122
physiognomic assessments, 20

pregnancy consultations, 54, *56*, 93, *94*
as *Régime* audience, 7, 94, 98, 101, 115, 119, 155
Régime inclusion purpose, 95, 132, 133
social status and authority, 54, 58–59, 93, 95–99, 96
with students, 34, *35*, 96, *96*, 107, *109*
teeth examinations, *95*
touch and, 54–57, *56*, *57*
training of, 99
physician's assistants, 95, 132
physiognomy, 20
Pierre of Roubaix and Herzelles, 128
Pitart, Jean, 73, 117
plagues, 73, 87, 89, 117, 142
plants, 11, 20, *22*, *23*
Poulet, Quentin, 79
Practica (Arderne), 112, *113*
practitioners
hair care featuring, *13*, 25
medical treatments and touch of, 57–60
social status and authority of, 57, 125
touching of patients, 57–58
training methods, 98
types of, 95, 98, 132
vomiting assistants, 39, *39*, 123, *125*, *126*
women as cupping, 13, *59*, 107, 113, 133, *133*, 134, *135*, *136*
See also apothecaries; barbers and barber-surgeons; physicians; surgeons
prayer books, 66, 70, 72, *72*, 180n40
See also books of hours
pregnancy
historiated initials featuring, *10*, *84*, *86*, *144*
medieval practices, 43, 44
physician consultations, 54, *56*, 93, *94*, 141
Régime instruction on, 21, 101
procreation. *See* fertility
Proctor-Tiffany, Mariah, 5, 77, 88
Psalms, 118
Pseudo-Hippocrates, 81, 83, 85, 109, 115, 118
Pucelle, Jean: *The Hours of Jeanne d'Evreux*, 109, *111*
pulse-taking, 55
purging
household intimacy and scenes of, 134, 153
illustrated initials featuring, *74*, *152*, *153*
illustration style descriptions, 13
practitioner touching during, 58
pregnancy care and, 21
for preventative health care, 100
as *Régime* subject, 20
purification rites, 49

Queen Mary Psalter, 66

rabbits, *33*
Rawcliffe, Carole, 120, 122
recipes
descriptions, 130
dissemination of, 131
herbal medicinal, 113–14
in manuscript margins as ancillary notes, 7, 130
manuscripts with textual accompaniments of, 70, 73, 79, 83, 113, 115, 116, 117, 118, 119, 130, 149
medical texts featuring, 102, 113
as social status marker, 152
See also herbals
redactions, 20, 68, 70, 73, 81, 83, 85
Regalis dispositio (*Pantegni*) (Haly Abbas), 102, 103
Régime du corps (*Régime de santé, Livre de physique*)
audience of, academic readers, 7
audience of, diversity, 90–91, 94, 101, 115, 155
audience of, families and communities, 6, 118
audience of, physicians, 7, 94, 115
audience of, religious, 7
audience of, social status, 25, 127
audience of, women, 2, 4–8, 5, 67, 90–91, 130
audience of unillustrated, 10, 116–17
chapter organization, 101
composition and writing style of, 2, 5, 101, 129
content descriptions, 1, 2, 4, 15, 20, 132–33
dating of, 65
dissemination of, 5–6, 63–67, 78, 83, 89, 90–91, 157–58
extant copies of, 1, 8–11, 67, 169–73
genre associations, 4, 15, 17–18, 27–37, 112–13, 114, 115, 125, 126, 129
genre descriptions, 5, 15, 93
illustrations of, 11, 190n82 (*see also* historiated initials of *Régime du corps*)
other titles of, 1
ownership as social status marker, 93, 127
patronage and commission, 2, 3, 64, 65, 75
popularity of, 2
prologue of, 100
scholarship on, 2–3, 4
size and dimensions, 26
text and image relationships, 20–25
textual accompaniments to, 115–19, 128
textual sources for, 2, 25, 99, 100, 101–3, 104, 105
translations of, 2
See also specific manuscript copies
Regimen Almerie (Arnau de Vilanova), 105

Regimen for the King of Aragon (Arnau de Vilanova), 105, 185n37
regimen literature
audiences of, 83, 92, 93, 104, 105–6, 106, 113, 117–18, 126, 128
foundational texts for, 99, 100, 101–3
genre descriptions, 93, 103
health care focus of, 100
historical development of, 103–5
for military campaigns, 105
patronage popularity of, 104
as *Régime* genre category, 5, 15, 93
in women's book collections, 129–30
Regimen sanitatis (Bernard de Gordon), 105
Regimen sanitatis (Maynus de Mayneriis), 185n41
Regimen sanitatis ad inclitum regem Aragonum (Arnau de Vilanova), 105, 185n37
Regimen sanitatis salernitanum (*Salerno Regimen of Health*), 104
relaxation, as preventative health care factor, 100
religious texts, 118–19
remedies ("simples")
herbal medicinal, 113–14
home, for self-managed health care, 121
manuscripts with textual accompaniments of, 83, 113, 115
as *Régime* section, 20, 21, 23
See also herbals; medical treatments
Rennes 593 (Bibliothèque municipale de Rennes), 77–78, 181n52–53
Reynolds, Catherine, 89
Rhazes, 100, 102, 184n12, 190n81
rice, *80*, 152
Richard, Duke of York, 78, 79
Richard de Fournival, 115
Richard of Cornwall, 65, 72
Riddy, Felicity, 132, 137, 138, 150, 153, 154–55
Robert I of Naples, 103
roger male branche redaction, 20, 81, 83, 85
romance literature, 13–14, 28, 105, 147–48
Roman de la Rose (Jean de Meun), 28, 128
Rouen (France)
artists of, 81, 83, 182n70
as book production center, 88, 89
book production in, 78, 81
Rouse, Mary A., 87–88
Rouse, Richard H., 87–88
royalty and royal courts
defecation as parody on, 153–54
household descriptions, 131, 137–40
manuscript collections, 79, 85, 140
patronage and commissions, 6, 66, 67, 70, 73, 83, 85, 175–76n11, 180n33
Ruskin Hours, The, 28, *31*

Sanchia of Provence, 65, 66, 89, 91, 132
Sandler, Lucy Freeman, 87
scientific texts
astrological, 85
astronomical, 68, 75–77, *76*, *77*, 116
copulation scenes in, 28
popularity of, 78
Scott, Kathleen, 79, 182n62
Scott, Margaret, 141
Secret of Secrets, 115
Serapion, 100
Sewright, Kathleen, 3, 118
sex. *See* copulation
silver, 140
simples. *See* remedies
skin care, 28, *30*, *142*
slavery, 44
sleep, 11, 20, 21, 100, 106, 126, 137, 150
Sloane 6 (British Library), 112, 134, 135, *135*
Sloane 1611 (British Library), 118–19, 172
Sloane 1977 (British Library)
apothecary shops, *36*, 111, *112*
audience of, 111–12
breast disease consultation, 35, *37* , 45
Christ-as-physician imagery, 28
dating of, 35
dissemination of, 68, 70
historiated initials in, function of, 32, 112
illustration content and narrative style, 35, 111, 112
male practitioners and touching taboos, 178n71
production location, 35
surgical scenes with biblical themes, 35, *36*, 45
texts of, 111
Sloane 2401 (British Library)
audience of, 83, 91, 118
cider and vinegar production, 11, *12*
coats of arms featured in, 83, 91
compound remedies in, 149
copulation, 53, 55
dating of, 8, 67
herbal recipes, 113
historiated initials in, statistics, 83
historical context, 78
illustration style descriptions, 27, 83
manuscript models for, 182n79
manuscript summary, 161
newborn care and lying-in scenes, 49, *50*
pregnancy, *84*
production location, 8, 83, 87
provenance, 9, 83, 155
scenes depicted in, overview, 163–68
texts of, 83, 130
Sloane 2435 (British Library)
animals in, 31, *33*
artist of, 8, 68
bathing, 68, *69*

bloodletting, 1, *3*, 4, 11, 97
BnF Fr. 12323 manuscript comparisons, 61, 73, 75
cheese, 61, *63*
clothing styles in, *23*, *94*, 96, 97, 141, 142, *142*
copulation, 28, *28* , 52–53
cupping, 13, 58, *59*
dating of, 8, 65, 67, 68
food production and consumption, 151
historiated initials in, 1, 68
hybrid creatures, *142*
location of, 1
manuscript summary, 161, 169
marginal figures as anxiety representations, 45, *46*, 49, 51
materiality of, 1, 26, 68
mulberries, 23, *23*, 97
patronage theories, 68
physicians in, 54, *94*, 96, 142, *142*
pregnancy, 93, *94* , 96
production location, 8, 68, 72, 75
purging, *152* , 153
scenes depicted in, overview, 163–68
skin care (complexion), 28, *30*, *142*
texts of, 20, 68, 75, 77
vomiting, 39, *39*, 123
wet nurse selection, 17, *18* , 40, *46*, 47, 51
wheat, *22*, 23
wine production, 11, *11*
Sloane 3525 (British Library), 57, 101, 117
social status
of apothecaries, 148
book ownership as marker of, 29, 67, 93, 126, 127, 128, 129, 140, 146, 148, 155, 166
clothing styles as markers of, 26, 51, 93, 97–98, 127, 140, 142, 144–45
copulation and gender, *28*, 52–54, *53*, *55*
figure positioning indicating, 51
food and drink as markers of, 25, 127, 139–40, 151–52
foods with lower-class associations, 63
gesture indicating, 17, *18*, 19, 40, *42*, 51
health care and disregard for, 19–20
historiated initials indicating, 38
household and gender, 125–26
household furnishings as markers of, 49, 137, 140
jewelry as markers of, 140, 141, 147
knowledge acquisition as indicator of, 92
lying-in rites indicating, 49
manuscript content reinforcing owners', 93, 95, 127
manuscripts communicating ideals of, 127
physician access as marker of, 93, 127
of physicians, 54, 58, 93, 95–99, 119–20
of practitioners, 57, 97–98, 125
touch indicating, 58
wet nurse selection and, 17, *18*, 39, 40, *42*, 43, 44, 51–52
spices, 23, *23*, 25, 151
Sponsler, Claire, 151
St. John's College Oxford MS 68, 181n56
stags, *33*
Stanton, Anne Rudloff, 139
Stones, Alison, 68, 70, 72, 88
students, medical, 34, *35*, 96, *96*, 107, *109*
sumptuary laws, 129, 141
sun cycle diagrams, *77*, 116
surgeons
attributes of, *9*, 142
barbers compared to, 111
as bloodletting administrators, 4
breast disease consultations, 55, 57, *57*
Christ-as-physician healing themes, 28, *36*
influential, 73, 102, 111, 181n45
medical references used by, 102
medical roles and procedures of, 109
as practitioner type, 95
surgical scenes with, *36*
training expectations, 99, 111
See also barbers and barber-surgeons; physicians
surgical texts and treatises
apothecary shops, *36*, 111, *112*
breast disease consultations, 35, *37*, 45, 54, 55, 57, *57*
cupping, 112
historiated initials, function of, 32
illustrations in, function of, 112
illustrative narrative style of, 35, *36*
phlebotomy, 112
as *Régime* text accompaniments, 117
surgical scenes, 35, *36*, 45
surgical tools, 112, *113*
women as cupping practitioners in, *136*
See also *Chirurgia* (Frugardi); Sloane 1977

Tacuinum sanitatis (Ibn Buṭlān), 104, 125, 145–49, *147*
teeth, *95*
theriacs, 148, *149*
Thwayte, John, 81
Thwaytes, Thomas, 182n68
touch
copulation and, 52–54
lying-in scenes and, 51
medical treatments and, 58
physicians and, 51–52, 54–58, 97, 178n71
practitioners and, 58–60
status associations, 51
wet nurse selection and authority of, 51–52

Tractatus de herbis, 176n24
Treasury of the City of Ladies, The (or *Le livre des trois vertus*) (Christine de Pizan), 125, 127, 128, 129
Très riches heures (Limbourg Brothers), 147
Trinity College Library, Cambridge
  MS B.11.22, 153–54, *154*
  MS O.2.5, 116, 186–87n74
Trota, 117
Trotula, Quant Dex nostre Seignor, 101, 117, 130
Tyers, Theresa L.
  health manuals and audience theories, 83, 106, 113, 117–18, 128, 155
  recipe collections, 113
  scholarship contributions of, 3, 7

Universal Diets (Isaac Judaeus), 2
Universitätsbibliothek Leipzig Cod. Haen. 3478
  barber-surgeons featured in, *9*, 97, 142
  breastfeeding, 40, 47, *48*
  dating, 9
  ear treatments, *9*, 97
  gloves featured in, 96, *96*, 142
  illustration program of, 9–10
  manuscript summary, 162, 169
  physicians featured in, 54, 96, *96*, 142
  production location, 9
  scenes depicted in, overview, 163–68
University of Montpellier, 103, 105
University of Paris, 88, 108
University of Pennsylvania LJS 55, 75, 106, 116, 173, 181n55
urine
  as diagnostic tool, 108
  flasks as physician attribute, 54, 107, *109*, *111*
  treatises and texts on, 7, 105, 117
  wheels and charts, 108–9, *110*, 116

Vale, Malcolm, 137, 139
Valls, Helen, 32, 55–56, 112
Vatican Reg.lat.1256 (Biblioteca Apostolica Vaticana), 9, *10*, 118, 162, 163–68, 171
veins, diagrams of, 106, *107*
venison, 151
vernacularization, 5, 15, 25, 63, 103–6, 120
Vienna Dioscorides, 114
vinegar production, *12*
Visconti, Giangaleazzo, count of Milan, 146, 149
Visitation, The
  prayer book visual traditions of, 28, *31*
  skin care conversation model, 28, *30*
  surgical manuscript featuring imagery of, 35, *36*
  as wet nurse selection model, 39
vomiting
  household intimacy and scenes of, 134, 153
  narrative content and imagery selection, 38–39
  patient's hat styles featured in scenes of, 144, *144*
  with practitioner assistance, 39, *39*, 123, *125*, *126*, 134
  practitioner touching during, 58
  for preventative health care, 100
  single-person compositions, 39, 123, *124*

Waleran II, 180n40
Wallis, Faith, 25, 185n37
Walloon (French dialect), 5
watermelon, 147, *148*
Wellcome Library
  MS.546, 101, 117–18, 172, 186–87n74
  MS.8932, 116, *117*
wet nurses
  breastfeeding, 40, 47, *48*
  as health guide topic, 21, 44, 47
  narrative content and image selection, 39, 51
  practice of using, 43–44
  as practitioner type, 95
  selection process and anxiety representations, 45, *46*, 49, 51
  selection process and touching, 51–52
  selection process descriptions, 13, 17, *18*, *42*, 44, 45, *46*, 47, 133
  social status and employment of, 43, 44
wheat, *22*, 23
Whittington, Karl, 35, 112
William of Saliceto, 57, 102
wine production, 11, *11*
Winer, Rebecca Lynn, 44, 47
women
  agency of, as theme, 4, 16
  as apothecary customers, *112*, 148–49, *149*, *150*
  authority through touch, 52
  book collections of, 126, 129
  book dissemination through, 5–6
  books on historical significance of, 128
  breast disease consultation, 35, *37*, 45, 52, 54, *55*, *57*
  childbirth, 21
  as childbirth assistants, 134
  courtesy manuals for, 128
  as cupping practitioners, 13, *59*, 107, 113, 133, *133*, 134, *135*, *136*
  health care knowledge transmission, 130
  household authority of, 125
  household health care roles of, 5, 7, 16, 125, 132, 134
  household management guides for, 100, 125, 127–28

literacy of, 13, 130
as lying-in caregivers, 39, 49–51, *50*, *51*, *52*
male practitioners' restrictions on touching, 57–58, 178n71
as medical text audience, 7
medieval gender studies and roles of, 5
as newborn caregivers, 39–40, *40*, *41*, 51, *52*, 134
physician behavior protocols and touching, 57–58, 178n71
as regimen literature audience, 83, 106, 113, 117–18, 128
as vomiting assistants, 123, *126*, 134
See also childbirth; fertility and procreation; pregnancy; wet nurses

Yale Medical Library, MS 28 (Paneth Codex), 34, *35*

Zodiac Man, 116, *117*